Elizabeth Scannell–Desch, PhD, RN, is a retired colonel in the U.S. Air Force Nurse Corps. For 25 years, Dr. Scannell-Desch served her country, holding many key leadership positions, including command nurse executive for the entire Air Force Reserve at Headquarters, USAF, the Pentagon; command nurse executive for the Air Force Material Command, Wright Patterson AFB, Ohio; chief nurse officer for the 48th Fighter Wing Hospital, RAF Lakenheath, United Kingdom; chief nurse officer at Robins AFB Hospital, Georgia; assistant chief nurse officer at Mather AFB Hospital, California; clinical positions as a flight nurse with the Second Aeromedical Evacuation Squadron covering Europe, the Middle East, and Africa; and USAF air transportable hospital chief nurse, emergency room charge nurse, medical inspector general's staff, nursing practice coordinator—surgical, oncology nurse and clinical nurse specialist, and medical-surgical nurse. She served as the consultant to the USAF surgeon general for oncology nursing and nursing research. She holds the tenured rank of professor of nursing at Mount Saint Mary College, Newburgh, New York, and served as the chairperson of the Division of Nursing from 2004 to 2010. She is an active member of the Eastern Nursing Research Society, Sigma Theta Tau International (Xi and Mu Epsilon chapters), American Nurses Association, American Association for the History of Nursing, and Air War College Alumni Association. She has authored many research and clinical articles that have been published nationally and internationally. Dr. Scannell-Desch has presented her research throughout the United States and internationally at scientific meetings in Dublin, Ireland; London, England; and Vienna, Austria. During the summer of 2001, she was a visiting professor at the University of Medicine and Pharmacy, Cluj-Napoka, Romania. Her military decorations and nursing awards are numerous.

Mary Ellen Doherty, PhD, RN, CNM, is an associate professor in the Department of Nursing at Western Connecticut State University in Danbury, Connecticut. Dr. Doherty teaches in the graduate and undergraduate programs. She also serves on the university's Institutional Review Board, which governs all faculty and student research. For more than 25 years, she has been a certified nurse-midwife and has practiced in a variety of settings. Always a pioneer, Dr. Doherty was Founder and President of Concord Nurse-Midwifery Associates, with delivery privileges at Emerson Hospital in Concord, Massachusetts. Other advanced practice roles in her career have included being a family nurse practitioner and a maternal-child clinical nurse specialist. She is a member of the American College of Nurse-Midwives; the Association of Women's Health, Obstetric, and Neonatal Nurses; Eastern Nursing Research Society; Sigma Theta Tau International Honor Society of Nursing (Alpha Tau, Mu Epsilon, and Kappa Alpha chapters); the International Childbirth Education Association; the American Nurses Association; and the American Association for the History of Nursing. Dr. Doherty has authored numerous research and clinical articles on midwifery, widowhood during pregnancy (9/11 and war), therapeutic alliance, and birth-plan decision-making. She is a reviewer for the *Journal of Midwifery and Women's Health* and the *Journal of Perinatal Education*. She has presented her research throughout the United States and at international conferences in Dublin, Ireland; London, England; and Vienna, Austria. Since 2002, she has served the legal system as an expert witness on cases involving maternal and newborn health.

Nurses in War

Voices From Iraq and Afghanistan

Elizabeth Scannell–Desch, PhD, RN
Mary Ellen Doherty, PhD, RN, CNM

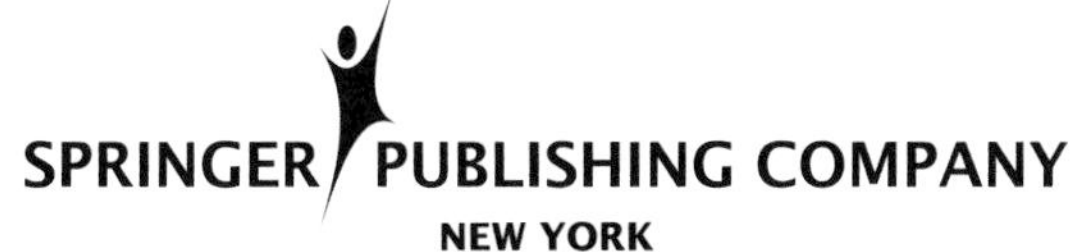

Springer Publishing Company, LLC
11 West 42nd Street
New York, NY 10036
www.springerpub.com

Acquisitions Editor: Allan Graubard
Production Editor: Lindsay Claire
Composition: Manila Typesetting Company

ISBN: 978-0-8261-9383-4
E-book ISBN: 978-0-8261-9384-1

12 13 14 15/ 5 4 3 2

Library of Congress Cataloging-in-Publication Data

Scannell-Desch, Elizabeth.
Nurses in war : voices from Iraq and Afghanistan / Elizabeth Scannell-Desch, Mary Ellen Doherty.
p. ; cm.
Includes index.
ISBN 978-0-8261-9383-4—ISBN 978-0-8261-9384-1 (e-ISBN)
I. Doherty, Mary Ellen. II. Title.
[DNLM: 1. Military Nursing—United States—Autobiography. 2. Afghan Campaign 2001—United States. 3. Iraq War, 2003—United States. 4. Nurses—psychology—United States. WZ 112.5.N8]
LC classification not assigned
610.69—dc23

2012009725

Printed in the United States of America by Bang Printing

This book is dedicated to all nurses who have served in the United States military. Through their steadfast personal commitment, untiring devotion to duty, and selfless dedication to the ideals of our nation, military nurses have provided the highest quality of nursing care in peacetime and in war. Their caring and humanitarian aid to victims of war and disaster all over the globe embodies and exemplifies the spirit and essence of the nursing profession.

Also, this book is dedicated to our mother, Marie Murphy Scannell, who has been our role model as a woman, as a caring and involved person, and as an educator and scholar. Her belief in her twin daughters always knew no bounds. We are eternally grateful for her support, her confidence in us, and her love.

Contents

Foreword

I can still recall how thrilled I was in early 2011 when I learned my friend and Air Force colleague, Elizabeth "Beth" Scannell-Desch, was going to be writing a book on military nursing along with her twin sister, Mary Ellen Scannell Doherty. I felt so honored when she asked me if I would consider writing the book's foreword. We agreed I would be sent each chapter of the manuscript as it was written to better enable me to write a meaningful foreword. I was enthralled after reading the first chapter, which gives a concise overview of military nursing through the ages. In the second and subsequent chapters, as readers, you meet the 37 nurses who participated in one, two, or all three of the research studies done by the authors.

Waiting for each chapter and the opportunity to learn about the additional nurses involved in the studies and learn more about their experiences and feelings reminded me of my childhood. It felt like I was a child during summer vacation anxiously waiting for the mailman to bring the latest issue of the *Weekly Reader*. I couldn't wait to receive and read each new chapter of *Nurses in War: Voices From Iraq and Afghanistan.* The nurses are so articulate at vividly describing what they were experiencing and feeling while deployed. After reading it in its entirety, I feel privileged to share some introductory thoughts with you in the foreword to this book.

After 40-plus years as a nurse, it has been my experience that the vast majority of nurses and society as well do not understand how military nursing—in particular, combat nursing—is unequalled. Even though the knowledge, skills, and abilities are constant, the combat setting adds additional and distinct stressors to the delivery of nursing care.

Military nursing is a unique career. Their love of country is first and foremost the reason why many individuals choose to make the military a career. When commissioned into one of the military services, certain rights and freedoms are forgone to assure these same rights and freedoms for citizens and residents of our great nation.

Nurses in War provides valuable insights into what separates military nursing from civilian nursing. The mission of each of the military services is to support and defend the United States of America against all enemies, foreign and domestic. Military nurses care for patients and provide nursing care in military settings similar to most civilian nursing settings. This peacetime delivery platform allows military nurses to maintain their knowledge, skills, and abilities for their combat-readiness mission should our country find itself at war or in a conflict. It is the unusual setting in which care is provided that sets combat nursing apart from nursing provided in peacetime military and civilian settings.

Most books written about military nursing in past wars and conflicts like Vietnam and World War II were published a decade or more after the war ended. This book is being published while our country is still involved in the Afghanistan war and just months after our country marked the 10th anniversary of the start of the wars in Iraq and Afghanistan. *Nurses in War* is extremely timely. The evidence from these research studies will be beneficial to every level of military nursing and the health care system. From chief nurse officers to staff nurses, this book will enable any nurse to be better prepared to deploy and/or to support those nurses who will or who have deployed.

As the 12th chief nurse of the Air Force Nurse Corps and the past director of medical readiness for the Air Force Medical Service from 1995 to 2000, I can personally attest to the importance of this book to health care leaders, in particular, military leaders. It is a book every nurse should read, especially military nurses. For nurses who will be deploying, it will give accurate information regarding what to expect while deployed. For those nurses who have not deployed, it will provide you with a realistic understanding of what family, friends, and colleagues who have deployed or will deploy will be experiencing. It will enable the reader to be more supportive when nurses who have deployed transition back into the peacetime health care delivery system post-deployment.

Nurses in War embodies the core values of each of the military services and is a personal testament to the integrity, excellence, selflessness, devotion to duty, courage, and commitment that exemplifies military nursing. The compelling first-person accounts of the challenges of combat nursing are readable and extremely informative. The authors' layout of the book coupled with the lived experiences of these 37 nurses will make an indelible impression. It is a step-by-step portrayal of the deployment experience. It starts with the assignment process to Iraq and Afghanistan and ends with the transition process back to the United States. It addresses every aspect of deployment comprehensively but not in a boring or repetitive manner. As a reader, this is as close as you will probably ever come to experiencing combat nursing unless you deploy to a war zone or an area of conflict. It is a realistic portrayal of nurses in war.

There is a growing body of nursing literature based on research addressing military nursing. Nursing research is not the passion of all nurses, nor does it excite every nurse. But Beth's and Mary Ellen's sharing of their three research studies in this book is unlike most published nursing research. Their book is an enjoyable and an extraordinarily interesting read. I guarantee it will be a book you will finish, and you will always remember some of these personal and moving vignettes. If you are a nurse, it will make you extremely proud of your chosen profession. And if you also chose to serve our great nation by wearing the uniform of one of the military service branches, it will make you even more proud of your decision to make military nursing one of your career choices.

In closing, I know *Nurses in War: Voices From Iraq and Afghanistan* made me proud of both of my career choices, nursing and military service. This book should be in every nurse's personal library. It has a well-deserved place of honor in my own nursing literature collection.

Brigadier General Linda J. Stierle (Retired)
United States Air Force

Preface

They came from the plains of west Texas, the commuter suburbs of New York City, or the heartland of Iowa. Some were parents with young children, whereas others were recent college graduates. A few were of Italian American descent, whereas others were African Americans or Irish Catholics. A few grew up in blue-collar industrial neighborhoods, whereas others were reared on Cape Cod. What did this mix of human diversity have in common? What was the glue that bound them together? They were all nurses. Most of them were women. They all took an oath to support and defend their country and to wear America's uniform. Most importantly, they all answered their country's call to serve in peacetime and in wartime. They were U.S. military nurses. Since 2003, these nurses have found themselves in places like Mosul and Tikrit, Iraq, or in Mazer-e-Sharif and Kandahar, Afghanistan. Although they were nurses, they carried weapons to defend themselves and protect their patients. They had no immunity to the horrors and dangers of war. As mortars and rockets landed in their hospital compounds, they continued to provide nursing care to wounded soldiers, enemy insurgents, and burned and maimed local nationals caught in the chaos of war. This book is their story.

More specifically, this book derives from three qualitative research studies examining the lived experience of military nurses in the Iraq and Afghanistan wars from 2003 to 2010. In the first study, 37 U.S. military nurses voluntarily told their stories of deployment; experiences of living and working in the war zone; and homecoming and readjustment to their families, stateside work environments, and communities. The sample for this study included 33 female and 4 male nurses. Within this sample, 18 nurses were from the Army Nurse Corps, 15 were from the Air Force Nurse Corps, and 4 were from the Navy Nurse Corps. All four male nurses were from the Army (Scannell-Desch & Doherty, 2010).

The second study focused on 24 female nurses' health and hygiene experiences during deployment to Iraq or Afghanistan. We wanted to explore the topic of women's health and hygiene because most deployed nurses were women, and the findings of the first study suggested that this was an area of concern for the nurses. The sample of 24 nurses was a subset of participants from the first study. Because the second study was conducted a year after the first study, several women from the first study were no longer available. Several were redeployed. Others had moved on to overseas assignments or could not be located because of reassignment or retirement (Doherty & Scannell-Desch, in press).

The third study examined the experience of parental separation for nurse-parents deployed to Iraq or Afghanistan. Again, we wanted to explore parental separation because it was an aspect of deployment from the first study that warranted further focused research investigation. Twenty men and women from the first study indicated that they were parents and agreed to be interviewed for the third study. Eleven were from the Army Nurse Corps, six were from the Air Force Nurse Corps, and three were from the Navy Nurse Corps. Sixteen nurse-parents were women, and four were men.

We used Colaizzi's (1978) phenomenological method to guide discovery of the lived experience of military nurses in all three of our research studies. Phenomenology is the study of human experience from the perspective of those experiencing a particular phenomenon. The phenomenon could be, for example, the experience of working in a combat support hospital, taking care of war-injured children, or losing a friend or colleague in a terrorist attack. Phenomenologists appreciate the importance and value of looking at the world through the variety of phenomena in human experience. Phenomenology seeks to describe the essential structures embedded in the phenomena under study (Husserl, 1970). Colaizzi's (1978) method includes elements of both descriptive and interpretive phenomenology.

The population in the first study consisted of male and female deployed military nurses. The second study on health and hygiene concerns only included a sample of deployed female nurses. The third study only included a sample of male and female nurses who were parents. Nurses in all three studies served in the Army, Navy, or Air Force in Iraq or Afghanistan during the war years 2003 to 2010. This included nurses assigned to aeromedical evacuation aircraft as well as those serving on mobile surgical teams, in combat support hospitals, in Iraqi or Afghan hospitals, and in hospitals for detainees. Sampling criteria included that study participants be: (a) a registered nurse; (b) able to read, write, and speak English; (c) a current or former member of the Army, Navy, or Air Force Nurse Corps; (d) able to recall experiences as a military nurse, and (e) willing to discuss war experiences. This group included active-duty and reserve Nurse Corps members. Contact information for all nurses who met these criteria was not centrally available, so a purposive sample was drawn using "snowball sampling" (Polit & Hungler, 2000) and calls for voluntary participation.

One researcher was acquainted with two nurses who met the sampling criteria, and both agreed to participate. These nurses contacted other nurses who met the criteria, and more nurses agreed to participate. This researcher also knew an Air Force nurse assigned at headquarters, who sent out an electronic synopsis of the study aims and a call for potential subjects. This electronic message yielded more potential subjects. The second researcher knew an Army Nurse Corps reservist and a retired active-duty Army nurse. She contacted these nurses, and both provided contact information for more potential study participants. Successive respondents were selected for participation in these studies while data collection and analysis progressed. These procedures served to broaden the scope, range, and depth of information (Denzin & Lincoln, 2000).

Interview settings were chosen by participants. Locations included residences, offices, parks, and restaurants. Interviews ranged from 45 to 90 minutes. Most interviews were conducted face to face. Owing to geographical constraints, several interviews were conducted by telephone. All face-to-face interviews took place in the eastern United States, whereas most telephone interviews included nurses in the western United States.

Data-generating open-ended questions guided the interview process in all three studies. We used an interview guide of four questions for the first and third studies and five questions for the second study. Follow-up questions were asked to clarify thoughts, feelings, and meanings of what was expressed, and to gain a deeper understanding. Reflective questions were asked, whereas suggestive questions were avoided.

The three study proposals were approved by institutional review boards where the investigators were employed, as well as by the funding agencies. Before commencing interviews, participants were mailed written explanations of the purpose and nature of the study. Once informed consent forms were returned, an investigator contacted potential participants by phone; verbally discussed the purpose of the study, informed consent, and study withdrawal procedures; and set up a date and time for the interview. Participation was voluntary and could be withdrawn at any time. Participants were informed of immediate availability of a mental health nurse practitioner, if needed, because of possible emotional upset due to recall of war experiences. Procedures about how data would be collected, analyzed, used, and stored were explained. Interviews were audio-recorded for transcription and analysis. Data collection for each study took place over a 5-month period for 3 consecutive years and continued until saturation occurred without discovery of any new themes.

Data for all three studies were analyzed using procedures adapted from Colaizzi (1978). Tapes were listened to several times by both investigators to gain familiarity with content, feeling, and tone. After verbatim transcriptions were made, respondents' descriptions were reviewed. Significant statements were extracted and categorized into thematic clusters for each study. Findings were integrated by the investigators into a thick exhaustive description of the lived experience. Although all experiences and interview content were appreciated and valued, within the confines of this book, it was not possible to include all interview statements. Because there was redundancy within answers to the research questions, statements that best captured the essence of an experience in our judgment were those we included in this book.

The reader will be introduced to each of the 37 nurses in the first half of the book, whose stories vividly relate the emotional, clinical, physical, and experiential stresses and strains of living and working in a war zone thousands of miles from the comforts and safety of home and family. They impart their roles in the austere and harsh environments where they provide combat casualty care. Some were volunteers for these roles, whereas others were deployed when their units were mobilized for war. Their stories capture the essence of the hardships, emotions, sounds, sights, and casualty care milieu found in a wartime nursing environment. Their stories form a tapestry of nursing experience within these two wars.

Because this book is representative of three research studies, the names and some of the demographic details about each nurse have been changed to maintain the anonymity of our research study participants. All study participants signed informed consent documents and agreed to have their interview comments repeated in scholarly presentations of this research as well as published in print media such as nursing journals and books. Any statement enclosed in quotation marks was recorded in a formal interview and represents that individual's recollection of events leading up to, during, and after their deployment to Iraq or Afghanistan. The quoted statements are the opinions and recollections of the people who expressed them. They do not constitute an official position of the Department of Defense or the military services.

For every military nurse who served in Iraq or Afghanistan during the war years 2003 through 2010, there is a story. Their stories contribute to the history of U.S. military nursing and add to the developing body of knowledge about nursing in war. This book gives the nurses a voice.

We are grateful to the nurses who shared their personal accounts with us. We acknowledge and respect their courage, dedication, and commitment as they ventured into harm's way to provide timely life-saving care to those injured by explosive projectiles and gunfire. The care they provided stretched across cultural and ideological boundaries to include U.S. and coalition troops as well as contractors, insurgents, detainees, local villagers, and children.

At Springer Publishing, we thank Allan Graubard, executive editor, for championing the need and demand for this book. His thoughtful advice along the way is greatly appreciated.

We are indebted to Brigadier General Linda Stierle, USAF, NC (ret.), and Major General Melissa Rank, USAF, NC (ret.), for review of our manuscript and many helpful suggestions. Our heartfelt thanks go to Colonel Jennifer Wilber, USA, NC (ret.), and Colonel Linda Kisner, USAF, NC (ret.), for their help in advertising our research studies to potential participants. We also want to thank our family—Len, Chris, Meaghan, Marie, Sadie, and Max—for their patience, support, and belief in us and in this book. We acknowledge support of the granting agencies, Connecticut State Universities/American Association of University Professors and Foundation of New York State Nurses in funding the three research studies defined in this book.

It is our hope that the nursing voices of the Iraq and Afghanistan wars will contribute to future improvements and training for those who will follow. We believe that the nurses' stories will inspire and guide future generations of nurses.

REFERENCES

Colaizzi, P. (1978). Psychological research as the phenomenologist reviews it. In R. Valle, & M. King (Eds.), *Existential-phenomenological alternatives in psychology* (pp. 48–71). New York, NY: Oxford Press.

Denzin, N., & Lincoln, Y. (2000). *Handbook of qualitative research.* Thousand Oaks, CA: Sage.

Doherty, M. E., & Scannell-Desch, E. A. (in press). Women's health and hygiene experiences while deployed in Iraq and Afghanistan during the war years 2003–2010. *Journal of Midwifery and Women's Health.*

Husserl, E. (1970). *Crisis of European sciences and transcendental phenomenology.* Evanston, IL: Northwestern University Press.

Polit, D., & Hungler, B. (2000). *Essentials of nursing research: Methods, appraisal and utilization.* Philadelphia, PA: Lippincott, Williams and Wilkins.

Scannell-Desch, E. A., & Doherty, M. E. (2010). Experiences of U.S. military nurses in the Iraq and Afghanistan Wars, 2003-2009. *Journal of Nursing Scholarship, 42*(1), 3–12.

1

Historical Roots of U.S. Military Nursing

Although this book tells the stories of U.S. military nurses in Iraq and Afghanistan during the war years of 2003 to 2011, it is important and timely to provide contextual and historical information about the roots of military nursing. To do so, we must start with the world's most famous war nurse, Florence Nightingale.

Florence Nightingale is most prominently known and revered for her work in caring for British soldiers in the barracks hospital in Scutari, Turkey. In March 1853, Russia had invaded Turkey. Britain and France, alarmed about the growing imperialism of Russia, went to Turkey's aid. This conflict became known as the Crimean War (Kalisch & Kalisch, 2004). The Crimean War was the first distant war covered by British war correspondents. News from the Crimean region marked the first time the British public was regularly informed of the actualities of war. War correspondents for British newspapers reported the deplorable and neglectful treatment of wounded and sick British soldiers. They described how, soon after the British soldiers arrived in Turkey, they began contracting cholera and malaria. Within a few weeks, an estimated 8,000 soldiers were suffering and dying from these two infectious diseases. These reports so angered the people of Britain that there was a public outcry for British intervention (Hobbs, 1997).

In early October 1854, Florence Nightingale, a woman from a prominent British family, who had trained as a nurse in France with the Sisters of Charity and in Germany with the Protestant Deaconess nuns, offered her services to the British War Office after being contacted by her friend, Sidney Herbert, the British Secretary for War. Nightingale was promised full support from the War Office and the British Army if she accepted the challenge to lead a group of British nurses to the British Army Garrison in Scutari, Turkey (Bostridge, 2008). On October 21, 1854, Nightingale and her group of 38 female volunteer nurses, many of them Roman Catholic and Anglican nuns, began their travel to Turkey to take over nursing responsibilities in the Scutari barracks hospital (Donahue, 1985).

These women found the conditions at the hospital in Scutari truly appalling. The soldiers were kept in open bays without beds; blankets; towels; clean bandages; medicine; and sufficient amounts of uncontaminated food, eating utensils, and clean water (Kelly & Joel, 1995). Soldiers were still clad in their service uniforms, which were filthy from the dirt of the battlefield. Open wounds and bodies enveloped with cholera or malaria were infested with vermin. The barracks hospital reeked of rotting flesh, infected tissue, and human excrement (Dossey, 2000).

Nightingale and her band of volunteer nurses worked diligently to bring order to the chaos they found at the barracks hospital. They instituted measures to clean up the environment by improving hospital sanitation practices through boiling water, opening windows and doors to allow for improved ventilation, and securing cooking utensils for meal preparation (Bostridge, 2008). Nightingale instituted wound-cleaning measures, established schedules for bandage changing and hot-meal preparation, and introduced proper waste disposal and disinfection of hands and other surfaces using soap and water. She also began recording the measures she took to improve conditions at the hospital and the results in terms of infection rates and other hospital statistics. The sanitary measures she employed dramatically reduced the hospital infection rates and overall mortality rates (Donahue, 1985).

Army commanders and military physicians opposed Nightingale's views on reforming and improving the barracks hospital. They interpreted her comments about the deplorable conditions and the measures she enacted to improve the health and hygiene practices at the hospital as an assault on their competence to manage the hospital and to provide care for their soldiers. As a result of this friction between Nightingale and the military hierarchy in Scutari, Nightingale and all of the nurses were made to feel unwanted and unappreciated (Kalisch & Kalisch, 2004).

Although Nightingale and her team had cleaned up the barracks hospital and added many sanitary and quality-of-life improvements for their soldier-patients, broad-based change did not happen overnight. The British War Office, at the urging of Nightingale, ordered the sanitary commissioners at Scutari to carry out immediate reforms, including revamping and unclogging the hospital's defective sewers and improving sick bay overcrowding and ventilation. By June 1858, the death rate had declined from 42% to 2% (Bostridge, 2008). Although Nightingale cannot be credited solely for the dramatic decline in the death rate, her efforts to improve the sanitation, hygiene, nutrition, and quality-of-life of the soldier-patients at the barracks hospital certainly contributed significantly to this end (Hobbs, 1997). After her tour of duty at Scutari, she went on to assist the British War Office with improvements in other war hospitals. Later, when she returned to England, she expanded her involvement by starting a nursing school, serving in health- and nursing-related posts, and authoring several texts for nurses.

The Crimean War emphasized the significant work of Florence Nightingale and her team serving the British Army in a war zone. This work led to the development and implementation of modern nursing methods and practices throughout the world and served as a foundational step in formalizing military nursing for the future.

EARLY NURSING IN THE UNITED STATES

The historical roots of military nursing in the United States can be traced back to before the founding of our nation. When the fight for independence began in 1775, untrained nurses served on the battlefield as wound dressers and water bearers (Donahue, 1985). General George Washington needed to provide for the medical care of his wounded soldiers, and there were too few men available to serve as nurses. Washington found meaningful work for the wives, mothers, daughters, and sisters of his soldiers who followed their encampments. The Continental Army offered these women employment as nurses, cooks, laundresses, and water bearers, thereby releasing male soldiers to fight. The Continental Army medical corps was authorized to employ one nurse for each 10 sick or wounded soldiers. Since most medical care at the time was provided in the home by women, training programs for nurses were nonexistent in the colonies. Therefore, whatever skills these women brought to war came from home experience or were learned as needed on the battlefield. These nurses were paid a few dollars per month and a daily ration of food and water (Kelly & Joel, 1995).

THE WAR OF 1812

The War of 1812 was fought between the United States and the British Empire. The United States declared war for a variety of reasons. The most prominent included U.S.-preferred expansion into the Northwest Territory, trade restrictions imposed owing to Britain's ongoing war with France, and British support of U.S. Indian tribes against U.S. territorial expansion. The war was primarily naval in scope, although ground troops were also involved (Donahue, 1985).

Female assistance in the War of 1812 was limited to making bandages, preparing meals, and tending to sick and wounded sailors. Untrained nurses served on Commodore Decatur's ship, the United States, caring for wounded sailors. This was the first time women nurses served on a naval vessel. Nurses employed by the Navy were generally wives and widows of sailors (Donahue, 1985).

THE U.S. CIVIL WAR

As we know, the main cause of the Civil War was the practice of slavery in the southern states. Politicians and slave owners in the South became angered at the antislavery factions in the North, especially because of northern attempts to block expansion of slavery into the Western territories. Southern slave owners believed that restrictions on slave ownership violated states' rights. The election of President Abraham Lincoln resulted in declarations of secession from the United States by slave states of the Deep South and their formation of the Confederate States of America. Fighting began in April 1861 when Confederate forces attacked Fort Sumter, a major fortress held by the United States on land claimed by the Confederacy (Kalisch & Kalisch, 2004).

When the Civil War began, there was no organized system within the Union or Confederate armies to care for wounded and ill soldiers. When calls came out from the two respective armies for volunteers to perform nursing duties, women rushed to join (Kelly & Joel, 1995). The Union Army secretary of war appointed Dorothea Lynde Dix, a former schoolteacher and advocate for human rights and mentally ill persons, as superintendent of Women Nurses for the Union Army (Kalisch & Kalisch, 2004).

By 1862, large military hospitals were being built by both the Confederate and Union armies. Since construction took considerable time, buildings of opportunity such as schools, churches, plantation homes, and factories were used as interim hospitals. Women provided casualty care for Union and Confederate troops at field hospitals and on the Union Hospital Ship Red Rover. Those serving included prominent women such as Dorothea Dix, Clara Barton, Mary Bickerdyke, and Louisa May Alcott, who organized nurses and provided support to Union Army casualties, and Walt Whitman, who served as a battlefield wound dresser (Kelly & Joel, 1995). Around 6,000 women performed nursing duties for the Union and Confederate forces. It is estimated that some 181 Black nurses served during the war in Union Army hospitals. Harriet Tubman and Sojourner Truth were notable Black women who provided care for Union soldiers (Carnegie, 1986).

Many women served as nurses in the hospitals of both the Union and Confederate Armies, often venturing out onto the battlefield to perform the humanitarian service of bringing water to the soldiers or bandaging their wounds. These women earned the utmost respect and gratitude of those they served so bravely and unselfishly. After the end of the Civil War, many training programs for nurses were established at U.S. hospitals, so the era of using untrained personnel to provide military casualty care ended (Kalisch & Kalisch, 2004).

THE SPANISH–AMERICAN WAR

This war originated in the Cuban struggle for independence from Spain that began in 1895. The 1898 conflict between Spain and the United States started after the mysterious sinking of the Maine, a U.S. battleship, in the harbor at Havana, Cuba. Prior to the sinking, there had been considerable friction and mistrust in the relationship between Spain and the United States for decades, and the Cuban people had revolted numerous times against Spanish rule of the island. The United States sent an ultimatum to Spain demanding it relinquish control of Cuba. The ultimatum was not accepted, and Spain declared war on the United States (Donahue, 1985).

While the importance of trained female nurses had been demonstrated in U.S. hospitals for several decades after the U.S. Civil War, there were still many physicians and military leaders who questioned whether a field hospital was an appropriate place for a woman. However, the Army surgeon general knew that women would be needed at military base hospitals to serve as nurses and dieticians. Therefore, he appointed both men and women nurses as civilian contract employees for the U.S. Army. At the same time, Dr. Anita Newcomb McGee, vice president general of the Daughters of the American Revolution (DAR), offered to examine all applications referred by the government from women seeking to serve. All applications were forwarded to Dr. McGee, who was permitted by the government to set her own standards. To be considered eligible, a nurse had to be a graduate of a nurse training school and have the endorsement of the school's superintendent. The age limit for these nurses was 30 to 50 years, but exceptions soon needed to be made because of the huge demand for nurses (Kalisch & Kalisch, 2004).

Several Catholic Sisters of Mercy from Baltimore served as nurses at Camp Thomas and the Chickamauga Park Camp in Georgia. The Sisters of Charity from Emmitsburg, Maryland, also provided over 200 nursing nuns to care for the sick and wounded (Donahue, 1985). By August 1898, there were almost a thousand nurses under contract with the demand still growing, owing to the dreadful epidemic of typhoid fever that erupted that summer in the military camps (Kelly & Joel, 1995). Although the military hierarchy had once again been reluctant to employ women nurses in battlefield hospitals and on naval vessels, by the end of the war, nurses proved their value once again (Donahue, 1985). The war with Spain established the essential need for trained nurses as hastily built army camps for more than 28,000 members of the regular army were overcome by diarrhea, dysentery, typhoid, and malaria. These infectious illnesses took more of a toll on the troops than did enemy gunfire (Kalisch & Kalisch, 2004).

The Spanish-American War marked the United States' entrance in the world scene as a global power seeking to expand its influence. U.S. forces quickly overcame the Spanish in the Philippines and then moved on to Cuba. Within months, they overwhelmed the Spanish, and Theodore Roosevelt gained the prominence that would lead him to the U.S. presidency (Alger, 1901).

Nursing under wartime conditions required professional competence, physical stamina, courage, personal discipline, and mental toughness. The nurses employed by the U.S. government became known as *contract nurses*. Between 1898 and 1901, more than 1,500 female nurses signed government contracts. Contract nurses served in the United States, Puerto Rico, the Philippines, Hawaii, China, briefly in Japan, and on the hospital ship, Relief. Fifteen nurses died of febrile illnesses while serving (Kalisch & Kalisch, 2004). Owing to the exemplary performance of contract nurses during the Spanish-American War, the U.S. military realized that it would be helpful to have a corps of trained nurses, familiar with military ways, available on an on-call basis. This led the way to the establishment of the Army Nurse Corps and Army Reserve Nurse Corps (Kelly & Joel, 1995).

U.S. ARMY AND NAVY NURSE CORPS ESTABLISHED

On February 2, 1901, the U.S. Army Nurse Corps became a permanent corps of the Medical Department under the Army Reorganization Act passed by Congress. Nurses were appointed to the Regular Army for a three-year period, although they were not actually commissioned as officers in the Regular Army during that period. The appointment could be renewed provided that the applicant had a satisfactory record of nursing performance, professional conduct, and good health. The law directed the surgeon general to maintain a list of qualified nurses who were willing to serve on an emergency basis as a reserve unit of the Army Nurse Corps. On March 25, 1901, Dita H. Kinney, a former Army contract nurse, was officially appointed the first superintendent of the Army Nurse Corps, a position she held until she resigned in July 1909 (Sarnecky, 1999). In October 1908, the Army Nurse Corps consisted of an initial core group of 20 nurses. Many of them had previous experience serving as Army contract nurses with the military. The Navy Nurse Corps was established in 1908 with 20 women selected as the first members. Esther Voorhees Hasson served as the first superintendent of the U.S. Navy Nurse Corps from 1908 to 1911 (Kalisch & Kalisch, 2004).

WORLD WAR I

Although the assassination on June 28, 1914 of Archduke Ferdinand of Austria, the heir to the throne of Austria-Hungary, was the immediate cause of the war, larger issues tied to imperialism also contributed. Simply, the ambitions of the great powers—Germany, France, Russia, Great Britain, and Italy—to control lands beyond their borders and to harvest their human and material capital, played a key role in fueling the winds of war (Goodspeed, 1985). The Archduke's assassination by a Yugoslav nationalist resulted in the Habsburg ultimatum against the Kingdom of Serbia. Several alliances formed over previous decades were invoked. Within weeks, the major powers were at war, and conflict soon spread around the world (Chickering, 2004).

The United States initially followed a strategy of nonintervention. When a German submarine sank the British ocean liner Lusitania in 1915, with 128 Americans aboard, U.S. President Woodrow Wilson demanded an end to attacks on passenger ships. Initially, Germany complied with this request. Wilson repeatedly warned that the United States would not tolerate unrestricted submarine warfare in violation of international law and human rights. In January 1917, Germany resumed unrestricted submarine warfare. After the sinking of seven U.S. merchant ships by submarines, President Wilson called for war on Germany, which the U.S. Congress declared on April 6, 1917 (Chickering, 2004).

When the United States entered the war, military nursing strength was very low. Only 403 Army nurses were on active duty, including 170 reserve nurses who had been ordered to duty in 12 Army hospitals in Texas, Arizona, and New Mexico. The United States stepped up its recruiting efforts, and more than 400 nurses sailed for France for service with the British Expeditionary Forces in May 1917. By 1918, more than 12,000 Army nurses were on active duty serving at 198 bases worldwide. During the course of the war, 21,480 Army nurses served in military hospitals in the United States and overseas (Sarnecky, 1999). More than 1,476 Navy nurses served in military hospitals stateside and overseas. More than 400 military nurses died in the line of duty during World War I (Kalisch & Kalisch, 2004). The vast majority of these women succumbed from a highly contagious form of influenza known as the Spanish flu, which swept through crowded military camps, hospitals, and ports of embarkation. Several nurses received wartime wounds, but none died because of enemy action (Sarnecky, 1999).

In May 1918, the Army School of Nursing was authorized by the Secretary of War. Courses of instruction began at several Army hospitals in July 1918. Annie W. Goodrich was appointed as Chief Inspector Nurse for the Army. She also became the first Dean of the Army School of Nursing. During World War I, Army nurses did not have officer status. They were not commissioned but appointed into the ANC. Appointment, rather than commission, meant that a nurse lieutenant received less pay than a male infantry commissioned lieutenant (Sarnecky, 1999).

WORLD WAR II (1941–1945)

As we know, World War II began in September 1939 when Germany invaded Poland. There were subsequent declarations of war on Germany by France and the British Commonwealth. The war extended into much of Europe and North Africa. In June 1941, Germany and the Axis powers launched an invasion into the Soviet Union (Adamthwaite, 1992). On September 11, 1941, U.S. President Franklin Roosevelt ordered the Navy and Army Air Corps to shoot on sight at any German war vessel. On December 7, 1941, the United States was attacked by the Japanese in a daring surprise assault on the Pacific fleet at Pearl Harbor, Hawaii. President Franklin D. Roosevelt and the U.S. Congress swiftly declared war on Japan. The German government discontinued diplomatic relations with the United States and declared war on the them on December 11, 1941 (Adamthwaite, 1992).

When the United States entered World War II in December 1941, U.S. military nursing assets were at peacetime diminished strength. There were fewer than 1,000 nurses in the Army Nurse Corps and 700 in the Navy Nurse Corps; all were women. Over the next six months, their numbers grew to more than 12,000. Throughout the duration of the war, more than 60,000 Army nurses served in the United States and overseas in every theater of U.S. military operations (Sarnecky, 1999). Sixty-seven Army nurses were captured by the Japanese in the Philippines in 1942 and were held as prisoners of war for over two and a half years (Frank, 1985). More than 14,000 Navy nurses served in the United States and overseas on hospital ships and at naval bases (Link & Coleman, 1955). Five Navy nurses were captured by the Japanese in Guam and held as prisoners of war for 5 months before being exchanged. A second group of 11 Navy nurses was captured in the Philippines and held for 3 years (Norman, 1999).

Military nurses were wounded by enemy fire on the beaches at Anzio, Italy, during the Allied beachhead landings. Nurses were killed in air evacuation flights and spent time behind enemy lines. They worked closer to the front lines than ever before. Army nurses were on Omaha beach just a few days after the D-Day invasion of Normandy and in North Africa caring for casualties from the tank battles (Hastings & Stevens, 1985).

Although carrying injured soldiers by airplane had been discussed and tried between the World Wars, the usefulness of this means of patient transport became a necessity in World War II. Use of air transport to move injured U.S. troops introduced the advent of a new nursing specialty, flight nursing. The first class of Army Air Corps flight nurses trained at Bowman Field, Kentucky, and graduated in February 1943. Their 6-week course included a curriculum of air evacuation nursing, air evacuation tactics, survival training, altitude physiology, mental hygiene in relation to flying, aircraft loading procedures, cargo aircraft interior reconfiguration procedures, and field bivouac (Link & Coleman, 1955). Following graduation, they quickly began flying aeromedical evacuation missions aboard C-47 transport aircrafts in the European, African, and Pacific theaters of operation. Flight nursing was considered the most dangerous nursing duty, and 17 flight nurses were killed during the war (Donahue, 1985). The war in Europe ended on May 8, 1945, and the war in the Pacific ended on September 2, 1945, with the surrender of Japan (Hastings & Stevens, 1985).

During World War II, the Army Air Corps became a significant, highly specialized, and sophisticated fighting force. Following the end of World War II, the Army Air Corps became a separate service, named the U.S. Air Force, in 1947. Later, in 1949, the Air Force Nurse Corps was established. A segment of the Army Nurse Corps, many of them flight nurses, transferred to the newly formed Air Force Nurse Corps (Barger, 1991). The Army–Navy Nurse Act of 1947 made the Army Nurse Corps and the Women's Medical Specialist Corps part of the Regular Army and gave permanent-commissioned-officer status to military nurses. This legislation put an end to relative rank and the full-but-temporary ranks granted during the middle of World War II. The law also granted military nurses permanent ranks and commissions in the Regular and Reserve Corps equal to the ranks of male officers (Sarnecky, 1999).

THE KOREAN WAR (1950–1953)

As we know, the Korean War was a military action between South Korea and North Korea. South Korea was backed by the United Nations (UN), and North Korea was supported by the People's Republic of China (PRC), along with military ordinance and weaponry supplied by the Soviet Union. The war was a result of the physical division of Korea by agreement of the Allied forces at the end of the Pacific fighting in War World II (Halberstam, 2007).

Following Japan's surrender in 1945, U.S. occupational forces divided the Korean peninsula along the 38th parallel, with U.S. troops occupying the southern part and Soviet troops occupying the northern part. The 38th parallel increasingly became a political border between the two Koreas, with frequent border attacks by the two sides. The situation escalated into open warfare when North Korean forces invaded South Korea on June 25, 1950. The United Nations, principally led by the United States, came to the aid of South Korea in repelling the invasion. The U.S. Army, Navy, and Air Force were employed to aid the South Korean military (Foot, 1985). At the beginning of the conflict, the U.S. Army Nurse Corps active-duty strength was below 3,500 persons, and that of the U.S. Navy Nurse Corps was below 2,000 nurses. The newly established Air Force Nurse Corps yielded fewer than 1,200 nurses (Kalisch & Kalisch, 2004). Many U.S. nursing leaders expected a mass exodus of civilian nurses to join the military, but this exodus never occurred. From 1950 until the end of the Korean War in 1953, the Army Nurse Corps membership rose to a modest 5,500, while the Navy Nurse Corps increased to about 3,200 nurses, and the Air Force Nurse Corps to about 1,800 members (Clarke, 1951; Kalisch & Kalisch, 2004).

During the Korean War, Navy nurses were assigned to hospital ships and at overseas and stateside bases. Three hospital ships, the Consolation, Repose, and Haven, rotated as main seaborne hospitals in Korean waters. Two hundred Air Force flight nurses were quickly engaged in providing air evacuation of wounded soldiers to base hospitals away from the fighting. Although Army Air Corps nurses served as flight nurses in World War II, the specialty of flight nursing really expanded and matured during the Korean War. The Korean War also provided the first real test of the usefulness of the helicopter and the Army's Mobile Surgical Hospital (MASH), a concept that had been born out of assessment of World War II casualty evacuation needs (Kalisch & Kalisch, 2004).

The typical MASH unit included about 15 physicians, 16 nurses, and 120 enlisted medical personnel. The nursing staff comprised 2 nurse anesthetists, 4 operating room nurses, and 10 nurses working on preoperative and postoperative wards. A helicopter unit was assigned to each MASH to provide rapid transport from the area of battle. Once patients were treated, they were either held at the MASH for recovery or, if their injuries would require longer-term care, evacuated by helicopter or air evacuation transport plane to a hospital further to the rear.

As was the case in World War II, Army nurses served in the war zone close to the extremely fluid front lines. As a rule, nurses were the only military women allowed into the combat theater. Nurses served in MASH units, in field hospitals, on hospital trains, and on Army transport ships and Navy hospital ships at the beginning of the war. Once again, nurses found themselves treating casualties on foreign shores and in the air aboard C-47 and C-54 cargo aircrafts. Army nurses staffed MASH units and standard hospitals in Japan and Korea. Navy nurses served on hospital ships in the Korean theater of operations as well as at Navy hospitals stateside. Air Force nurses served stateside, in hospitals in Japan and Okinawa, and as flight nurses in the Korean theater. Nurses found themselves on the forefront of battlefield medicine, playing a major role in the treatment of wounded UN forces within mere minutes or hours of the wounds being inflicted (Holm, 1982; Hovis, 1992). One Army nurse, 11 Navy nurses, and 3 Air Force nurses were killed during Korean War service (Donahue, 1985).

In 1953, the war ended with an armistice that restored the border between the Koreas near the 38th parallel and created the Korean Demilitarized Zone, a 2.5-mile-wide (4.0 km) buffer zone between the two Koreas. Minor outbreaks of fighting continue to the present day.

Following the end of the Korean War, male nurses were accepted into the Army and Air Force Nurse Corps in 1955. It was not until 1965 that men were accepted into the Navy Nurse Corps (Donahue, 1985).

THE VIETNAM WAR (1965–1973)

There was no fixed beginning for U.S. involvement in Vietnam. The United States entered that war incrementally in a series of steps between 1950 and 1965. In 1950, President Truman authorized a modest program of economic and military aid to the French, who were fighting to retain control of their Indochina colonies, including Laos, Cambodia, and Vietnam. When the Vietnamese Nationalist Viet Minh army defeated the French forces at Dien Bien Phu in 1954, the French were forced to agree to the creation of a Communist Vietnam in the north at the 17th parallel while leaving a non-Communist portion of Vietnam south of that line. The United States refused to accept the arrangement. U.S. President Eisenhower feared the spread of communism throughout Vietnam and sent military advisers to train the fledgling South Vietnamese Army (Lewy, 1977).

In 1961, U.S. President Kennedy sent 400 Special Operations Forces-trained Green Beret soldiers to teach the South Vietnamese how to fight what was called a "counterinsurgency war" against Communist guerrillas in South Vietnam. When Kennedy was assassinated in November 1963, there were more than 16,000 U.S. military advisers in South Vietnam. President Lyndon Johnson committed the United States more deeply to the war. In early 1965, Johnson authorized the sustained bombing of targets north of the 17th parallel, and in March, he dispatched 3,500 combat Marines to South Vietnam (The Pentagon Papers, 1971).

The fundamental reason for U.S. involvement in Vietnam was rooted in the fear that the Viet Minh, then the National Liberation Front (NLF), and the forces of Ho Chi Minh would become agents of global communism. U.S. administrations after the end of World War II through the late 1960s bought into the domino theory, which held that if one nation fell to communism, other nations would follow like dominos lined up on end. U.S. policymakers viewed Vietnam as the first domino in Southeast Asia (Lewy, 1977).

Before the current wars in Iraq and Afghanistan, the Vietnam War was the longest war fought by the U.S. military. Although this was an undeclared war, active U.S. military participation began in 1961 and lasted until early 1973 (Santoli, 1985). Humanitarian military aeromedical evacuations were flown into and out of Vietnam until April 1975 (Scannell-Desch, 1996; Schimmenti & Darmoody, 1986). A total of 2.6 million U.S. military personnel served in Vietnam (Frye & Stockton, 1982), of whom over 250,000 were seriously injured or wounded (Cook, 1988) and over 58,000 were killed or listed as missing and presumed dead (Jones & Janello, 1987).

According to U.S. Department of Defense estimates, between 1962 and 1973, approximately 7,500 U.S. military women served on active duty in Vietnam (Walker, 1985). About 80% of these women were members of the Army, Navy, or Air Force Nurse Corps (Marshall, 1988). Among the more than 58,000 names carved on the wall of the Vietnam Veterans Memorial in Washington, D.C., are those of eight female and two male military nurses. Their names are preserved on the wall along with the sailors, soldiers, airmen, and marines they cared for and died with (Scannell-Desch, 2000a).

The Vietnam War was fought with no discernible front lines, safe places, or clear rules of engagement. Much of the enemy forces did not wear uniforms, and in some situations, it was impossible to distinguish the enemy from pro-U.S. or neutral villagers. These circumstances added a dimension of deception and confusion to the fighting (Gault, 1971; Schwartz, 1987), and soldiers on patrol rarely saw the enemy they were attempting to kill (Freedman & Rhoads, 1987; Santoli, 1981).

In April 1965, with the rapid buildup of American forces in Vietnam, Army nurses were dispatched with medical units to support the fighting forces. The 8th Field Hospital, Nha Trang, had been the only U.S. Army hospital in the country for three years. The 3rd Field Hospital, Saigon, was the first to arrive during the buildup (Freedman & Rhoads, 1987).

Because there were no front lines or consistently secure road systems in Vietnam, the helicopter became the primary means of evacuating casualties from combat to medical facilities. Helicopters, known as "dust-offs," delivered wounded troops to hospitals or aid stations within minutes of injury (Cook, 1988). As a result of this rapid evacuation, many patients who would have died in previous wars were kept alive by pressure dressings, intravenous fluids, emergency tracheotomies, and a short flight to immediate surgical care (Freedman & Rhoads, 1987; Schwartz, 1987). As Holm (1982) pointed out, "the record of the Vietnam War in terms of saving the lives of the wounded was unparalleled in the history of warfare. Less than 2% of the casualties treated died as a result of their wounds" (p. 233).

The first Navy hospital opened in Saigon in 1963 (McVicker, 1985). As the war progressed, the Navy established hospitals in Danang and near Cam Ranh Bay (Marshall, 1988). The Danang hospital was completely leveled by an enemy rocket in 1965, injuring several nurses (Donahue, 1985; Martin, 1967). The majority of Navy nurses assigned to the Vietnam theater of operations were stationed aboard two hospital ships, the U.S.N. Repose and the U.S.N. Sanctuary, which sailed off the coast in the South China Sea. These ships followed the intensity of the fighting up and down the coast, usually between Danang and the demilitarized zone in the north (Marshall, 1988). The U.S.N. Repose, for example, was 520 feet long and could accommodate up to 750 patients. The ship was completely air-conditioned and superbly equipped with intensive care units and operating rooms. Battle casualties needing immediate surgery were evacuated to these floating hospitals by dust-offs, sometimes within 5 minutes after injury (Martin, 1967). Navy nurses went on to serve in the Provincial Health Assistance Program at Rach Gia from 1965 to 1968 and at the station hospital at Danang from August 1967 to May 1970. The Danang hospital became the Navy's largest land-based combat casualty treatment facility, with 600 beds and admissions of 63,000 patients (Holm, 1982).

Air Force nurses worked in large evacuation hospitals, such as the 12th USAF Hospital, Cam Ranh Bay, Vietnam, and at smaller hospitals, called *casualty staging flights*, such as those at Phan Rang, Danang, and Tan Son Nhut Air Base (Martin, 1967). The hospital at Cam Ranh Bay usually operated at a bed capacity of 650 but could be expanded to up to 1,200 beds when necessary. It consisted of 18 Quonset hut wards, most of which were air-conditioned (Marshall, 1988). Air Force flight nurses cared for wounded troops on in-country aeromedical evacuation flights, using the C-7 Caribou, the C-123 Provider, and the C-130 Hercules aircraft. These planes were propeller or turbo-prop cargo aircraft, which were reconfigured to carry patients in litter stations within the rear fuselage. Additionally, the planes could perform in a short takeoff and landing configuration and could safely land on a short dirt strip. When under enemy fire, loading of patients could be accomplished in 1 to 3 minutes as the plane stayed in a slow taxi or takeoff roll. These planes could take off under fire with the back doors still open. This type of loading was referred to as *hot loading* by most flight and aeromedical crews (Scannell-Desch, 1999, 2000b).

Strategic aeromedical evacuation missions carried the more seriously wounded or ill patients out of Vietnam to medical facilities at Clark Air Base, Philippines; Yakota Air Base, Japan; Kadena Air Base, Okinawa, or back to the continental United States (Marshall, 1988; Schwartz, 1987). The aircraft used for these long-range missions was the C-141 Starlifter, which could accommodate up to 77 litter patients in the wartime configuration of 5 patients per tier. Routinely on in-country and strategic aeromedical evacuation missions, a flight nurse served as senior medical authority aboard the aircraft. Physicians rarely served on air evacuation missions (Scannell-Desch, 1996, 1999, 2005).

Flight nurses airlifted more than 400,000 patients between 1964 and 1973. During the height of the Tet 1968 offensive, about 11,000 casualties were airlifted per month (Schimmenti & Darmoody, 1986). Additionally, when Saigon was falling in April 1975, flight nurses airlifted more than 1,000 homeless infants and refugees as part of Operations Babylift and New Life. The last military nurse to die in Vietnam was an Air Force flight nurse, Captain Mary Therese Klinker. She was killed while caring for Babylift children when her C-5 Galaxy aircraft experienced a catastrophic decompression and crashed shortly after takeoff from Tan Son Nhut Air Base, Vietnam (Scannell-Desch, 1996).

The Army sent more nurses to Vietnam than the other services combined. The Army established 27 field, evacuation, surgical, and convalescent hospitals on the coast and at inland locations within the Republic of South Vietnam. Many of these medical facilities were close to the fighting. Inflatable rubber shelters known as MUSTs (medical unit, self-contained, transportable) were shipped to Vietnam for the Army Medical Services; however, the lack of a safe road system severely hampered the mobility of these medical units. These hospitals, therefore, could not follow and support tactical troop movements and other ground operations, so most were converted to fixed permanent medical installations (Donahue, 1985).

Thousands of U.S. Army nurses served in Vietnam between 1962 and 1973. The largest number for any single year was 900 in 1969. Several were wounded, and nine Army nurses and one Air Force nurse died while serving. One Army nurse, 1st Lt. Sharon A. Lane, was killed by hostile fire. The other seven female nurses and two male nurses died in the line of duty in Vietnam (Bigler, 1996). On March 29, 1973, the last of more than 5,000 nurses departed from the Republic of Vietnam, two months after the ceasefire (Freedman & Rhoads, 1987).

CHANGES IN U.S. POLICY AFTER THE VIETNAM WAR

By the mid-1970s, policy changes relating to women serving in the military were long overdue. These policy changes finally paved the way for equal treatment for women serving on active duty with minor children as family members. In late 1974, the U.S. Supreme Court ruled that inequities in benefits for the dependents of military women were unconstitutional. Until then, military women with dependents were not authorized housing, nor were their dependents eligible for benefits and privileges afforded the dependents of male military members, such as medical, commissary, and post exchange availability. In 1975, the Department of Defense finally reversed its policy and provided pregnant service women with the option of electing discharge or remaining on active duty. The previous policy required that women be discharged upon pregnancy or the adoption of children (Holm, 1982).

THE PERSIAN GULF WAR (1990–1991)

The invasion of Kuwait by Iraqi troops that began on August 2, 1990, was met with international condemnation and brought immediate economic sanctions against Iraq by members of the UN Security Council. President George H. W. Bush deployed U.S. forces to Saudi Arabia and urged other countries to send their own forces to the Persian Gulf. A wide assortment of nations joined the deployment of coalition forces. The majority of the military forces in the coalition came from the United States, Saudi Arabia, the United Kingdom, and Egypt.

The Persian Gulf War (August 2, 1990–February 28, 1991), commonly referred to as the Gulf War, was waged by a UN-authorized coalition force from 34 nations led by the United States against Iraq in response to Iraq's invasion of the sovereign nation of Kuwait. The mobilization buildup of coalition forces was known as Operation Desert Shield, whereas the actual fighting after mobilization became known as Operation Desert Storm. Operation Desert Storm commenced with aerial bombardment of Iraqi troops and bunkers on January 17, 1991. Once targets were softened by airborne assault, the ground war followed on February 23, 1991 (Schwartzkopf, 1992).

Some 40,000 U.S. military women were deployed during Operations Desert Shield and Desert Storm. By January 17, 1991, when the air campaign began, 2,265 Army nurses were serving in the Persian Gulf. At the conclusion of the ground war on February 28, 1991, 2,215 Army Nurse Corps officers were on duty in the Persian Gulf region. As of April 1991, the required strength of the Army Nurse Corps in the Persian Gulf theater was 2,211, and 2,214 Army nurses were assigned there (Sarnecky, 2010). The Army Medical Department mobilization in support of Operation Desert Shield/Desert Storm was enormous, complex, and very challenging. At this time, the Army was converting from its Vietnam-era MUST hospital configuration with updated deployable medical system equipment and tentage. Many of the units deploying to the Persian Gulf had the MUST equipment. Deploying medical personnel soon discovered that the desert environment severely tested the efficient operation of those medical units that went to war with the MUST setup, and this forced a fast-track substitution of deployable medical systems in many of the Army's medical units (Sarnecky, 2010).

In addition to updating medical material and equipment assets with deployable medical systems, the Army Medical Department was also transitioning to a new doctrine and concept of operations, called Medical Force 2000, at the time of Operation Desert Shield/Desert Storm. Two important changes included far-forward surgical care and enriched psychiatric support. It used forward surgical teams (FSTs), exceedingly mobile portions of the MASH, to provide initial care close to the combat area. The FSTs operated separately from their units of origin by moving with the combat forces to provide far-forward surgical treatment. An FST usually had a staff of 10 officers and 10 enlisted medics. The officer staff usually included two nurse anesthetists, an operating room nurse, one medical–surgical nurse, one critical care nurse, three trauma surgeons, an orthopedic surgeon, and one field medical officer. The enlisted component usually included four emergency medical technicians, three surgical technicians, and three practical nurses. To enhance psychiatric capability, the Army employed combat stress teams staffed by psychiatric nurses, psychiatrists, psychologists, social workers, and chaplains to assess, treat, and efficiently return troops with combat stress symptoms to the battlefield (Sarnecky, 2010).

When the air campaign began, the Air Force had deployed 972 nurses on active duty, of whom 19 were flight nurses, and 872 nurses from the Air Reserve Component, of whom 613 were qualified as flight nurses. This was the largest Air Force medical deployment since the Vietnam War. The Air Force medical deployment in support of Operation Desert Shield began in August 1990. Air Force medical teams were the first medical assets in the Gulf, arriving on the Arabian Peninsula just two days after combat units. The Central Command surgeon controlled one 250-bed contingency hospital, 15 air-transportable hospitals, 31 air-transportable clinics, and several aeromedical staging facilities in the Persian Gulf theater of operations. The European Command Surgeon controlled four contingency hospitals, three in England and one in Germany, in preparation for potential casualties that needed to be moved out of the combat theater for more extensive and definitive treatment (Lindberg, 1999).

Shortly after Iraqi troops invaded Kuwait, Navy medical personnel deployed to Saudi Arabia. Navy corpsmen accompanied Marine units in the combat zone. Three days after forces were committed to support Operation Desert Shield on the Arabian Peninsula, deployment orders went out to the Navy hospital ships, the U.S.N. Comfort and U.S.N. Mercy. Both vessels were immediately activated, manned, and supplied. They were on station and ready in the Persian Gulf by September 23, 1990 (*United States Navy*, 1991).

After being treated by a corpsman in the field, sick or injured personnel could be rapidly moved to battalion aid stations, where a physician could assess their condition in a safer environment with ample time to accomplish a more definitive examination. The next step up the medical ladder of care was a medical battalion surgical support company or a casualty receiving and treatment ship, where patients were treated by teams of medical personnel with more sophisticated medical facilities, including pharmacy and laboratory facilities, holding wards, and more specialty surgical capability. Casualties requiring even more extensive treatment were transported to either a combat zone fleet hospital or a hospital ship. The scope of treatment available at the combat fleet hospital or hospital ship mirrored fully staffed hospitals in the United States (*United States Navy*, 1991).

Although the casualty toll on the coalition forces was light in the Persian Gulf War, the U.S. and coalition medical forces stood ready to handle a much more robust onslaught of injured troops and civilian casualties. The coalition ceased their advance and declared a cease-fire 100 hours after the ground campaign started (Schwartzkopf, 1992). The medical concept of operations in war had evolved from the Vietnam era of mostly fixed medical facility assets to a much more fluid and mobile set of small facilities tailored to follow the fighting. This concept has been carried forward into the current wars in Afghanistan and Iraq.

THE WAR IN AFGHANISTAN

In December 1979, the Soviet Union deployed occupying troops to Afghanistan. Shortly after the invasion, like thousands of Muslims throughout the world, a wealthy Saudi Arabian named Osama Bin Laden traveled to Afghanistan to join the Afghan resistance. Osama Bin Laden and his comrades viewed it as the duty of all Muslims to repel the Soviet invasion. Bin Laden helped finance and take command of about 20,000 Muslim freedom fighters from around the world. The conflict lasted almost 10 years and ended with a Soviet force withdrawal. Later, Bin Laden left Afghanistan but became increasing militant toward the west, especially the United States (Cole, 2004; Feifer, 2009).

The United States went to war in Afghanistan because the global intelligence community determined that Osama Bin Laden, a known terrorist whose global organization was called Al Qaeda, was behind the September

11, 2001, attacks on the United States, and that he was being sheltered in Afghanistan by the Taliban. After several unsuccessful attempts to negotiate the surrender of Bin Laden to U.S. security forces, the United States launched bombing attacks on Afghanistan, specifically on the Taliban. Later, Osama Bin Laden was killed in Pakistan in a daring surprise raid ordered by U.S. President Barack Obama and carried out by a U.S. military special-forces unit on May 2, 2011.

Several coalition countries, including the United States, deployed forces to Afghanistan to engage the Taliban and Al Qaeda on the ground. In 2003, the United States began assigning military nurses and other medical personnel to formerly Russian-built hospitals in Bagram and Kandahar, Afghanistan. These personnel were housed in tents or primitive plywood structures called "B-huts." The medical mission was to support U.S. and coalition forces deployed in Afghanistan at the time. From 2003 through 2010, the number of nurses deployed to Afghanistan increased, as did the number of combat forces.

THE WAR IN IRAQ

On another front, the March 2003 invasion of Iraq was considered a continuation of the Gulf War of 1991. The 1991 Gulf War, known as Operation Desert Storm, started several months after Saddam Hussein invaded Kuwait. Hussein's forces were subsequently defeated by coalition forces, led by the United States and the United Kingdom, after short-lived combat operations. Following Hussein's defeat, the Iraqi government had agreed to surrender or destroy several types of weapons, including missiles and chemical and biological weapons caches. In early 2003, the U.S. government, led by President George W. Bush, believed that Iraq was still hiding some weapons of mass destruction. As a result, in March 2003, Operation Iraqi Freedom, with a combined force of troops from the United States, the United Kingdom, and smaller contingents from Australia and Poland, invaded Iraq and toppled the regime of Saddam Hussein, which concluded with the fall of Baghdad.

After the fall of Baghdad, the second phase of the Iraq War lasted until August 31, 2010. The second phase was marked by urban warfare in the cities, intermittent ground operations, convoys being blown up by improvised explosive devices, construction to restore Iraqi infrastructure by provisional reconstruction teams, and many military and civilian casualties. The third phase of the war began on September 1, 2010, and consisted of a drawdown and redistribution of U.S. and coalition forces into a training mode to support the Iraqi military and police forces. This third phase ended 12/31/2011 when the last U.S. troops were withdrawn from Iraq by U.S. President Barack Obama.

The first contingent of military nurses supporting the U.S. invasion of Iraq was sent to Kuwait in February 2003. When the U.S. invasion began in late March, nurses assigned to FSTs and mobile hospitals moved into Iraq and quickly set up to receive the first casualties. It was not long before an intermittent stream of the injured and dead began to ebb and flow into triage areas and a hastily set up morgue (Ruff & Roper, 2005). The U.S. military and its nurses had embarked on a long journey that would test its resolve as well as its nursing readiness for war.

CURRENT STATUS OF AFGHANISTAN AND IRAQ WARS

U.S. military nurses and nurses from multinational coalition forces served in the Iraq and Afghanistan war zones. All U.S. military personnel left Iraq by December 31, 2011. Many of these nurses are from the military services of the United Kingdom, Australia, Germany, Denmark, Poland, South Korea, and Spain, as well as the U.S. Army, Navy, and Air Force. These nurses are members of their respective military services and are providing care for their own forces as well as forces of other coalition countries, local civilians caught in the crossfire of war, and insurgents brought to their hospitals for care.

In 2009, the death toll of U.S. forces deployed to Iraq and Afghanistan surpassed 5,000. Estimates place the number of physically injured U.S. personnel at over 35,000, and no estimate of those psychologically injured is available. The number of military nurses deployed to Iraq and Afghanistan from 2003 through 2009 is not available, nor is the number of nurses injured in these wars. To date, one Army nurse has been killed in Iraq, and no U.S. military nurses have been killed in Afghanistan. Very little has been written about the U.S. military nurse experience in the Iraq and Afghanistan wars.

REFERENCES

Adamthwaite, A. P. (1992). *The making of the second World War.* New York: Routledge.

Alger, R. A. (1901). *The Spanish-American War.* New York: Harper & Brothers.

Barger, J. (1991). Preparing for war: Lessons learned from U.S. Army flight nurses of World War II. *Aviation, Space, and Environmental Medicine, 62*: 772–775.

Bigler, P. (1996). *Hostile fire: The life and death of First Lieutenant Sharon Lane.* Washington, DC: Vandamere Press.

Bostridge, M. (2008). *Florence Nightingale: The woman and her legend.* London: Viking Press.

Carnegie, M. (1986). *The path we tread: Blacks in nursing 1854–1984.* Philadelphia: Lippincott.

Chickering, R. (2004). *Imperial Germany and the Great War, 1914-1918.* Cambridge, United Kingdom: Cambridge University Press.
Clarke, A. (1951). Draft nurses: A new war and old theme, *R.N., 14*(3), 24-25.
Cole, S. (2004). *Ghost wars: The secret history of the CIA, Afghanistan, and Bin Laden, from the Soviet invasion to September 10, 2001.* New York: Penguin Press.
Cook, J. L. (1988). *Dust Off: The Vietnam War.* New York: Bantam Books.
Donahue, M. P. (1985). *Nursing, the finest art: An illustrated history.* St. Louis, MO: C.V. Mosby.
Dossey, B. M. (2000). *Florence Nightingale: Mystic, visionary, reformer.* Philadelphia: Lippincott, Williams & Wilkins.
Feifer, G. (2009). *The great gamble: The Soviet war in Afghanistan.* New York: Harper.
Foot, R. (1985). *The wrong war: American policy and the dimensions of the Korean conflict, 1950-1953.* Ithaca, NY: Cornell University Press.
Frank, M. E. (1985). *Army and Navy nurses held as prisoners of war during World War II.* Washington, DC: Department of Defense, Office of the Assistant Secretary of Defense, Manpower, Installations and Logistics.
Freedman, D., & Rhoads, J. (Eds.). (1987). *Nurses in Vietnam: Forgotten veterans.* Austin, TX: Texas Monthly Press.
Frye, J., & Stockton, R. (1982). Discriminant analysis of post-traumatic stress disorders among a group of Vietnam veterans. *American Journal of Psychiatry, 139,* 52-56.
Gault, W. (1971). Some remarks on slaughter. *American Journal of Psychiatry, 128*(4), 450-451.
Goodspeed, D. J. (1985). *The German Wars 1914-1945.* New York: Random House.
Halberstam, D. (2007). *The coldest winter: America and the Korean War.* New York: Disney Hyperion.
Hastings, M., & Stevens, G. (1985). *Victory in Europe.* Boston: Little, Brown, & Co.
Hobbs, C. A. (1997). *Florence Nightingale.* New York: Prentice Hall.
Holm, J. (1982). *Women in the military.* Novoto, CA: Presidio.
Hovis, B. (1992). *Station Hospital Saigon.* Annapolis, MD: Naval Institute Press.
Jones, B., & Janello, A. (1987). *The wall: Images and offerings from the Vietnam Veterans Memorial.* New York: Collins.
Kalisch, P. A., & Kalisch, B. J. (2004). *American nursing: A history* (4th ed.). Philadelphia: Lippincott, Williams & Wilkins.
Kelly, L. Y., & Joel, L. (1995). *Dimensions of professional nursing.* New York: McGraw Hill.
Lewy, G. (1977). *America in Vietnam.* New York: Oxford University Press.
Lindberg, C. (1999). *The history of the U.S. Air Force Nurse Corps from 1984-1998.* Maxwell AFB, AL: The Air War College, Air University.
Link, M. M., & Coleman, H. A. (1955). *Medical support of the Army Air Forces in World War II.* Washington, DC: Department of the Air Force, Office of the Air Force Surgeon General.
Marshall, K. (1988). *In the combat zone: An oral history of American women in Vietnam.* Boston: Little, Brown, & Co.
Martin, L. G. (1967). Angels in Vietnam. *Today's Health, 8,* 17-22, 60-62.

McVicker, S. J. (1985). Invisible veterans: The women who served in Vietnam, *Journal of Psychosocial Nursing, 23*(10), 13–19.

Norman, E. (1999). *We band of angels: The untold story of American nurses trapped on Bataan by the Japanese.* New York: Simon & Schuster.

The Pentagon Papers: The Defense Department history of United States decision making on Vietnam. (1971). Boston: Senator Gravel Edition.

Ruff, C. L., & Roper, K. S. (2005). *Ruff's War: A Navy nurse on the frontline in Iraq.* Annapolis, MD: Naval Institute Press.

Santoli, A. (1981). *Everything we had: An oral history of the Vietnam War by thirty-three soldiers who fought it.* New York: Ballantine Books.

Santoli, A. (1985). *To bear any burden: The Vietnam war and its aftermath.* New York: E. P. Dutton.

Sarnecky, M. T. (1999). *A history of the U.S. Army Nurse Corps.* Philadelphia: University of Pennsylvania Press.

Sarnecky, M. T. (2010). *A contemporary history of the U.S. Army Nurse Corps.* Washington, DC: The Borden Institute.

Scannell-Desch, E. A. (1996). The lived experience of women military nurses in Vietnam during the Vietnam war. *Image: Journal of Nursing Scholarship, 28*(2), 119–124.

Scannell-Desch, E. A. (1999). Images and relationships forged in war: A study of women nurses who served in Vietnam. *Journal of Psychosocial Nursing, 37*(8), 32–42.

Scannell-Desch, E. A. (2000a). Hardships and personal strategies of Vietnam War nurses. *Western Journal of Nursing Research, 22*(5), 526–545, 548–550.

Scannell-Desch, E. A. (2000b). The culture of war: A study of women military nurses in Vietnam. *Journal of Transcultural Nursing, 11*(2), 87–95.

Scannell-Desch, E. A. (2005) Lessons learned and advice from Vietnam War nurses. *Journal of Advanced Nursing, 49*(6), 601–607.

Schimmenti, C., & Darmoody, M. (1986). Taking flight. *American Journal of Nursing, 86*, 1420–1423.

Schwartz, L. S. (1987). Women and the Vietnam experience. *Journal of Nursing Scholarship, 19*, 168–175.

Schwartzkopf, N. H. (1992). *It doesn't take a hero.* New York: Bantam Books.

Tilghman, A. (2011, September 12). Our decade at war. *Air Force Times*, p. 3.

United States Navy in Operation Desert Shield/Desert Storm: Summary Report from the Chief of Naval Operations. (1991). Washington, DC: U.S. Naval Historical Center.

Walker, K. (1985). *A piece of my heart.* New York, NY: Ballantine Books.

2

Deploying to War: An Uncertain Future

Nurses found themselves traveling to a war zone. There was an atmosphere mixed with fear, adventure, and uncertainty. Some deployed with their active-duty units from Army, Navy, or Air Force hospitals, whereas others in reserve forces units were activated. Still others volunteered as individual augmentees and joined units already in Iraq or Afghanistan or scheduled for deployment. Some nurses served on mentoring teams to help Afghan military medical and nursing personnel learn modern patient care procedures. Their reasons for joining active or reserve forces were as diverse as the nurses themselves. A handful came from military families. Others secured Reserve Officer Training Corps (ROTC) college scholarships. Some joined to pay back student loans for their nursing education. Others wanted to supplement their income or to meet a new network of people. Many said they wanted to do something for their country. Several felt a resurgence of patriotism and unity after the terrorist attacks on the United States on September 11, 2001. Some were volunteers for deployment; others did not volunteer but traveled with their military units to Iraq or Afghanistan. None knew what the future would bring.

SOME VOLUNTEERED

Commander Josie

Josie joined the Navy as a hospital corpsman after graduating from high school. She was adventurous and wanted to see more of the world. After several years as a corpsman caring for patients on medical-surgical nursing units, Josie was selected to attend college to obtain a bachelor's degree in nursing. Once she received her degree, she was commissioned as an ensign in the Navy Nurse Corps. Her first assignment was at a large medical center in Southern California. She worked on a medical-surgical floor. She enjoyed the challenges and opportunities of being a nursing officer. In later assignments, Josie found herself on the coast of Virginia, on the island of Guam, and in Hawaii, South Carolina, and Maryland. She asked for sea duty after her children were grown, but an assignment aboard ship always eluded her. When an opportunity to deploy to a war zone afforded itself, Josie was first in line to volunteer.

Josie related, "I volunteered for Afghanistan. I had been in the Navy for 26 years. Many people had said to me, 'I bet you've been on this ship, and that ship, since you've been in the Navy for a very long time.' Well, I had never been on a ship or seen a war. It was a little embarrassing to be in the Navy for that length of time and never served in a war or served on a ship. I called M-5 at BUMED [Bureau of Medicine and Surgery] and said, 'I'm probably not the most competent nurse in the world because I've not done patient care since 1997, but I want to deploy. Do you have anything out there for me?"

Josie continued, "I thought I could help the Navy by not sending another nurse since some nurses were on their second or third deployment. I thought if I could prevent someone from having to go on another deployment, it would be worth it. They found me a position in northern Afghanistan in a place called Mazar-e-Sharif, where I would be mentoring a senior nurse executive at the regional national Afghan army hospital. I mentored the director of nursing services at this Afghan army hospital. He was a lieutenant colonel in the Afghan army. I was the only U.S. military nurse on the FOB [forward operating base] when I got there. I was there in an imbedded medical training team of 12 mentors from the U.S. military. Most of our patients were Afghan national police or Afghan national army troops. The police in that country were the ones who were engaged in knocking doors down, fighting the Taliban, and keeping the nation secure. The Afghan national police did search, seizure, and urban warfare, not the National Army. This Afghan army hospital was built by the U.S. in 2006 and was one of four regional Afghan army hospitals in Afghanistan. It was one of only several buildings in Afghanistan that had air-conditioning and hot and cold running water."

Major Diana

Diana has been a nurse in Dayton, Ohio, for over 20 years. She received her bachelor's and master's degrees in nursing from two large Midwestern universities. She was employed in preoperative and surgical nursing in a large Dayton-area medical center. After being out of college for a few years, she joined the Air Force Reserve to enhance her income and serve her country. Dayton is home to the U.S. Air Force Museum and the large sprawling Wright-Patterson Air Force Base. It is a pro-military and pro-Air Force city. Many folks in the local area are Air Force retirees, active-duty personnel, or reserve forces personnel. Diana said she welcomed the professional and social interactions afforded in her military environment as well as the educational opportunities to advance her career. Diana described herself as someone who was always ready for a new challenge or adventure. Although she had deployed for two humanitarian missions in South America, she had never been in a war zone.

Diana stated, "I have been in the Air Force Reserve for 19 years. Every deployment we have ever had, I have volunteered for. I guess you could describe me as patriotic and adventurous. We went into what they call 'the bucket,' meaning that our reserve unit was up for deployment. We had certain specialties they needed, and if your specialty was needed, you could volunteer for deployment. From my unit, some people went to Iraq, some went to Kuwait, and some went to Germany. They needed nurses in my specialty in Iraq, so I volunteered for Iraq. My unit was an ASTS, an aeromedical staging transport squadron. That means we assessed the patients and got them ready for air evac. We provided care while they were in a medical holding area."

Captain Vanessa

Vanessa is from a small town in Long Island, New York. She graduated from a small church-affiliated college and then went to work in a large New York City medical center. After a few years working in medical-surgical nursing, Vanessa was selected to attend a critical care nursing course and transferred to a position in the medical intensive care unit (ICU). She said although she did not know much about the military or military nursing, she thought joining the reserves would be a good balance between her civilian employment and actively supporting her country. Because no members of her family had any military affiliation, Vanessa said it really did not matter to her which military service she joined. Vanessa described herself as a New Yorker who was affected by the terrorist attacks in New York. She just knew she wanted to serve and to make a positive difference.

Vanessa reported, "I joined the Army Reserve after the 9/11 attacks. I'm a lifelong democrat. After 9/11, I was single, in good health, with no dependents, and I thought it was time that I did something for my country. I called all three branches of the military, the Army, the Navy, and the Air

Force, and decided whoever called me first would be my primary choice. The Army called first, so that is how I ended up in the Army. We were told from the get-go that deployment was very possible. It was pretty much a threat at every drill weekend. We were told, 'Get ready, we are going to be deployed; get ready, we are going to be deployed.' I didn't know what to believe. When I joined the unit, I was told that I had joined the worst unit in the Army. This unit never went anywhere for years, and the Army probably wouldn't send us anywhere. We were a hopeless case with a terrible reputation, so the Army wouldn't take us anywhere. We weren't quite 'dress right, dress,' as they say. When we got deployed, we had a false start 6 months earlier. I was deployed to Abu Ghraib prison, just outside of Baghdad."

Vanessa explained, "After about 6 months at Abu Ghraib, I heard they needed a nurse to temporarily go to Tikrit, Iraq. This would be for 8 weeks, until another cadre of active-duty nurses arrived. I jumped at the chance to get out of detainee care, even if it was for only 2 months. The hospital in Tikrit was small. I worked on the intermediate care ward. We had 20 beds and a 7-bed ICU. We took care of coalition forces, Iraqi employees, government contractors, British soldiers, Iraqi police, local civilians, and children. It was a good change of scenery for me, but it was rough duty as far as the trauma care. Some of the injuries were just so devastating, especially when that happened to 19-year-old soldiers or little kids."

Lieutenant Commander Clare

Clare grew up in a large African American family in Northern California. Her older brothers had served in the Marine Corps. Her father was a Vietnam-era Navy veteran. Clare joined the Navy a few years after graduating from college. She said she had a desire to travel and to be part of something bigger than herself, felt bored, and wanted a change from her civilian nursing job. She was single at that time. There were no other responsibilities to keep her from joining. Clare also liked the educational opportunities advertised by the Navy. She took advantage of several, including advanced trauma and critical care courses. Prior to her deployment, Clare worked as an ICU and senior trauma nurse at a large Navy medical center in Virginia. Earlier in her career, she was assigned in South Carolina, Japan, Maryland, and California. She said she looked forward to testing her leadership and clinical skills in a war zone.

Clare stated, "I volunteered to go to Iraq. I went to an area in Anbar province where mostly Marines were deployed. They needed some more senior nurses to go, so I volunteered because I wanted to provide critical trauma care to our injured troops. They were mostly sending junior nurses, and they needed a handful of senior-ranking nurses to go to provide the nursing leadership and expert trauma care. I was there from February 2006 through June 2006. I was the senior shock-trauma nurse in a mobile field surgical hospital. We had an ICU, three inpatient units, and a medevac holding area. Most of our medevacs went out by helicopter, but we did have a flight line for C-130s."

Lieutenant Colonel Judd

Judd joined the Army when he graduated from high school in the late 1960s, before he probably would have been drafted. He went to Vietnam as an infantryman when he was just 18 years old. He described life in Vietnam as rough but a valuable personal growth experience. He said he became a man and an adult while serving in Vietnam. When he left active duty in the early 1970s, he said he missed the bonding and esprit de corps of being in a military unit. Later, after he graduated from nursing school in Boston, Massachusetts, he joined the Army Reserve as a medical-surgical nurse. After several years of nursing practice in the Army Reserve and in civilian hospitals, Judd returned to school to become an adult health nurse practitioner.

Judd describes himself as someone who was deeply affected by the attacks on the United States on September 11, 2011. "First of all, I volunteered. I didn't wait to get activated. I wanted to do this. I figured it is the last time I am going to have this opportunity in the military before I am too old. I will turn 60 next year. They said if I am considered a critical asset, they could keep me on past 60 years of age. If the government needs me, they can call me back. I wanted to go to Iraq. Some of the people that got activated were moaning and groaning. They got pulled out of civilian jobs, and they got pulled from their families. My wife understood. She was in the military for 21 years. She retired a few years before I deployed. I asked her what she would do. She said she would do exactly what I did; she'd volunteer. Yeah, she didn't like me being gone. Yeah, she was lonely, but she understood. I was administratively attached to another unit, but I heard that this other unit was going to be activated for deployment to Iraq, so I volunteered. The unit also used me as an instructor. I taught trauma nursing skills, BLS [basic life support], and things like that. Since I am a nurse practitioner, they said they needed me to run sick call, so I deployed with 1 week's notice."

Judd further reported, "We had to train as a unit at Fort McCoy in Wisconsin for 4 months before we deployed to Iraq. With the training time, plus the year in Iraq, we were pulled from our jobs and families for 15 months. The reserves and National Guard have long training periods before deployment. It usually works out to 15 to 18 months away from home, as opposed to the active-duty folks, who are usually deployed for 12 months straightaway. When we trained in Wisconsin, we practiced how to set up a field hospital. We did physical training. We went to some classes on the Middle Eastern culture. We also did a lot of medical training, since our enlisted people usually do not work in the medical field in their civilian jobs. They could be secretaries, mailmen, truck drivers, or something else. On the other hand, our nurses usually work in nursing areas in their civilian jobs. So, for almost 4 months, we are trying to get the enlisted folks up to snuff on how to work in a hospital."

Judd continued, "When I got to Iraq, I was assigned to a combat support hospital in Mosul, which is in northern Iraq. Therefore, our FOB was in the middle of the city of Mosul. For my first 3 months, I ran sick call every day in Mosul. Then I was sent to an Army hospital in Tikrit, where I ran the orthopedic clinic there for another 3 months. Lastly, the Army sent me to their brand-new hospital in the desert at Anbar Province, which is southwest of Baghdad. I thought I was going to be running sick call again, but they needed me in surgery as first assistant in the operating room. I spent a year in Iraq, with my time divided between hospitals in Mosul, Tikrit, and Anbar Province."

MOST DID NOT VOLUNTEER BUT SERVED

Most nurses were not volunteers for the war zones but willingly went to war to honor their commitments. Some were active duty, whereas others were reserve forces.

Captain Tina

Tina grew up in an Air Force family. Her father was an Air Force pilot. Tina lived in Japan, England, and Germany as well as California and Texas as a child. She went to college on an Air Force ROTC scholarship and was commissioned as a second lieutenant upon graduation. Tina's first assignment as an Air Force nurse was in Maryland, working on a busy medical-surgical unit. It was while on her second assignment in Texas at a large Air Force medical center that she found a large cadre of personnel from her hospital being deployed to Iraq. Later in her career, Tina was deployed to a small base in Afghanistan.

Tina recalled, "I have been deployed twice. In the early part of the war, I was deployed with a large group of people to Balad Air Base in Iraq. The hospital in Balad was the largest U.S. military medical facility in Iraq. A few years later, I deployed to FOB Salerno in Afghanistan. I left in January 2007 for Afghanistan and came home in May 2007. FOB Salerno was in a southeastern province in Afghanistan, near the city of Khost. Salerno was a joint base with mainly Army troops and Marines but some Air Force assets as well. When I got there, our small hospital had just converted from being a tent hospital to being a semifixed facility. We had medical-surgical care, a small ICU, and an ER [emergency room]. We took care of military personnel, Iraqi civilians, and insurgents."

Captain Marie

Marie was raised in an Italian Catholic family in Providence, Rhode Island. Marie and several of her friends joined the Army Reserve after high school. They wanted to earn extra money and meet a wider circle of young people. Marie married her high school sweetheart a few years later. They waited to start a family because they wanted to establish themselves in their careers. They had two small children when the attacks of September 11, 2001, occurred. Marie seriously contemplated resigning from the Army Reserve at that time. Marie recalled, "I had been in the Army Reserve since 1987. I started out as an enlisted soldier and then got my Bachelor of Science degree in nursing and was commissioned as an officer in 1998. When the twin towers fell in 2001, I had two babies. I said to my husband, 'I think I better get out of the reserves.' He said 'I don't think you need to do that right away.' So I didn't think about it for a while. I could see things happening down the road, and I said, 'I think it is time to get out before I get mobilized and go over to Iraq.' I had 17 years in at that time. My husband was very encouraging that I should continue and see what happens. He reminded me I had only 3 more years till retirement. I would be crazy to let that go. However, I just didn't understand how it would work, if I got deployed. I just didn't understand how he would be able to stay home with the kids. Logistically, I just wasn't sure how it would work out and how everyone would be on time and get where they were supposed to go. How could they live without me? I voiced 'a mother's concern.' I said, 'Okay, I'll stay as long as you can tell me what your plan would be.' I asked him again, and he said I was trying to put him on the spot. He said, 'I'll ask my brother to come and sleep over.' I said, 'That is not going to work.' His brother is a recluse. Finally, I said to speak to his employer to see what they can do."

Marie continued, "My husband's supervisors were very supportive. They said he could come in late to work. He works as a law enforcement officer. They let him sell off some of his shifts so other people could work. Therefore, he only had to work three shifts a week. Since I had only worked part time, my Army pay was going to increase my salary substantially. Therefore, he formulated a plan with three shifts a week and going in late on those three days, so the kids could get off to school. At that point, we had to go with it. By that time, my unit had been mobilized. I got promoted to captain just as I was writing my resignation letter. Therefore, I stayed and accepted the promotion to captain. We got mobilized right after that. In the end, the plan my husband formulated worked out great."

Marie described the training before her unit deployed. "We went to Fort McCoy, Wisconsin, for 4 months of training. That was not just medical training but Army combat training, too. It was requalifying on the M-16 rifle, doing convoy training in case you get attacked on a convoy and have to react, and some medical training because we are a combat support hospital. We went out to the field, set up MASH [mobile Army surgical hospital] tents, and took care of fake casualties. They had observer–controllers, who are Army nurses or doctors. They watched how we treated the 'casualties' and how we reacted to things like simulated chemical attacks or a heavy influx of patients. They critiqued us and tried to help us improve our triage and treatment skills. We'd have fake scenarios and fake casualties coming through our camp. In all honesty, it was hell because it was trying to cram a whole Army's worth of training into 4 months. You'd get up in the morning and train and practice day after day for 4 months. It was kind of frustrating because you knew that after 4 months of training, you were going to Iraq for 12 months. You would not see your family for a total of 16 months."

NURSE SPECIALISTS IN DEMAND

Commander Rita: Nurse Anesthetist

Rita grew up in the suburbs of Philadelphia, Pennsylvania. Several years after joining the Navy, Rita was selected to attend nurse anesthesia training. She received a master's degree as a nurse anesthetist. She had been assigned to shore duty as a certified registered nurse anesthetist in several naval hospitals and medical centers as well as sea duty aboard a large ship before she found herself deploying to Iraq. Rita was a career officer in the Navy and retired from naval service shortly after returning from Iraq.

Rita explained how some specialties were in great demand and short supply in the war zone. "It was the beginning of 2003. As a nurse anesthetist in the Navy, you are highly deployable. When there is a deployment, it is just a matter of who is going and when are they leaving. In late 2002, before the war started, I got a call saying that my deployment status was going to change from a shipboard deployment to a ground deployment supporting the Marines. Therefore, now I'm thinking, 'We are going to go to war, the Marines are usually the first to go, and I may be going with them.'

In January 2003, we found out that we were going to have a meeting of all the people from up and down the east coast that were assigned to my deployment platform. We met during the 3rd week in January, and at the meeting, we would find out who was going to deploy. It was actually on my birthday when the meeting occurred. I found out that I was going to deploy with the Marines when they invade Iraq, but nothing was set in stone. Within 48 hours of this meeting, I got tapped on the shoulder by one of the nurses in the operating room. She said, 'I have something to tell you. You are going to be leaving.' I said, 'For sure?' And she said, 'Yes, for sure.'"

Rita continued, "I knew I had to get moving on preparing my family. Therefore, I had my sister and my family come down to my house in November. I had been notified in October that my deployment platform [status] had changed. I had my family go through all my personal stuff that I stored in my firebox. I just reviewed everything with them. I wanted them to know where all my stuff was, if I was going to be deployed. I had everything catalogued for them with account numbers. Therefore, I got that taken care of ahead of time. I was glad because when I got the tap on the shoulder, I had exactly 7 days before I left. I left on January 28, 2003. President Bush had given the State of the Union the night before. I remember lying on my sofa watching it. It was over about 9 o'clock. I was to leave at 3 o'clock the following morning. I never went to bed. In addition, that's how I remember that day with the State of the Union; he said that we are going to go to war. He said that, and I was leaving in 6 hours to go down to Camp Lejune to get ready to go over to Kuwait. That morning at 3 o'clock, I drove over to the Naval Hospital to meet up with about 70 of us that were going to deploy. We gathered there, and they issued us our Geneva Convention cards, new sets of dog tags, and some of our gear. Then we said our good-byes. Families were there. My family was still up in Pennsylvania, but my good friend and her husband were there to say good-bye. She was a classmate of mine in anesthesia school."

Rita described her trip to Iraq. "We boarded a United Airlines charter flight to Kuwait. The flight attendants on our flight were our age, probably 45 to 65 years old. They were just wonderful. They were all volunteers because they were flying into a war zone area. United Airlines did not tell anybody they had to fly this trip; they asked for volunteers. The plane was red, white, and blue on the inside and on the outside. They had American flags up in the cabin and in the galleys. In addition, oh my God, did we get first-class treatment. I still get chills when I talk about those flight attendants. It couldn't have been any better. They were so accommodating, and they kept us pumped up the whole way over there. We stopped in Germany to refuel, and the Red Cross was set up to give us little packets with snacks and toothbrushes and some cold drinks."

Rita further explained, "When we landed in Kuwait, things moved quickly. They got all our gear off the plane, and then the plane quickly took off. They were not allowed to refuel in Kuwait. Therefore, the plane had to go on to Turkey, where they had permission to refuel. As we were flying into Kuwait, they had all the lights off and the window sun visors down because they didn't want us to be a target. We landed in the middle of the night. They had us off that plane so quickly. Then we had to show our military ID cards and give our thumbprints. We had our guns on us, our backpacks, and we each had two C-bags in the cargo hold. One C-bag was any personal stuff you wanted to bring, and the other was military gear. Once we were off the plane, we went to a staging area. We all congregated in this barbwire-enclosed area and sat for about 4 hours. It was the middle of the night, and it was cold. We got on buses and were transported in a convoy with tanks and snipers sitting up high on the tanks. We were kept in the middle of two tanks in this convoy. We started to drive to Camp Guadalcanal. As we kept going, it got dustier and dustier, and you couldn't see anything out the windows. There was sand on the inside of the bus and sand on the outside of the windows as well. When the sun came up, all you could see against the horizon was sand and more sand."

Rita found that once her deployment cadre arrived in Iraq, the mission plans they were briefed on in the United States prior to deployment changed. She recalled, "The original plan, which was formulated at Camp Lejeune, was to form surgical teams. There would be four teams—Alpha, Bravo, Charlie, and Delta. They were going to have an even number of folks on these four teams—so many orthopedic surgeons, so many general surgeons, so many critical care nurses, so many anesthesia folks, and so many hospital corpsmen. From the original plan, I was going to be on Bravo Surgical team. During the 2 weeks we were in Kuwait prior to invading Iraq, we got the rest of our gear and uniforms. We practiced shooting our weapons and practiced setting up our forward hospital. We had classes on escape and evasion, how to handle it if you were captured as a prisoner of war, how to handle ambushes, how to treat scorpion bites, and how to handle an emergency back home. They told us, 'You are in a war zone, forget it, you are not going home. They may not be able to get you out to go home."

Rita further described, "We went from A to Z in our training. Those of us in anesthesia were a very small community. We would get our anesthesia group together. We would go over to the hospital and sit down as an anesthesia group. We would discuss the types of anesthesia we were going to use, the drugs we had available to us, what we didn't have available to us, and supplies. No one knew when we were going to get supplies or how we were going to get supplies. We were going to reuse syringes, and we were going to mark syringes as 'EPW' [enemy prisoners of war] or 'US' [U.S.

soldier] because we didn't know if we would get any more syringes. Those syringes that we would draw up medicines with, we would just use on the EPWs or on Iraqi civilians. On our guys, we would use the same syringes and endotracheal tubes. We washed the ones for our guys and then reused them on our troops. What we didn't want to happen was to use an endotracheal tube that we used on an Iraqi to be reused on our guys. Our guys were immunized for smallpox, anthrax, and lots of other diseases, but we didn't know what immunizations the Iraqis had. We tried to keep everything as clean as possible."

Rita continued, "We discussed antibiotics and decided that wounded folks would be on triple antibiotics. We discussed fluid management because we were only given so many bags of Ringer's lactate and saline. We didn't know how, or when, we would be resupplied. We discussed blood transfusions, and of course, the blood transfusions would be from the walking wounded and other Marine troops. We would get whole blood from these troops. We discussed at what point we would stop giving transfusions to a patient. We are limited as to how much blood we can give. Our whole idea of these surgical platoons was to patch up, stop the hemorrhaging, and get them out to a combat support hospital or hospital ship for more sophisticated and long-term care. We were going to be moving with the Marines as they moved forward to Baghdad."

Rita continued to explain, "Once we arrived by convoy to Camp Guadalcanal, we met up with Forward Surgical Team Charlie, which had left the states a few days before we did. It was there we learned all this great talk about having four surgical teams wasn't going to work. We learned the supplies that were supposed to have arrived in Kuwait, well, some of them never arrived. Therefore, they condensed us down to three teams—Alpha, Bravo, and Charlie. Only Bravo and Charlie surgical teams moved forward because there were so many casualties on the Iraq-Kuwait border, with bombings, mortar attacks, and oil fires. The Navy Medical Department left Alpha team right there on the border between Kuwait and Iraq to deal with all the injuries."

Rita recalled, "We had trained so much and practiced so much. We were like a well-oiled machine. Everyone knew their job, how to tear down and put up the tent hospital, and all the equipment and gear that went into the hospital. When we finally hit the dirt running, we moved into Iraq. We took people from our bases up and down the eastern U.S. who had never worked together and threw them into a horrific environment. We were so well rehearsed, it was like a symphony. No one was panicking because we had done it so much before. We had rehearsed it at night, in the wind, and during a simulated attack. Honest to God, it worked, and it worked perfectly!"

Major Christina: Flight Nurse

Christina joined the Air Force after working in Memphis, Tennessee, for several years as a critical care nurse in pediatric and adult ICUs. She was single at the time she entered active duty and looked forward to travel, adventure, and furthering her education. After critical care assignments on the East coast and the West coast, Christina was chosen to attend flight nurse training at the School of Aerospace Medicine, Brooks Air Force Base, in San Antonio, Texas. Following graduation from the fight nurse course, Christina returned to her ICU position.

She was later deployed to Germany. After the Germany deployment, she received reassignment orders to be a flight nurse in an aeromedical evacuation squadron. As a flight nurse, Christina had to quickly acclimate to a mobile lifestyle.

Christina remarked, "I've been deployed four times, twice to Germany, once to Iraq, and once to Afghanistan. My first deployment was to Landsthul Hospital in Germany at the beginning of the war. My last three deployments, I went as a flight nurse. I was deployed once to Germany to crew aeromedical flights from Germany back to the U.S. for 4 months. Then I was deployed to Balad Air Base, Iraq, to fly air evac missions inside Iraq and Iraq to Germany. My last deployment was to Afghanistan to fly air evac missions inside Afghanistan and occasionally from Afghanistan to Germany. I am going to be deployed for a fifth time next month. In my four deployments, I would say that I have had about a month's notice that we are going to deploy. Since I'm assigned to an aeromedical evacuation squadron, I am more used to deploying on shorter notice than nurses assigned to a hospital. As a flight nurse, I am used to being gone since that is really our mission, to go wherever we are needed."

Christina further reported, "During the months while I was serving as a flight nurse in Iraq, I had a 6-week special assignment to teach a course for some Iraqi nurses about flight nursing and aeromedical evacuation. We took them on some Iraqi C-130 Hercules aircraft that the U.S. gave them. The U.S. Air Force had completed a lot of the training for their pilots and other aircrew members to increase their capabilities to move patients. I worked with an Iraqi physician to teach this course. This physician and I met on several occasions to develop the course. I wrote this course with him, and we had it translated. Three other flight nurse instructors and I organized the course and then taught it for 14 Iraqi nurses. Those 14 represent about one third of the Iraqi medical service providers who are not physicians. It was fun and a very worthwhile experience. Before that, I didn't have any positive experiences with Iraqis. Therefore, it's good to have these additional opportunities to have good interactions. It's a once-in-a-lifetime chance. It was really good, very fruitful."

Major Millie: Operating Room Nurse

Millie grew up in a small town about 40 miles outside of Chicago, Illinois. Following graduation from nursing school, Millie worked as an operating room nurse in a large Chicago hospital. After working in Chicago area hospitals for over a decade, she joined the Army. Because Millie had a wealth of experience before she joined the Army, her first active-duty assignment was as an assistant operating room nursing supervisor in California. Then she was transferred to another hospital in Texas.

Millie recounted some details about her deployment. "I was an alternate for another nurse who had gotten into some legal difficulties, and she was not able to deploy. Therefore, I gave them a hard time, saying 'Now I have to go because she got into some things she shouldn't have.' In the end, it was all fine and dandy. We left in August 2004 for Iraq and came back in July 2005."

Millie continued, "I've been an operating room nurse for 27 years. I found out about 3 weeks before the deployment that I would be a substitute on this deployment. Eighty members of my stateside Army hospital were going to be deployed to Iraq. I worked at the main hospital in the operating room. I knew there were a few nurses who were forward deployed to very small tent hospitals on small FOBs, but that was not my situation. I was actually in a semifixed facility that had a few areas of air-conditioning, which I understand is a big plus. I would consider my hospital one of the better ones in Iraq for which the U.S. Air Force actually had responsibility. Much of the base was run by the Army, but the Air Force had the lead for the hospital compound. The hospital staff was a mixture of Air Force and Army medical personnel."

Millie recalled, "In the operating room [OR], we cared for just about any type of trauma injury you could imagine. It reminded me of when I worked downtown [Chicago] on a Saturday night. We would get in gunshot wounds, stabbings, people burned in house fires, and lots of serious car accidents. However, Iraq was a real challenge, even for an old OR nurse like me. A lot of the young nurses had never really seen trauma like this before. I got to mentor a lot of the younger, less experienced nurses. The volume of patients when the choppers came in, or if an in-country air evac plane landed, took some getting used to. You had to prioritize, prioritize, and prioritize. It kept us all on our toes."

Captain Meaghan: Critical Care Air Transport Team (CCATT) Nurse

Meaghan hailed from the suburbs of St. Louis, Missouri. Her older brother was in the Army and had served a tour of duty in Iraq as an intelligence officer. Meaghan joined the Air Force while her brother was serving in Iraq. She described her family as patriotic, with relatives serving in all branches of the military over the years. Meaghan said that she always wanted to be a nurse since she was a little girl. Her aunt had served as an Army nurse during the Korean War. Meaghan said she is especially close to her aunt. However, Meaghan said she chose to join the Air Force because she wanted to be a flight nurse. She thought the challenge of taking care of patients in the airborne environment would be a unique and different experience that would test her clinical skills.

Meaghan had been on the waiting list to attend the flight nurse course when her hospital was notified of its pending deployment. There was a need for CCATT nurses, so Meaghan volunteered to fill that role. She reported, "I was notified about 2 months prior to deploying to Afghanistan. I was told I would be going to Bagram Air Force Base in Afghanistan and that I would be there for 6 months. It turned out that I was there for 7 months. I am a CCATT nurse, which stands for Critical Care Air Transport Team. I took care of critically injured patients aboard aeromedical evacuation planes. Therefore, I flew air evac missions out of Bagram Air Force Base into different locations in Afghanistan. I brought patients back to the hospital at Bagram or on to the big hospital at Landsthul, Germany. It was a very challenging deployment, and I took care of the most critical patients on those flights. Our CCATT team was composed of a critical care physician, a respiratory therapist, and me. We had some close calls, but we never lost a patient in flight during my deployment. You had to be on top of your game as far as reading cardiac monitors, performing physical assessment, carrying out clinical procedures, and calculating and administering intravenous medications. It was a very special and unique assignment for me, and I absolutely loved the experience. Our team was just the best group of people you could ever have to work with. Each team member was selected because of their strong clinical skills and ability to work cohesively with others. It was truly an honor to be on this team."

Lieutenant Colonel Victoria: Nurse Executive

After college and getting some civilian nursing experience, Victoria thought joining the Army Nurse Corps would broaden her horizons. She had worked in an adult ICU for 14 months prior to joining the Army. Her first assignment in the Army was in California, and from there, she was transferred to Hawaii. While on her first assignment, she had the opportunity to become an obstetric nurse because that area was short-staffed at her hospital. Victoria worked her way up to becoming proficient in the labor and delivery area, caring for laboring mothers through their newborn's delivery. She found obstetric nursing to be a gratifying clinical specialty. Like most obstetric nurses, Victoria had the opportunity to deliver several babies when the physician was not present. By the time she was deployed with a portion of the staff from her third hospital assignment in Texas, Victoria was an experienced medical-surgical, obstetric, and ICU nurse.

Victoria recalled, "I have deployed twice to Iraq. The first time I deployed was in March 2003 to a combat support hospital. I was working as the head nurse of the labor and delivery unit in an Army medical center in Texas. I was notified on a Friday afternoon that on the following Monday I was going to report to the combat support hospital for training. About 4 weeks later, we flew to Kuwait. We spent about 3 weeks in Kuwait. This was at the very beginning of the war. They had three mobile combat support hospitals in theater sitting in Kuwait. Some of us had equipment, and others were waiting for equipment. I was slotted to be the charge nurse of an intermediate care ward in an 84-bed combat support hospital. They were short an experienced ICU nurse, so I moved into that slot as we entered Iraq. We actually convoyed all the way through Iraq. We spent 23 hours in the back of a 5-ton truck with all our gear strapped on, and then we stopped in the middle of the desert in the middle of the night. We woke up to see Bedouin sheepherders wandering close to our area. This was not a good thing, so we packed up and spent another 8 hours in the back of the truck. We finally arrived in Mosul, which was where we were supposed to be located. Getting there was quite an experience. We got to Mosul right before the unit we were supporting, the 101st Airborne. We were told we needed to have the operating room, emergency treatment area, and ICU set up to receive casualties by nightfall. We were literally in the middle of a farmer's field. We set up our chemically protected hospital by that night. I was only in Iraq for 4 months because I had been selected by the Army to go to midwifery school."

Victoria further reported, "My second deployment was very different than my first. My chief nurse sent out an email message to all the lieutenant colonels in the region, saying they were looking for a lieutenant colonel or colonel to volunteer to go as an assistant chief nurse for one of the combat support hospitals that was going to deploy to Iraq in the spring of 2007. I came home that night, and my husband and I sat and talked. I felt that I had unfinished business from my first deployment because it was only for 4 months. I left everybody I deployed with there to come back and get an Army-sponsored master's degree. I had left my group in July 2003, and they were all there till February 2004. I felt like I hadn't done my part. Therefore, I had a conversation with my husband and the kids. I felt that if I went again now, they wouldn't tap me for another deployment for a couple of years. Therefore, I went back to talk with the chief nurse. I reminded her that I had just been promoted, so I was the most junior lieutenant colonel in the Army Nurse Corps and that I was a nurse midwife and not a nurse administrator. I said that I would go if they needed somebody. She said, 'If I send your name forward, you will go.' She sent my name forward, and I went back to Iraq. I went back in March 2007. On my second deployment, I knew I was going to be the assistant chief nurse for another 84-bed combat support hospital. This time, we were sent to Camp Bucca, Iraq, which is a large detention facility. When I was there, we started out with 14,000 detainees and then peaked at about 22,000 detainees because this was during the troop surge. I was there about 2 weeks when they announced that all deployments were being extended from 12 to 15 months. I had a hospital commander, who kept saying that it wouldn't be us. However, I kept telling my troops that they would be in Iraq for 15 months. We were there for 15 months. It was hard for me to do 15 months because I knew I'd miss my son's entire senior year of high school and his graduation. I returned from Iraq 2 days after his graduation."

Lieutenant Colonel Heidi: Nurse Researcher

Heidi was raised in the suburbs of Spokane, Washington. She attended a large university on the west coast and joined the Army Nurse Corps within a year of her graduation. Heidi had assignments in Kansas and North Carolina before the Army selected her to attend graduate school to obtain a master's degree in adult health nursing. Later, after assignments in Germany, Texas, and Washington, DC, Heidi was competitively chosen to get a doctoral degree in nursing research. It was while she was working as a research nurse that a unique opportunity presented itself.

Heidi explained, "I am a doctorally prepared nurse researcher, and I also have nursing field experience. I've been in the Army for 21 years and have always felt that my primary mission was the health care support of a combat mission. Over the years, I have been relatively disappointed in a way that we have been at peace, and I haven't gotten the opportunity to deploy in a war zone. I've gone on a lot of field training exercises, but training got old after a while, and I really wanted the real thing. When September 11th happened, I was in a medical readiness training position. The tradition is that if you are a training instructor, when something like that kicks off, your slot gets frozen, and you can't go to the front because you have to gear up to train more people. I had a whole cadre of folks just like me who wanted to go to the front, and now they are kind of stuck and have to stay where they are. I stayed there and finished out my tenure in the training position. Then, I got selected for school to get my PhD. When you are in school, you can't deploy either. You are actually frozen or 'safe,' so to speak, in that kind of position. My instructors would say, 'How likely is it that you are going to have to go?' I'd say to them, 'You're a reservist. It's much more likely that you will go, than me.' Well, that's what happened. Several of my instructors got pulled out to deploy. After that, everyone settled into a comfortable rotation. The shock of 9/11 had passed. We thought everything would be over quickly. We thought, 'Let's get some nurses over there, get the job done, and then they'll all come home.' Then the reality of a long war set in, and we had more predictable rotations. Our bosses started to adopt the philosophy that it shouldn't be a surprise if you go. We should take volunteers first, and everyone should go for a first time before people go for a second time. Then I was asked. I had a lot of personal control over my situation. I was offered a job by name to take the first team into Iraq that conducts research. I was to be the human subject's protection administrator."

Heidi continued, "I looked at my family situation. I had just come out of school, started a new job, and we had just moved. My kids were still quite young, and I was trying to start a program of research. I had a Triservice Nursing Research proposal application submitted. I thought it was not good timing for me and not good timing for my family. Therefore, I actually said, 'I don't want to go.' My bosses respected that and said they'd find a volunteer. Then, I saw everything unfold, and I thought, 'I need to go. Everyone needs to go at least once.' It made sense for me to go as a researcher. It would not have made sense for me to go back to the bedside and have to relearn skills I had lost. I volunteered, and I could not volunteer fast enough. I wanted the job bad. I got the job, and I went to Iraq."

Heidi described her deployment. "I deployed with a combat casualty team of six people. We were deployed out of the ISR [Institute of Surgical Research] stationed next to Brooke Army Medical Center in San Antonio, Texas. We went under the auspices of wonderful trauma surgeons. They had a vision of how we could do research in the combat theater of operations, while adhering to all the regulations as U.S. researchers and military personnel. We were starting to think about how we could do research. We have all the usual civilian human subject regulations as well as military regulations. We hammered out a process, but we also needed boots on the ground in Iraq to execute it. I was deployed as the human subjects' administrator on the ground. I had the responsibility of overseeing the human subjects' protection rules for about 60 research protocols in the combat theater while I was there. It was like the Department of Clinical Investigations in a combat zone. I was the facilitator for identifying potential studies and investigators or having them referred to me for consultation."

Heidi continued, "I helped researchers through the process. Most of the investigators in theater were clinicians. For example, a combat surgeon, who was going to be in Iraq for 6 months, wanted to look at using a near-infrared system to detect how well an extremity perfused after a vascular repair. This surgeon may have never done a study before and needed help. Therefore, we'd get him CITI [Collaborative Institutional Training Initiative] training. We'd help him rewrite the research protocol, and I'd pay particular attention to the protection of human subjects. We'd pass the project through the whole chain of command so that everyone was aware of approval by the nonmedical and nonclinical people who were there. The research data obtained there had to be generated in the war zone. We could not interfere with any combat operations in the conduct of our research. I would facilitate that, and the protocol was put on a template and sent for scientific review. I did not review any studies. They went back to the States. Subject matter experts did the scientific review. The investigators would answer the reviewers' questions, but many of them did not have any experience with that, so I would help them. I ran a spreadsheet and kept time hacks on all studies. I had a very good track record getting studies approved in a timely manner."

Heidi recalled, "At the Institutional Review Board [IRB] in Texas, studies received a high priority because they were Iraq studies. Sometimes approval only took 3 to 4 days. This was the best job I've ever had. It was so rewarding, partly because of the quick turnaround time. You really felt like you were doing something that really mattered. I could not have done it on my own, but I had two offices standing behind me in the States propping me up and supporting me. We had good connectivity. It felt so good to know my email sent at 10 p.m. by Iraq time would be the first email they would answer in the morning. They would come to their job and search their inboxes for anything from me. I'm talking about two full offices of people. Anything with my name on it was the first priority and the first email they would answer. It was really good."

Major Derek: Critical Care Nurse

Derek was an Army reservist from Westchester County, New York. He joined the Army Reserve to get money to help pay for nursing school. After graduating, he started working in a large medical center that was a major trauma center for the Hudson Valley of New York. Derek worked in the trauma ICU, the medical ICU, the coronary care unit, and the emergency room.

Derek reported, "I was in a unit attached to a combat support hospital, and the combat support hospital was deployed to Iraq. I was the aide-de-camp to the commanding general of the entire Army Reserve division, but by specialty, I was a registered nurse. I took the aide job to have a better chance to be selected for promotion. I thought it would be interesting to do something out of the medical chain of command for a year or two. I figured I would learn a lot about how the combat arms in the Army are organized, equipped, and mobilized. What happened was that I was asked to transfer back into the nursing staff of the combat support hospital for deployment. I transferred because I wanted to go to Iraq. The other units in our reserve division were not deploying."

Derek further explained, "I've been in the Army Reserve for 25 years. I was retirement-eligible when I went to Iraq. I was an LPN [licensed practical nurse] for the first several years. Then in 1997, I completed my RN and later received a commission. We were mobilized in June 2006, and we deployed to Iraq in September 2006. We trained at Fort McCoy in Wisconsin for 4 months before we left for Iraq. My job in the combat support hospital was charge nurse of an intermediate care ward. It was a medical-surgical ward, or a step-down unit to the ICU. Even though I was an ICU nurse in my civilian job, the Army wanted me in a charge nurse position because of my leadership expertise."

Derek recalled, "Before we deployed to Iraq, we went for training in Wisconsin. The General in charge was from Louisiana. He decided a few mobilization changes were going to be made. They created FOBs on the mobilization station. We would stay on our FOBs the whole time we were in training. He was trying to create the atmosphere and environment we would work and live in while deployed. Even during 4 months of training, we lived and trained in very primitive conditions. The training base proved to be worse living conditions than we found in Iraq."

Derek recalled, "I felt that there was a lot of unnecessary training before we deployed to Iraq as a hospital unit. They had us kicking down doors, engaging in urban combat maneuvers, escape and evasion, and throwing hand grenades. I said, 'I'm not going to be doing that in Iraq.' We didn't mind training on the weapons because we want to be able to protect our patients and ourselves if the enemy comes through the wire. The other stuff seemed to be a bit much. The average age of an infantry soldier is about 19, and the average age of a hospital reservist is in one's early 40s. I was the third-oldest soldier in the hospital unit. Therefore, you are making me train like the 19-year-old infantry soldier. We lost five lieutenant colonels in our unit before we deployed to Iraq because of training injuries. So we lost five critical people who couldn't deploy."

"We left for Iraq on June 7, 2005, and came back Memorial Day of 2006," *recounted Derek*. "Initially, we did split operations. The main contingent was at Abu Ghraib, outside of Baghdad, and we had another contingent down at Camp Bucca in the south, right on the border near Basra. So initially,

I was assigned to Camp Bucca. When I got to Camp Bucca, I was assigned as charge nurse of the intermediate care ward, even though I'm a critical care nurse. Camp Bucca was set up more as a long-term care facility for the detainees. They could convalesce at Camp Bucca from their injuries."

Major Yvonne: Brigade Nurse

Yvonne was raised in an Army family. Her father was a retired sergeant major, who had served in the Vietnam War and in the first Persian Gulf War. Yvonne was born in Germany at a U.S. Army hospital. As an Army brat, she and her siblings lived in many places and considered the Army their home. Yvonne said she attended four grammar schools and two high schools. In college, Yvonne received an Army ROTC scholarship to cover the expense of her last 3 years in college. After graduating, Yvonne was commissioned as a Second Lieutenant in the Army Nurse Corps. After general duty nursing assignments in North Carolina, Louisiana, and Italy, Yvonne was selected for an assignment that was unique for a nurse. She was selected to be on the brigade staff of an infantry unit as the brigade nurse.

Yvonne recalled, "My deployment was to Afghanistan. I was with an Airborne Infantry Brigade. It was really an interesting deployment because there had never been a nurse in that unit before. It was a new concept to put a registered nurse in a combat brigade. We did not have a hospital attached to the brigade. I was the only nurse in the entire brigade. I went to Afghanistan in 2005 till 2006. As a brigade nurse, I was very, very lucky. It is a very proud, very historic, well-known unit and a very tough unit. They are famous from Vietnam. Their lineage goes back to World War II, and they are the only unit that had combat jumps in Vietnam and Iraq. To be associated with a unit of that quality was a huge honor for me. I feel that I was able to serve the nurse corps proud as a member of that unit."

Yvonne further reported, "My role with that unit was to make sure that the combat medics were trained and that they would keep current on their EMT [Emergency Medical Technician] qualifications. I worked a lot of medical readiness for 3,500 soldiers in the brigade. I made sure they had their shots, and I followed up to make sure they had their physicals, immunizations, and dental work so everyone was ready to go. I also did a lot of training with the infantrymen on first responder training such as self-aid, buddy-aid, how to apply tourniquets, and how to start IVs [intravenous] on each other. Combat life savers was the term used back then. Now, the Army calls it tactical combat casualty care."

Yvonne continued, "When I wasn't doing training with the guys from the airborne infantry brigade, I used to work at the nearby Air Force combat support hospital to keep my inpatient and ICU clinical skills current. They could pretty much plug me in to work in the ER, ICU, or any medical-surgical area except the operating room. I tried to do at least one day in the hospital each week."

Major Samantha: Critical Care Nurse

Samantha hailed from Michigan and attended college there. After 2 years of civilian practice in Michigan, she joined the Army Nurse Corps. She said she was influenced by her older brother, who attended college on an Army ROTC scholarship and was serving in a stateside armored tank unit. Samantha visited her brother in Texas and met some Army nurses while she was there. She found the nurses to be upbeat and career motivated. They appeared to like their jobs and the Army lifestyle very much. They, like Samantha, were single at the time and full of motivation and adventure. When Samantha was commissioned, her older brother administered the commissioning oath to her at their parents' home.

After assignments near Seattle, Germany, Kansas, and North Carolina and deployments to Somalia and Oman, Samantha was notified of her pending deployment to Afghanistan. Samantha recalled, "I was unofficially notified in November 2006, that I was going to deploy to Afghanistan. I was the fourth candidate contacted. Please forgive some of my cynicism, but I think it's an important point. The three people contacted prior to me had never deployed. We were distributed throughout the Western Regional Medical Command. The three other people ahead of me, who were asked to go, had a variety of reasons why they couldn't go. We all know that deployments never come at a convenient time. It is a stress for families and impacts a lot of people besides the individual. I was unofficially notified in November, and I was officially notified only 15 days prior to having to report to Fort Bliss in Texas for training and then deployment. I deployed in February 2007 with my combat support hospital and returned home in June 2008. I've been on active duty for 17 years. I was happy to go. I have been deployed before to Somalia for the Black Hawk Down situation and to Oman. Honestly, it was a privilege to go. Whether I retire at 20 years or 30 years, I'm glad I've done three deployments. However, I was very disappointed in my peers for a variety of reasons that they didn't feel they could go. It was stressful for everyone."

Captain Penny

Penny had been a nurse for 7 years and an Army nurse for 4 years when she deployed to Afghanistan. When she joined the Army, she was single, but she met and married her husband on her first assignment.

Penny described how she believed her pregnancy made her an unlikely candidate for deployment. "I was assigned to a forward surgical team [FST] in Washington state, which was a brand new unit at the time. There was one other FST already established at my hospital, and they decided to add a second one. It was just a few months before the September 11th terrorist attacks, and I had decided to take the position. I was pregnant at the time, and I remember thinking to myself, 'Thank goodness I'm pregnant because I probably won't have to go anywhere.' Little did I know, 10 months later, for the first time in the history of FSTs in the military, they actually deployed a unit. I left for Afghanistan with a 5-month-old baby at home."

Photo Courtesy of U.S. Air Force.

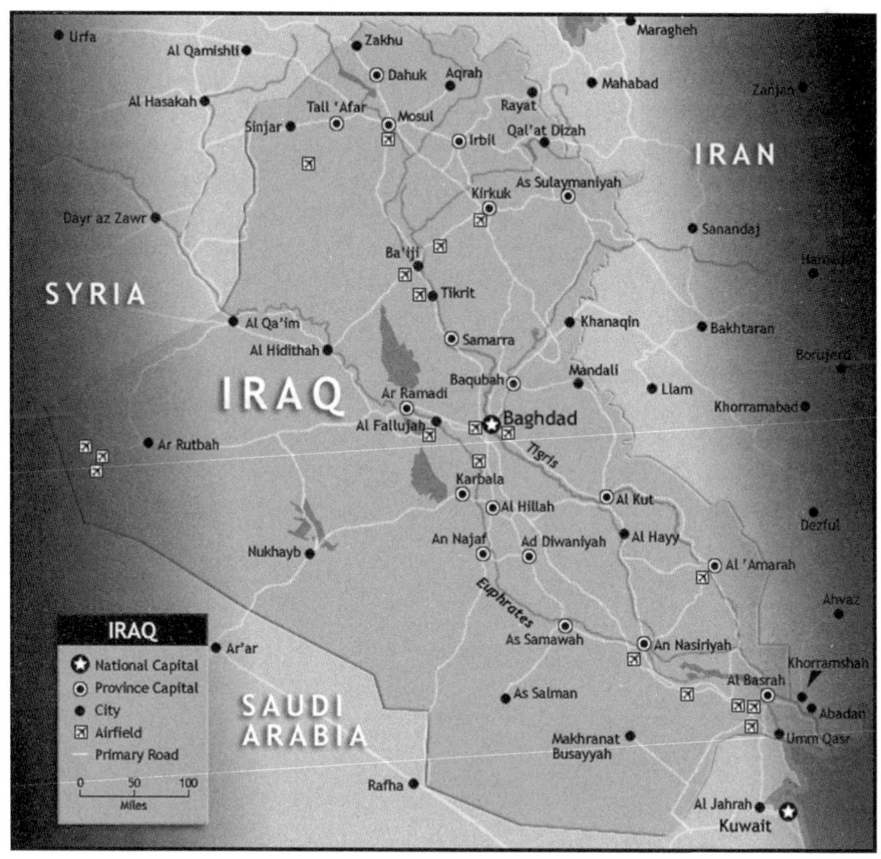

Map of Iraq.

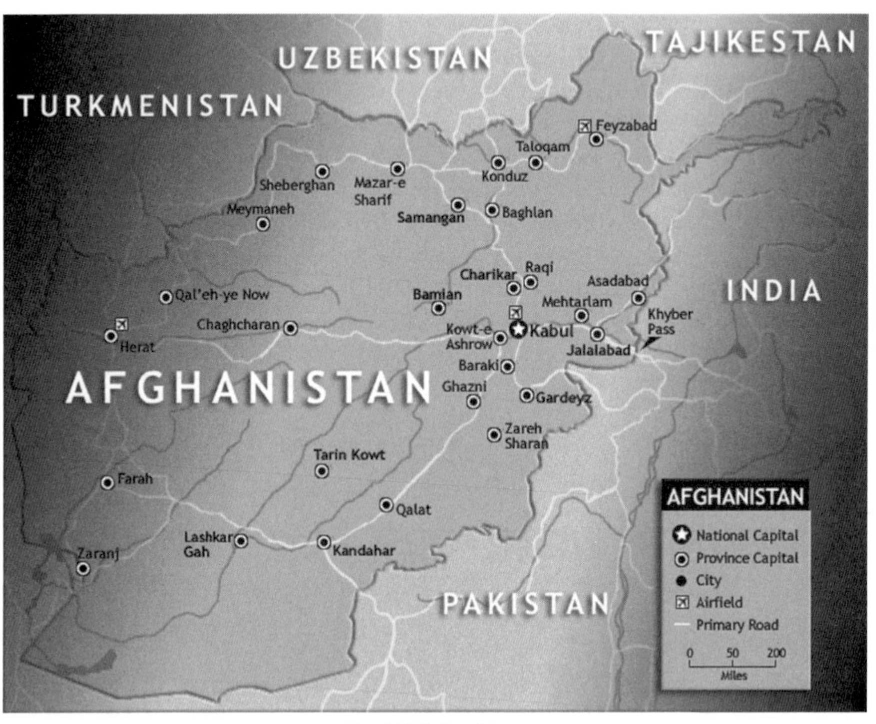

Photo Courtesy of U.S. Air Force.

Map of Afghanistan.

3

Nurses in Harm's Way: More Than I Bargained For

Nurses told of the dangers they faced in Iraq and Afghanistan. They described mortar attacks on their hospital compounds, the improvised explosive device explosion risk when participating in convoys, the dangers associated with humanitarian mission trips outside the wire to local villages, and the risks of insurgent attacks even within the perimeters of their bases. Two of the nurses in this research study were wounded in enemy attacks. From the moment the nurses arrived in Iraq or Afghanistan, they were almost constantly in harm's way because there were no safe places. Everyone is vulnerable in a combat zone. Luckily, the overwhelming majority returned home physically uninjured.

The dangers were real and ever present as nurses survived mortar and rocket attacks on their hospital compounds. The improvised explosive device detonation risk was great as slow-moving humanitarian aid convoys traversed the primitive road system outside the wire to transport nurses and other medical personnel to nearby villages to provide free clinics for the local population. Ambush was always another risk as nurses ventured into the countryside to provide humanitarian aid or when they participated in helicopter medical evacuation missions to pick up the injured. One of the nurses in this study was hit with shrapnel in her neck and jaw from a mortar attack on her hospital compound in Iraq. Another nurse was shot in the elbow by an AK-47 semiautomatic rifle round brandished by an insurgent dressed as an Afghan national army soldier. This nurse was lucky to be alive, as two of her colleagues lay dead at the scene from wounds sustained in the ambush attack.

Lieutenant Commander Clare

Clare, an active-duty Navy nurse assigned to a surgical hospital in Iraq, recalled, "I was hit by a mortar blast. I was hit with shrapnel in the neck and have right-sided hearing loss. I had just left the trauma unit and was walking through the galley when the compound was hit. I had surgery at my hospital, and the next day, I was airlifted to Germany in one of the Air Force's flying hospitals. I was in the military hospital in Germany for a few days before I was flown on the hospital plane back to the States for further care."

Commander Josie

Josie was a seasoned Navy nurse assigned to mentoring duty in Afghanistan. She recalled, "Four of us were jogging on an Afghan army base. An insurgent dressed in an Afghan army uniform opened fire on us with an AK-47 [semiautomatic rifle] from a security tower. First, I was shot in the arm. Then, my best friend and another jogger were killed. Our other running buddy was not hit. He took off to get help. It all happened so fast. I was only shot once, probably because I stayed down and lifeless. My best friend was hit in the thigh first, and she was moaning, so he shot her again twice in the back. The other jogger was shot in the head and probably died instantly because his brains were all over the grass."

First Lieutenant Leah

Leah hailed from New England. She joined an Army Reserve medical unit as an enlisted member while she attended college. Leah was deployed to Iraq as soon as she completed Army Reserve combat training in Wisconsin. This training commenced immediately after her college graduation. She was deployed with her reserve combat support hospital to Mosul, Iraq, for 15 months. Her first combat assignment was working in the intensive care unit (ICU) at the coalition hospital. She described mortar attacks at her base. "We were mortared in Mosul from the first week I was there. We actually had 17 hits in one night. One female took some shrapnel in the abdomen, another in the shoulder."

Leah went on to describe her environment in Mosul. "We had an airfield there. They bombed the airfield, they bombed the hospital, and they bombed the CHU [containerized housing unit], which is where we lived. These were like tiny dorm rooms in a trailer made of metal. I shared one with a nurse practitioner. A mortar actually landed in the CHU five sections down from us, and luckily, no one got hurt because it did not explode. It went through the roof, through the side, and landed in the dirt right outside. It was unexploded ordinance, and the ordinance disposal team [bomb squad] had to come remove it. I think they took it somewhere isolated and exploded it. Therefore, we were lucky because it landed right where people were sleeping. Sadly, I just read that in December, a doctor was killed right near where I was living, same exact hospital, because of mortar fire. They liked to mortar right around Ramadan, Christmas time, and around all the holidays. The doctor died on Christmas day."

Major Michelle

Michelle was raised in Columbus, Ohio, and attended college nearby. She joined the Air Force a year after she graduated from college. Michelle had been in the Air Force Nurse Corps for 12 years. In her first 6 years, she worked as an ICU nurse, with assignments in Maryland and California. She graduated with a Master of Science degree in nurse anesthesia care after completing her assignment in California. She has practiced as a nurse anesthetist for the last 6 years. Michelle served in Afghanistan on a medical mentoring team at an Afghan national army hospital. Her assignment was to mentor and teach anesthesia care to Afghan medical teams.

Although Michelle says that she loves working in an expanded nursing practice role, she admits to being frightened in the war zone and missing her family greatly. She believes that she was less fearful before she had children. According to Michelle, the responsibility of parenthood looms large in her life.

Michelle remarked, "I was scared. I always had my 9-millimeter handgun in my shoulder holster, even in the OR. I never took it off. Not only did I never take it off, I always had a clip of bullets loaded in it. Therefore, I had a loaded gun with me all the time. I never left it. It was always with me. Sometimes, we had to drive to the NATO hospital, which was 3 miles down the road; it was outside the wire in an unprotected area. You had to drive through a village to get to the hospital, and we were not authorized to have armored vehicles, so we were always very vulnerable to attack. Only if we were with a general officer could we have an armored vehicle. It was funny because when other units came to visit our hospital, like the Canadian forces, they always showed up in an armored convoy. Our vehicle to drive places was a pickup truck."

Michelle described security problems at her hospital and how she almost had a close call. "We were attached to the Afghan army hospital on an Afghan base, but we lived outside the wire on a small U.S. compound. The Afghans were our guards, but you couldn't trust them. The Afghans didn't screen people at the hospital entrance, so just about anyone could get in. One time, a guy came in with a long knife and said he was looking to kill the American women. It was no secret that Americans were working at the hospital. Luckily, all four of us women were back at our compound for lunch. It was rare for us to have lunch together because most days I was working through lunchtime in the OR. The Afghan medics did not kick this guy out of the hospital, and when we came back from lunch, he saw the four of us, and we got a look at him, too. Our hospital commander had a fit after he heard about this, and security got better."

Captain Trudi

Trudi, an Army reservist from New England, joined the reserves as an enlisted member when she was a licensed practical nurse. Several years later, when she completed a bachelor's degree in nursing, she was commissioned into the Army Nurse Corps. When she was deployed to Iraq, she was in her early 40s. She deployed to Mosul, Iraq, in September 2006 and returned home a year later. Her unit was moved to Anbar Province 6 months into their tour of duty. Trudi recalled, "It was very hard for people because the alarms would go off, and we would have to run to get our Kevlar helmets, weapons, and flak vests and sprint to the bunkers. The soldiers who protected the hospital would have to jump in their vehicles and head out to try to find the bad guys who were launching mortars into the compound. It was hard because in northern Iraq there are trees, and we had snow, so it was really unlike the desert. It was freezing, and it was snowing, and you had trees blocking views, and often you couldn't find the bad guys that were doing this."

Major Fran

Fran was raised in the suburbs of Chicago, Illinois. She attended parochial schools and graduated with a nursing degree from a large university in Chicago. Before joining the Air Force, Fran had worked in medical-surgical nursing and mental health nursing in Chicago. She had been a mental health nurse for 12 years. She was assigned to bases in Texas, Ohio, England, and California before deploying to Iraq. Fran was assigned as a mental health nurse and combat stress team leader in Iraq. She spent most of her tour of duty in the area around Tallil, Iraq. She enjoyed the challenges of mental health nursing and using what she had learned about combat stress.

Fran remarked, "It just got tiring after a while because you kept getting interruptions with your sleep. It was rough getting mortared. You wouldn't think that would be the case in a hospital area, but war is war, and we were certainly in harm's way. The attacks usually occurred after dark or right before dawn. This one attack was at about 6 o'clock in the morning. I went to the emergency room shortly after the attack. We had two dead troops and a third that was dying. I met with the commanders of the units that had lost troops and then went with them back to their units. Later that day, my team took the whole base through a kind of critical incident stress debriefing with the current model in use."

First Lieutenant Joy

Joy hailed from Idaho and joined the Air Force 4 years after she graduated from college. She had worked in a large San Francisco hospital on a trauma unit before joining the military. Joy deployed to Afghanistan with a cadre of about 100 people from a large Air Force medical center in California. Joy related, "We took rocket fire at our base probably weekly. I also went out to the FOBs outside the wire to run a clinic with a physician's assistant. These FOBs took a lot of random fire and some targeted fire, too. One FOB took a direct hit on the MWR [morale, welfare, and recreation] trailer. Luckily, there were no fatalities."

Captain Suzanne

Suzanne joined the Air Force in 2004 after 4 years of working on medical-surgical units in St. Louis, Missouri. Suzanne lived near a large Air Force base and had several friends who were Air Force nurses. She said she learned a lot about the Air Force from her friends and decided to join because she felt the military lifestyle would be compatible with her personal and professional goals. After assignments in Texas and Florida, Suzanne deployed to Balad Air Base, Iraq, with several colleagues from her hospital in Florida. She was assigned to the aeromedical staging facility at Balad Air Base. Suzanne recalled, "For some reason, we usually got hit a lot on Wednesday nights, when I was taking my trash out. One night, my team members told me I couldn't throw my trash out anymore because we usually always got a rocket attack on those nights."

Captain Olivia

Olivia was a 28-year-old nurse who was born in the Bronx, New York, and grew up in Massachusetts. Olivia recalls that for as long as she can remember, she wanted to be a nurse. She came from a family of five children, of whom she was the oldest. She believes that taking care of her younger siblings—feeding them, putting Band-Aids on their cuts and scrapes, and comforting them when they were sick or hurting—brought out her nurturing side and set the path to her later nursing career. Olivia joined the Future Nurses Club at her high school, where school field trips opened her eyes to what nurses did in hospitals and clinics. Olivia's parents did not have the money to send her to college. At the suggestion of her uncle, who was a retired Army sergeant major, Olivia applied for and received an Army ROTC scholarship to attend college as a nursing major. After 6 years on active duty, Olivia transferred to the Army Reserve. Olivia was sent with her reserve unit to the coalition forces hospital in Mosul, Iraq.

Some nurses were tasked with going out on helicopter missions to pick up casualties in the field. Olivia recalled, "Sometimes I'd have to go out in a helicopter to pick up injured troops. Soldiers provided cover so I could treat their wounded buddy in the field. One time, when I went to get a wounded soldier, they thought the area was secure, and we didn't see a vehicle coming up.There was a 'boom,' and I [went] flying in the air. I landed on my patient. He says, 'Are you O.K.?' He had a leg wound, so he was talking. I said, 'Yeah, I'm ready to go, are you?' His buddies helped me drag him to the chopper and throw him on a litter."

Olivia went on to describe another harrowing experience she had on a helicopter mission near Mosul, Iraq. She stated, "The fire fight could be like the length of two football fields away from me. We would land, and hopefully, if I was lucky, the injured person would be carried out of where the fighting was taking place and moved closer to me. I'd run to them, throw them on a litter, do what I can, and then throw them on the helicopter, and then work on them as we flew back to the hospital. I'd have one medic go with me on these missions. However, sometimes I wouldn't even know the medic till I got on the helicopter. I rarely got to fly with the same crew. Most of the crews and the medics were men. It was kind of hard for me. I had to earn their trust every time I went out there on one of these missions. I'd have to prove that I know what I am doing." *Olivia added,* "The soldiers provided cover for me, so I could treat their wounded buddy in the field and get him to the helicopter for medevac out of the fire zone. There were bullets flying over the medics and me. The soldiers in the field could only do so much to protect us. I was always warned if it was going to be a hot LZ [landing zone], and they couldn't go any further away because of the terrain. We had to quickly scoop up the injured and take off."

Captain Alice

Alice was born in Germany, the daughter of an Air Force Major and an elementary school teacher. Alice grew up on Air Force bases in Germany, Texas, California, and Florida. She graduated from a large university in Florida with a bachelor's degree in nursing. Following graduation, she worked on a medical-surgical floor of a large Veteran's Administration hospital in Florida for 3 years. Several of her nurse colleagues were former military nurses. Alice joined the Air Force in 2000. She was assigned to a large hospital in Texas. While there, Alice completed a critical care course and was reassigned to an adult surgical ICU. After a year in this ICU, she was reassigned to a large critical care unit in Ohio. When a large cadre of medical personnel from her medical center deployed to Afghanistan, Alice deployed as a critical care air transport team nurse.

Alice flew on air evacuation missions in Afghanistan and occasionally to Germany. She described landing on an FOB to pick up casualties. "We'd fly in the C-130 turboprop because it doesn't need a standard runway and is a STOL [short takeoff and landing] aircraft. We would frequently open the back ramp before we landed so we could get the patients aboard in 3 minutes or less, if the area was not secure. We'd take off as the back ramp was closing and get the hell out of there. A plane sitting on a runway makes a big target! Sometimes, we'd count the bullet holes in the fuselage after we returned to our base."

Major Diana

Diana was an Air Force Reserve nurse assigned to an aeromedical staging facility in Iraq. She described her work environment. "It was scary because you didn't know if you were going to be shot at or if we'd get mortared that day. It was scary not knowing what was going to happen from day to day. Every day was different. It was dark. I worked mainly at night, 7 in the evening until 7 in the morning, and I was always in the dark. We were loading patients for air evac in the dark; we were unloading helicopters on the helipad in the dark. You always had this 'doom' kind of feeling and wondered if we'd get mortared tonight. The helipad was encased by cement walls, but the mortars could come over the walls. We got mortared several times very close to the helipad."

Captain Abby

Abby grew up in Florida and attended college there. When she graduated with a bachelor's degree in nursing, she moved to Atlanta, Georgia, and started working as a medical-surgical nurse. After 3 years, she took a critical care course and moved to working in an adult ICU. Several years later, Abby was looking for a change in location. She decided to join the Air Force. Her first assignment was in California, followed by assignments in Germany and Texas. She continued to work in critical care and medical-surgical nursing, depending on the needs of the Air

Force. She deployed with a cadre of medical personnel from her hospital in Texas to Bagram Air Base, Afghanistan.

Abby reported, "At Bagram Air Base, I felt fairly safe; it was like a fortress there. However, when I went to the FOBs to help with clinics, we got mortared and bombed a lot, and I got really scared. I wondered if I was going to get hurt or killed. My first few months at Bagram were easy from a safety perspective compared to my last few months, when I was assigned to also do clinics outside the wire and on the FOBs."

Commander Rita

Rita was an active-duty Navy nurse anesthetist assigned to a fast-forward surgical team at the beginning of the war in Iraq. Rita reported, "It was rough doing surgery out in the field when you could hear shooting in the distance and knew our Marines were trying to keep a secure perimeter around our forward surgical team position. You wondered how many of the Marines would be injured or killed trying to protect our position so we could keep doing surgery. You concentrated on your work, you kept your weapon nearby, and you prayed."

Major Samantha

Samantha was a seasoned active-duty Army nurse assigned in Afghanistan. Samantha recalled, "Deployment was very difficult for many of the young people, let alone us older people. You don't sleep much, and at night, they will shoot rockets at the base, especially if there is a full moon. You may be walking home, and then all of a sudden, you have to run. You can hear the rockets, and you have learned how to distinguish the sound. You are always on alert and have become highly vigilant. This is especially true if there is a blackout where there are no lights at night. There is a sense of paranoia because you can't see, and you wonder if someone is behind you. When there is no moon, you can't even see your hand in front of you. You have to use a blue, red, or green light—you can't use a regular yellow flashlight because they can see it from afar, and you don't want to be a target for a sniper. It was very dangerous."

Captain Robert

Robert was an Army Reserve nurse assigned to combat support hospitals in Tikrit, Mosul, and Al Asad in Anbar Province, Iraq. Robert was from Maryland. He had been in the reserves for 9 years, first as an enlisted corpsman for 3 years and then as a registered nurse once he received his bachelor's degree in nursing and officer commission. When not involved with Army Reserve duties, Robert worked in Baltimore at a large medical center on a cardiology unit.

Robert summarized the sentiments reflected by many of the nurses. "There were really no front lines, and we all felt very vulnerable over there. You had to be on your guard all the time. You wondered how many local people who worked on your base by day were insurgents by night. It is not as if insurgents wear uniforms as we do. There have been attacks on a base from within the base, like the RPG [rocket propelled grenade] attack on a military mess hall in Iraq. An Army nurse was killed while jogging in the green zone in Baghdad. So, we were fearful, and we had to be alert all the time, but we were still able to do our jobs well and perform our mission."

4

Living Conditions: A Mixed Bag

Austere living quarters presented one more stressor for the nurses. Living conditions varied greatly depending on if a nurse was assigned to a fixed facility or a mobile one. Some found themselves living in tents, whereas others lived in B-huts or trailers. Those who deployed in earlier years of the wars described more primitive living conditions than those who deployed in later years.

In Afghanistan especially, nurses frequently lived in B-huts, simple structures built of plywood with tin or aluminum roofs. In the winter, the B-huts got cold, whereas any tent structures in Afghanistan or Iraq became stiflingly hot during the summer months. Air conditioning was a luxury in the living quarters, although most nurses' living areas did receive air-conditioning units later in the deployment cycle. All of the nurses reported having to travel outside their tent, trailer, or B-hut areas to use the bathroom and shower facilities. Port-a-potties or trailer latrines were the norm in Iraq and Afghanistan.

Another reality that added to the austerity of living and working in a war zone was a general lack of privacy while sleeping, showering, or even toileting. Tent and trailer toileting and shower facilities were generally communal. Cleanliness of latrine facilities was always a challenge owing to high-volume use and relying on local nationals or contractors to clean the facilities only about twice a day.

Commander Rita

As an active-duty Navy nurse anesthetist with a position on a fast-forward mobile surgical team that trained year-round for an austere combat environment, Rita would have said she believed she was trained and equipped for almost anything before she deployed to Iraq. However, following her tour of duty in Iraq, Rita admitted there were some surprises. "When the war started, we took on heavy casualties. I went without a shower for 11 days. The OR was like a litter box. We just scooped out bloody sand and other bodily secretions. We slept in tents or outside on the ground. I would lay a cot down outside the operating room tent. I preferred being outside. I didn't like sleeping in a tent. It was so bloody hot in the tents. I felt better outside. I have to have light when I sleep, so I stayed outside the tent to sleep. Over there, I felt that sleeping in a tent was like being in a coffin."

The variety and type of food available in Iraq and Afghanistan were location driven. Nurses assigned to mobile hospitals usually had much fewer choices of food, and much of the food consumed in the field was not hot food. Just like the sleeping accommodations, those assigned in the earlier war years usually had much more limited meal choices. Rita went on to describe dietary provisions. "We had very little food at the beginning of the war. We ate MREs [meals ready to eat]. Water was from a water buffalo. It tasted like chlorine and was always warm since it was 110 degrees outside. I brought Kool-Aid and Crystal Light packets with me to make the water more tolerable. After the first month of fighting in Iraq, we got some hot meals from the Seabees. It was good, maybe two or three hot meals each week. I lost 20 pounds while in Iraq."

Lieutenant Colonel Judd

Judd was a 57-year-old Army reservist who had been a young infantry soldier in Vietnam during the war. He described his living quarters in Iraq. "I lived in what the military calls a CHU [containerized housing unit]. You've seen containers on container ships. Well, you take a container and you put in two windows and a door. In one window, you put a combination heating-and-air-conditioning unit. Well, that is what we lived in. If you are under the rank of 0–5 [lieutenant colonel], two people lived in each CHU. For 0–5 and above, you got your own CHU. Compared to where I lived in Vietnam, the CHU was a five-star hotel. In Vietnam, I was in the field, in the mud, and slept in the field in a tent. I was comfortable in Iraq. Life was good! However, many nurses assigned to other places in Iraq still slept in tents, some of them in very large tents."

Many nurses found the heat in Iraq to be an added stressor in their living environment. Judd recalled, "On July 26th of 2007, it was 142 degrees in Iraq. We took a picture of the digital thermometer. It was 142 degrees! I sent my wife the picture. She called me up and said, 'But dear, it is dry heat.' I said, 'Okay, turn on the oven to 142 degrees, wait a half hour, and stick your head in it!"

Lieutenant Colonel Victoria

Victoria was an active-duty Army nurse who deployed to Iraq twice. The first time she deployed was in March 2003 to a combat support hospital near Baghdad, Iraq. Her unit spent about 3 weeks in Kuwait at the beginning of the war. Then they convoyed to where her hospital would be set up. Because they were the first combat support hospital to be set up near Baghdad, all their supplies, tents, and modular structures had to be brought in by truck convoy.

Victoria recalled, "The living conditions were deplorable. For our first 3 months, we ended up staying in a tent with 79 of our best friends. Doing shift work, living with your stuff, and of course, you had too much of your stuff with you, so our quarters were very, very tight. It was very challenging, extremely crowded, everyone was extremely cranky, and it was too hot. We arrived in theater in April. In southern Iraq, it's almost 120 degrees already! Later, we moved into our pods [small living areas]. Each pod was like a small trailer with not any more than 75 square feet of living space. If you didn't have a roommate whom you were compatible with, you were already challenged. That was a very difficult time for me."

Victoria found the living conditions much better on her second assignment in Iraq. Victoria reported, "Living in Iraq was a very difficult time for me. I think I would have been more successful in that assignment if I simply had more living space. I think most of my staff felt the same way, too. I didn't know how bad it was until I got to Camp Bucca, which is near Baghdad. When I went to Camp Bucca for my second deployment, I had almost 400 square feet of living space and a trailer all to myself! Therefore, the living areas are not equal from FOB to FOB by far."

Victoria recalled, "Part of the problem with the housing in Iraq is that I was there when they officially made the extension of tours of duty from 12 months to 15 months. Therefore, a lot of soldiers had to stay for another 3 months, and housing wasn't available. It just kind of went downhill. The biggest challenge for me over there was not being able to do a lot of the things that make me happy, like taking courses, like things outside of the normal humdrum of the job. Most of my staff felt that way, too. We tried our hardest to find the fastest computer in the hospital, and we'd take turns. We tried very hard to work around the conditions. It was my biggest challenge while there. It was very depressing."

Commander Josie

A seasoned Navy veteran, Josie described her quarters in Afghanistan. "I lived at a forward operating base [FOB] next to an Afghan national army base that housed the Afghan army hospital. I lived 'outside the wire' in a plywood structure at the FOB and walked every day to the Afghan hospital. There were 16 of us on this mentoring team to assist the Afghan military medical personnel. The hospital had indoor toilets and running water; however, where we lived did not. We'd have to walk outside to shower or use the toilets. They were located in a trailer that we called 'the Cadillacs.' I lived in a B-hut, which is a wooden shack. It was not insulated well at all. I was one of six women in our B-hut. I'm glad we got there in the summer. I enjoy the summer. I would rather be in 100 degrees than in 30-degree weather. In the winter, those B-huts were so ill equipped to handle snow. I think the roof was made of sheet metal. It gets cold there in the winter. You'd wake up in the middle of the night to pee and have to put your shoes on because there are rocks outside. Walking to the toilets to do my business and then coming back was a hassle and dangerous. Waking up in freezing weather and having to walk to the outdoor latrines was not fun! I remember cutting back on my fluid intake later in the evening so I wouldn't have to get up in the middle of the night to pee."

Major Diana

Diana was an Air Force reservist assigned in southern Iraq. She reported, "There were four of us in our trailer. What made this arrangement particularly difficult was that we had day-shift and night-shift workers living together. There were alarm clocks going off all the time. It was horrible. You could hear everything that was going on around you. You had no privacy. Those trailers were awful. I don't think I would have made it without earplugs. I'm glad I wasn't there more than 4 months. I must say that by the fourth month, you are into your routine. You are so exhausted by the end of the day. I could almost sleep through anything with my earplugs and eye mask. In the beginning, I had trouble sleeping because the flight line was right near the trailers. I could hear planes taking off and landing, especially those fighter jets that always left in pairs. Later, I just tuned them out because I was so exhausted."

Diana recalled, "It was miserably hot. We had it as high as 149 degrees. Most of the time we had air conditioning, but a few times, we would lose our power. We lived in these trailers that were like 20 feet by 10 feet. You had two beds in each cubicle. We could lift our beds up and put our trunks underneath. We had like a wall locker that we could put our stuff in. My roommate was another nurse. The trailers were small but okay. The heat, when we lost electrical power, was not okay."

Captain Meaghan

Most nurses who arrived in Iraq or Afghanistan in 2007 or later described improved living conditions. Meaghan, an active-duty Air Force nurse assigned to Bagram Air Base, Afghanistan, remarked, "The living environment was much better than I expected. I lived in a two-person trailer. The latrines were about 50 feet away. The showers were about 100 feet away. The huts we lived in were much better than the tents we expected to live in. I was very lucky at Bagram, Afghanistan, in 2008. We had a coffee shop and Dairy Queen. We had television, Internet, a library, a theater, and a gym. I didn't have trouble getting in touch with family like others in remote places."

Captain Vanessa

Vanessa, an Army reservist assigned to detainee care, remarked, "I cannot complain about my living conditions. We had better living conditions over in Iraq than we did at our training site in Wisconsin. The food in Iraq was better, too. I think the worst thing was trying to sleep. I was so wound up every day after work. It was such an intense experience. Trying to make sure that I would get enough sleep became an obsession for me. I would get off work, and I knew I had to get my rest for the next day of work. We were 12 hours on, 12 hours off, usually 6 days a week. If I didn't get the sleep I needed, the next day would absolutely kill me. I think that hurt me tremendously after I got home. It was hard to sleep when you are so wound up, and other people are snoring and tossing around."

Captain Tina

Tina was an active-duty Air Force nurse who arrived in Iraq shortly after the war began. Later in her career, she also deployed to FOB Salerno in Afghanistan. Tina reported, "My living conditions were better than I expected. At Balad Air Base in Iraq, we lived in trailers, and some were bigger than others. We had enough space. We had two bunk beds, so there were usually only two people to a room. It was sometimes three or four people to a room, when you were going through a transition with a new group of people coming in, and the other unit getting ready to return to the U.S. We had television, Internet access, and the ability to call home. The military provided us with many connections to the outside world. We had a lot of water, which was placed on pallets between the trailers. The showers were clean, although we didn't always have hot water. They had people from third-world countries cleaning the showers and toilets. We had a small library and theater. The only thing that was difficult was not being able to leave the compound. The living conditions were good for a war zone. We were comfortable for the most part."

Major Samantha

Samantha was an active-duty Army nurse in Afghanistan. She recalled, "We had air-conditioned living quarters, and our hospital was always air-conditioned. We also had Internet access. I could go to school online even though I was in Afghanistan. Sometimes the Internet would go down for a day or two, but it wasn't interrupted enough that I couldn't go to school or write to my family. It was nice to have the Internet. The food was also good in the mess halls, and we had several fast-food places on our compound. There was a little coffee shop that we liked to go to on our midmorning break. It was near the hospital."

Captain Marie

Marie was an Army reservist assigned to three locations in Iraq during her 12-month tour. At first, she went to the Air Force hospital on Balad Air Base, Iraq, to augment Air Force nurses at the largest U.S. hospital in Iraq. After 3 months, Marie's cadre of reservists moved to Mosul, Iraq. She spent the last 3 months of her deployment at the newly built U.S. hospital in Anbar Province, Iraq.

Marie described living in Anbar Province. "We slept in pods. They were like small trailers connected to one another. There were hundreds of these smaller trailers all lined up. We didn't have plumbing in the pods, but we did have air-conditioning. The pods had room for a bed, but mine didn't have a bed. I found a bed in a dump. I dragged it into my pod. It was like a bed frame. I found a spring-type mattress, and I put it up on cinder blocks. I had my own pod to myself because it was the last few months of my deployment. When we were leaving, we had to free up our pods for the new unit, so we moved into tent city. We had about 20 of us to a tent. It was tight quarters, but we were going home, so we didn't mind. They were temper tents, and they were air-conditioned. When we moved to Kuwait before going home, we lived in a very large tent. We had about 100 people to these big tents."

Marie did have a problem with the noise when she was assigned to the big Air Force base at Balad, Iraq. She stated, "The noise of living on an air base contributed to the stress of living in a war zone. It was very noisy. Helicopters, fighters, and transport aircrafts constantly taking off and landing all day and night. I worked in the ER sometimes. It was near the helipad where the Blackhawk helicopters would come in with patients. Apache attack helicopters would always be protecting the Blackhawk air evac helicopters when they flew into the base, so it was always very noisy."

Major Christina

Christina was an Air Force flight nurse. She reported, "Our flight quarters were quite good. We had two flight nurses to a trailer. They were air-conditioned, so we could get proper crew rest before each flight. The food was also good. I was there for the holidays, and they really went all out for us. We had Thanksgiving and Christmas dinner with all the usual trimmings. The folks working in the mess hall were truly wonderful. They had little Christmas trees and Menorahs displayed around the mess hall."

Christina added, "One thing that bothered me was that I couldn't escape the noise. Our trailers were near the flight line, so we had jets and helicopters taking off and landing all the time. When I was out on a mission transporting casualties, I wore earplugs. There was still the constant drone of the plane's engines. Noise stress was 24/7 for me while I was deployed."

Lieutenant Colonel Heidi

Heidi, an active-duty Army nurse researcher, remarked, "We had lots of food, which was not at all bad. There were meals around the clock because of shift workers. On Friday nights, we would have steak-and-lobster night, and we really enjoyed that. It really boosted morale. We had different dining facilities. This particular one was probably a mile walk from where I lived, but I was willing to make that walk for steak and lobster! It was something to look forward to in the week. I'd have to say that dining facility scored a very good rating on the food. They had a variety of vegetables, and they always had fruit for breakfast, which was huge for me. There was something for everyone."

Major Millie

Millie, an Army operating room nurse, remarked, "The food and the hospital itself in Iraq were a lot better than what I was prepared for. The food over there was good. I felt guilty because the food was good, and I didn't have to cook it. Our living conditions weren't bad either. We lived in trailers. The showers and latrines were a short walk down the path. My only complaint was that we didn't always have hot water for showers. It was really hit or miss some days in terms of hot water. We got window air conditioners after I was there for about a month. They worked fine as long as we didn't have a power failure."

Major Derek

Derek was an Army reservist who served at Camp Bucca and Abu Ghraib prison hospital in Iraq. Derek commented on his living conditions in Iraq. "The dining facility served a lot of food. It was the same routine every Monday. It was hot food. It was healthy food, and you could have as much as you wanted. No complaints from me, except for the lack of variety. You knew what they were going to serve by what day it was. I wish they varied the meals a bit. It was very, very hot in Iraq. I was sweating all the time over there. The blowing powdery sand just caked on[to] my sweaty skin. It was hard to sleep in that oppressive heat. Eventually, we got air conditioners in our sleeping quarters. The hospital buildings were air conditioned, but when we lost electrical power, it was terribly hot and smelly."

Captain Trudi

Trudi, an Army reservist from the Cape Cod area, joined the reserves as an enlisted member when she was a licensed practical nurse. Several years later, she completed a bachelor's degree in nursing and was commissioned into the Army Nurse Corps. When she deployed to Iraq, she was in her early 40s. She deployed to Mosul, Iraq, in September 2006 and returned home a year later. Her unit was moved to Anbar Province 6 months into their tour of duty. Trudi's clinical background in civilian life included medical-surgical nursing and emergency room nursing. Trudi remarked, "I think the food was amazing for being in the desert. We had Baskin-Robbins ice cream and desserts galore. The dining hall had Chinese night, lobster night, and Mexican night. These were specialties along with their good old regular sandwiches, burgers, and fries. Both places where I was stationed had good food. Probably Al-Asad in Anbar Province had more variety because it was easier to get the supplies there. I must say the food in Mosul was great, too. I remember they had milk shakes, so I could always get a strawberry shake. Maybe the selection was a little bit less, but everything was good. If you're on a base, the food for the soldiers is good. If you are out on the trail, you usually have to eat MREs. On the base, we'd have different specialty nights at least once a week. Ice cream was always available, so I gained weight in Iraq."

Trudi recalled, "The heat was a negative, but that was part of life. I usually enjoy the heat. If I have a choice between a hot place and a cold place, send me to the hot place. However, I just found temperatures over 120 degrees to be a little too hot for me. Luckily, the hospital had several air conditioners. After a few months in Iraq, we were able to get small window air conditioners for our trailers. It took some getting used to, but things over there could have been much worse."

Lieutenant Commander Clare

Clare was a Navy critical care nurse specializing in shock trauma care. Clare reflected, "When we first got to Iraq, we lived in tents. They were hot, crowded, and noisy. After about 2 months, we got trailers to live in. The trailers were two to four women to a trailer, depending on your rank. The trailers were air conditioned. It was a short walk to the latrine trailers and a little-bit-longer walk to the shower trailers. To preserve the hot water, we were told to take 3-minute showers. Most people complied because they didn't want to cut their colleagues short on water. The heat wasn't too bad for me because I grew up in California. We actually loved the weather out there. We planned our lives around it. So the weather in Iraq wasn't really an issue for me, but the housing and living space were in the beginning until I got used to it."

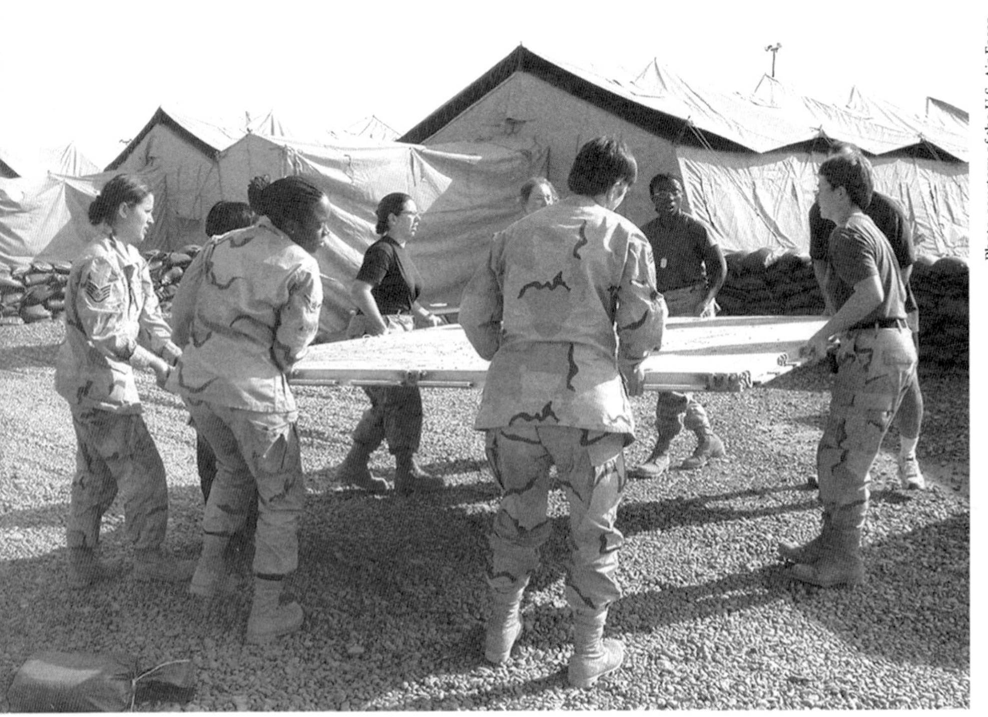

Photo courtesy of the U.S. Air Force.

Tent city at Balad Air Base, Iraq.

Photo courtesy of the U.S. Air Force.

Airmen and tents at Balad Air Base, Iraq.

Photo courtesy of the U.S. Air Force.

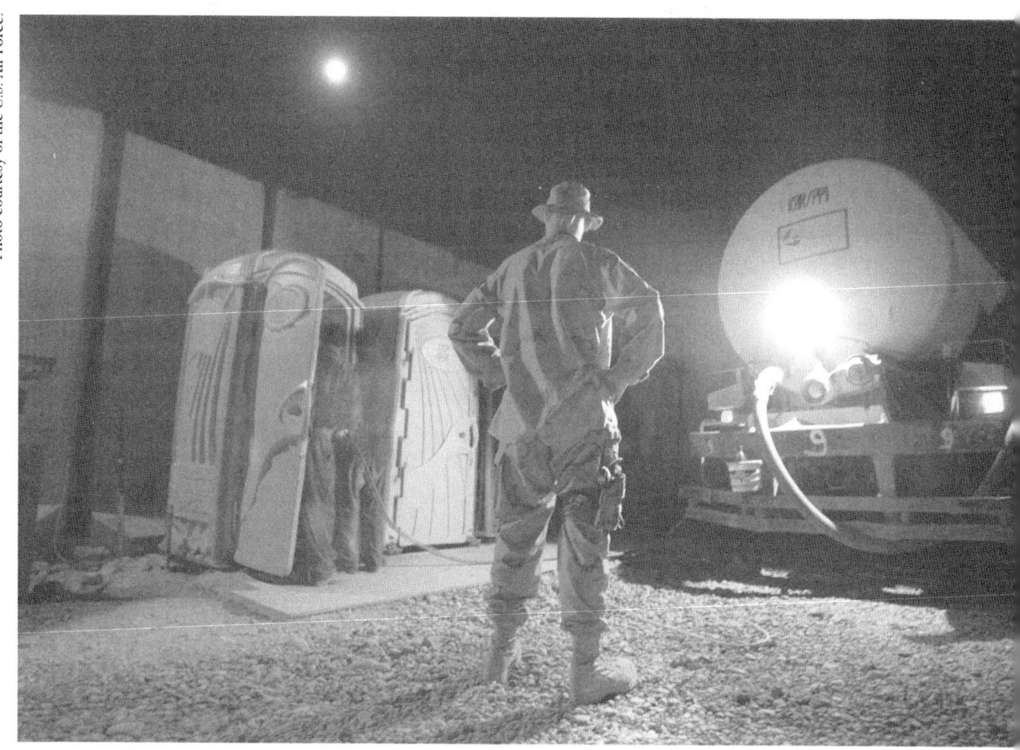

Pumping out port-a-potties, Balad Air Base, Iraq.

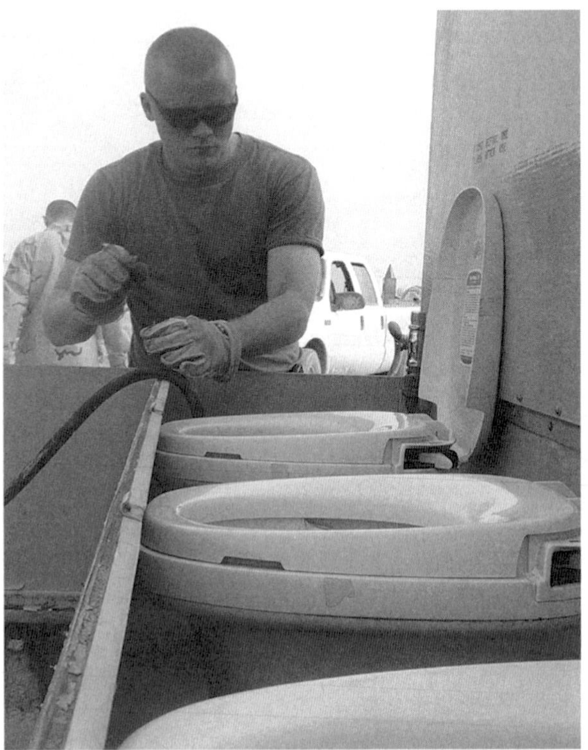

Photo courtesy of the U.S. Air Force.

"Three-hole latrine" at Tallil Air Base, Iraq.

5

My Work Place: A Plane, a Tent, or a Trailer

Nurses worked in many different capacities and physical locations in Iraq and Afghanistan. Some were assigned to combat support hospitals (CSHs), Afghan national army (ANA) hospitals, or combat stress teams. Others worked in mobile surgical hospitals or on fast-forward surgical teams (FFSTs) that moved with the ebb and flow of battle. Some found themselves caring for patients in detainee prison hospitals, aeromedical casualty staging units, or on aeromedical evacuation aircraft. A nurse's role was dictated by the mission of one's particular unit. Sometimes a nurse's role changed periodically, owing to nurse specialist shortages or purely out of necessity. For example, an emergency room (ER) nurse or an intensive care unit (ICU) nurse was frequently tasked to care for critically injured patients on helicopter medical evacuations from smaller medical facilities to larger theater CSHs. Army nurses were also detailed to stand guard duty, whereas Air Force nurses frequently provided humanitarian care to local nationals outside the wire. Both Air Force and Navy nurses told of mentoring duty with Afghan medical personnel.

FAST-FORWARD SURGICAL TEAMS

An FFST is a small mobile surgical unit of personnel and equipment that provides stabilization surgeries close to the fighting forces. Surgeons perform hemorrhage control on combat casualties within the "golden hour" of injury. Casualties can then be prepared for medical evacuation to a higher level of care. The FFST typically includes a very small cadre of surgeons, registered nurses, nurse anesthetists, and medics. This team operates out of mobile tent structures, which may be attached to one or more expandable Humvee vehicles. The mobile structure is self-contained. It provides its own electricity through portable generators and battery units.

Captain Penny

Penny, an Army nurse assigned to a fast-forward mobile surgical team, described her medical facility and its mission. "I was assigned to an Army FFST on the border with Pakistan in the northern part of Afghanistan. We were a small mobile team of two surgeons, an anesthetist, an operating room nurse, and a critical care nurse. We worked 12-hour shifts. However, by the time we finished everything, it was usually more than a 12-hour shift. We got patients right from the field. The only medical care they may have gotten before coming to us was from the field medics. I was on call 24/7 because we only had a small team of medical personnel there. I truly enjoyed the experience. All the injuries were fresh trauma, and we never knew what might be coming in to us. Casualties were either driven there by convoy or brought in by choppers. We got these troops in their most acute phase. The casualties were evenly split between American and Afghan soldiers. Somehow, the Afghans tended to arrive in worse shape. This might have been because the Americans usually got some treatment by the field medics. We got people who had just been in an IED explosion or just received a gunshot wound. We got quite a few coming in with head injuries. The surgeons knew there was nothing they could do that far forward for serious head injuries. They would do what they could, but many had to be sent out knowing they would probably die. If there was any way possible we could get the Americans to Bagram for neurosurgery, we would try very hard to do that."

Lieutenant Commander Rita

Rita, an active-duty Navy nurse anesthetist, described her FFST and her role in providing anesthesia care. "The concept of operations for the fast-forward surgical team was to patch up casualties, stop the hemorrhaging, and ship the patient out to a combat support hospital or hospital ship for more definitive care. My team moved with the Marines as they moved forward toward Baghdad during the invasion. We did whatever the casualties needed right away to keep them alive and to get them evacuated. That was our mission.

Rita continued, "There were no roads. We were out in the middle of the desert. It was very dangerous, especially when we moved forward in a small convoy behind the Marines. We were a team of two surgeons, one anesthesia provider,and one critical care nurse. We operated out of a Humvee ambulance that had a pop-up tent feature in the back that turned into a small operating room. When a soldier got shot, the field corpsmen would get him to us for immediate care. When we did surgery, we had these little electrical power generators to run the operating room equipment. Our anesthesia machine was a very basic field unit. The first 2 weeks of the invasion were very busy with lots casualties. Convoys were one of the most dangerous things to be on. When they were ambushed, and they frequently were ambushed, it was just a killing field. You are a sitting duck on those slow-moving convoys. We got a lot of casualties from the IEDs, mortars, and RPGs."

FORWARD MOBILE SURGICAL HOSPITALS

Forward Mobile Surgical Hospitals were a more modern-day version of the mobile Army surgical hospital (MASH). The MASH was first established in 1945 and was deployed during the Korean War and later conflicts. It was designed to get experienced medical assistance closer to the fighting so that the wounded could be treated sooner and with greater success. Casualties were first treated at the point of injury by a field medic or buddy care. Then they were routed through a battalion aid station or the newly established FFST for emergency stabilizing surgery. Finally, the casualties were transported to a MASH, or the newer forward mobile surgical hospital, or CSH for more extensive treatment. The last MASH unit was deactivated on October 16, 2006. The 212th MASH, based in Miesau Ammo Depot, Germany, was the first U.S. Army hospital established in Iraq in March 2003 supporting coalition forces during Operation Iraqi Freedom.

Major Olga

Olga hailed from Manchester, New Hampshire. After graduating from a large university in the Boston area, Olga worked as a medical-surgical nurse and eventually as a critical care nurse in a large Boston medical center. After several years of civilian nursing experience, Olga joined the Army Nurse Corps. Olga said she was looking for upward mobility and advanced nursing education. She was first assigned to Walter Reed Army Medical Center. Later, she had assignments in Germany, Hawaii, and Washington state.

Olga described her assignment with a forward mobile surgical hospital. "My first deployment was to Iraq in March of 2003 for the invasion. I was with the 212th MASH unit, and that was the last MASH unit in the U.S. Army. Everybody had to work together—nurses, doctors, and medics—because there were only 130 of us, and we moved as the battle environment geography changed. We had 37 trucks to drive, and everybody had to pitch in to set up the hospital each time we moved. That was such a great unit. We were very proud of our unit's distinguished history. We were deployed from Germany. I had been the head nurse of the critical care unit at a hospital in Germany just before the war kicked off. We got ready to go quickly. We really ramped up from 8 ICU beds to 20. Therefore, it was quite a busy time. After the invasion, we started receiving casualties, including coalition forces and local people who were injured. Most patients came to us by helicopter, Humvee, or truck. We did stabilization surgeries before moving patients away from the fighting. We got some patients from the fast-forward surgical teams, but sometimes they bypassed us and sent those patients by helicopter to the bigger hospital in Balad. We had many patients with blast injuries from IEDs or RPGs, gunshot wounds, traumatic amputations, and head wounds."

COMBAT SUPPORT HOSPITALS

A CSH is a permanent or semipermanent large field hospital usually located on or near an air base with an active runway. It is used to treat wounded soldiers, local nationals, and opposition soldiers wounded by U.S. military. The CSH is the successor to the MASH. The size of a CSH is almost unlimited because tents can be linked together. The CSH typically deploys with between 16 and 256 hospital beds. An 84-bed CSH is the most common configuration.

The CSH is climate controlled and has a pharmacy, laboratory, X-ray, dental unit, and CT (computerized axial tomography) scanning capability. The CSH provides its own power from generators. Most CSHs are structurally made of tents as well as hard-sided expandable trailers containing the ICU, surgical recovery area, and operating rooms. A fully functioning CSH produces surgical outcomes similar to that seen in fixed-facility hospitals and can do so in an austere environment. The CSH receives most patients via helicopter, convoy, or C-130 "in-country" air evacuation aircraft and stabilizes these patients for further treatment at hospitals in Germany or the United States. Ideally, the CSH is located as the bridge between incoming medical evacuation helicopters and outgoing Air Force air evacuation fixed-wing aircraft. The largest CSH has 624 military personnel to staff 256 beds. The Army, Navy, and Air Force have CSHs of varying sizes operating in Iraq and Afghanistan.

Captain Marie

Marie, an Army reservist assigned to CSHs, remarked, "I was assigned to three different combat support hospitals in Iraq. I was in Balad, then in Mosul, and then in Al Asad in Anbar province. In Balad, Iraq, I was at the Air Force hospital. I saw a lot. I saw a great amount of trauma because I was there right around Ramadan. We cared for a lot of burn casualties from explosions with multiple fractures and internal injuries. Some were our soldiers, and others were Iraqi civilians, including children. The hospital was very busy and had a high census. Balad was somewhat like the TV show MASH, except now the stretchers had wheels. The patients came in nonstop to the triage area in the ER. The beds were cots. We worked in a tent about 20 yards from where the helicopters land. The main way we received the wounded in Balad was by helicopter. You couldn't take report or hear anything on the telephone when the helicopters were coming in."

Marie continued, "We were assigned to Mosul, Iraq. It was probably one of the most dangerous places in Iraq because you have our tiny hospital compound in the center of a city. So, our FOB was surrounded by a city. You could look out and see people hanging out their clothes for the day. It was actually interesting culturewise, seeing their houses and way of life. At the same time, when they were trying to mortar you, they had very close access to the base. They could get very close. They were still authorized to be there because it was still their city. They would throw mortars or shoot projectiles into our compound and then run away. We were attacked with mortars seven or eight times every couple of nights when I was there. People in my unit were injured, but luckily, no one was killed. The unit we replaced had two women with serious shrapnel wounds to their chests and abdomens from the almost nightly attacks."

Lieutenant Colonel Victoria

Victoria, an active-duty Army nurse, described what it was like being one of the first units arriving in Iraq, "Well, things were pretty primitive. We came in as the first combat support hospital in Iraq. We had to sleep in a big tent, so your space was very limited. You didn't have much room with all your gear and your cot. The people that came after us lived in trailers, and now I hear the conditions are much better. The mess tent was more than a mile away. When I first got there, you had to walk there in 130-degree heat. Most people would eat snacks during the day, so they didn't have to walk there too many times each day. After a few months, we had buses to take us back and forth for meals. Of course, the heat was constant, as was the sand. When the sun would go down, it would be 120 instead of 130 degrees. We had air conditioners, but some did not work very well. About the coolest any place could get would be 98 degrees. You have to remember that we didn't have a commissary or PX [post exchange] when I got there. By the time I left, they were being built. We had a lot of young and inexperienced nurses. Some did well, but others struggled. We were mortared more than 100 times while I was there. I think some of the nurses were not prepared for this, and it really unnerved them. Others got ready to accept casualties without anyone having to tell them what to do after a while. They gained experience and confidence in themselves."

Lieutenant Commander Clare

Clare was an active-duty Navy critical care and shock-trauma nurse. She described her tent hospital. "The ICU was in a temper tent, it had seven beds, and each bed had a ventilator. We needed the space around the beds to maneuver the portable X-ray machine. There was a nurse's desk in the front and supply areas in the rear of the tent. The tent was connected to a Conex, which was a trailer containing more supplies. These supply trailers were parked in the rear of each temper tent that contained a ward, like the ICU or the intermediate care ward. We had three ICU beds on one side of the tent and four beds on the other. In the middle of the unit, they made some nice shelving out of wood. These must have been made by the unit before us. It was nice and convenient to store the suction machines there. The ventilators were from Germany, and they were awesome, but we still had old portable suction machines that made a loud racket. Next to our ward trailers, we had what we called a 'Wal-Mart' trailer that contained all the gifts and care packages we received from so many people. We could get socks, tee shirts, shaving kits, or whatever our patients needed from the Wal-Mart trailer."

Clare recalled, "The electricity in the hospital tents wasn't the best. Wires were strung toward the top of the temper tents. If you came in the back of the tent, there was a break area. If you put the microwave on, it would shut off the ventilators. So, if you were going to heat up a cup of tea, you'd have to tell your colleagues to bag the patient in bed number two."

Major Vivian

Vivian was an Air Force reservist from Wilmington, Delaware. She worked in a large ICU in Philadelphia specializing in trauma and burn care. She had earned a master's degree in critical care nursing soon after she joined the Air Force Reserve. She was qualified to work in the ICU, ER, and medical-surgical units. Vivian was deployed to Balad Air Base, Iraq, on her first deployment and to Afghanistan on her second deployment. She recalled, "I worked in an ICU tent in Balad, Iraq. They tried to send me to the ER to work, but I always wiggled my way out of it. I didn't want to go to the ER since they had raw trauma, and in ICU, at least they were bandaged. Balad was very much a MASH situation. We had lots of trauma coming in at all hours. Helicopters were flying in all the time, and fixed-wing jumbo jets were taking off for Germany every day. It was organized chaos."

Captain Abby

Abby was an active-duty Air Force nurse assigned at the joint theater hospital at Bagram Air Base, Afghanistan. She described her hospital. "The hospital was much nicer than I expected. Most of the equipment came from the States. We had regular hospital beds, oxygen tanks, and suction machines. The facility was made of old shipping containers hooked together with cement walls. Even though it was nicer than I expected, they still had lots of problems with heating, water, and sewage overflow and those sorts of things."

A nurse's schedule was dictated primarily by the nursing resources available and by the patient census at any given time. It was not unusual to be scheduled to work 6 days a week on 12-hour shifts. Abby described her schedule. "Our working schedule was usually 6 days of 12 hour shifts, then a day off, and 3 more days of 12-hours shifts. It was typical for the duration of our deployment. In the summer, people started taking leave to go home for their 2-week R & R [rest and relaxation] break in the middle of the deployment. Therefore, you'd have less staff. You'd have to go to 4 to 5 days of 12-hour shifts with 1 day off. We were pretty lucky because there were places in Afghanistan at the FOBs [forward operating bases] where people didn't get a day off for 2 to 3 months."

Abby continued, "At my hospital, the mornings were generally relatively slow in the ER because the clinics would open up and a lot of the 'sick call' stuff would go to them. Usually, at around 10 or 11 in the morning, we'd get busier when the medevacs started coming in. We didn't get a lot of fresh traumas. Most of the traumas we got were transfers from the FOBs where we had FFSTs set up who deal with the initial trauma. The FFSTs have a two- to four-bed holding capacity. They stabilize the patients and then evacuate them to us in Bagram. We were the largest, most advanced hospital in Afghanistan with specialized surgical capabilities. Usually, everyone who would be evacuated to Germany would come through Bagram. They would all come to us. If they were a bad trauma, they would come to the ER and be reassessed. Sometimes, we would send them out by air evac within 30 minutes to 1 hour. They would not be with us very long if they were real critical. I know that there were a few cases, two that I especially remember, that went right from the FOB to Germany, bypassing Bagram. Typically, that didn't happen because the flight was so long and the smaller bases did not have the airfield capability for the larger planes that could make the flight to Germany."

Abby related, "The conditions were harsh. We worked, on average, 6 days a week. It got a little bit better as time went on, but we never got 2 days off in a row. Days off weren't really days off over there. Where are you going to go? You get up, get dressed, get your weapon, eat, do your laundry, and catch up on sleep."

Captain Robert

Robert was an Army reservist assigned to hospitals in Tikrit, Mosul, and Al Asad, Iraq. Robert recalled, "It was rough, but it was also great. When we weren't busy with Americans, we were busy with Iraqi soldiers and civilians. Some of our staff resented having to use their great nursing skills and our great technology on Iraqis. Many thought they would only be caring for American and coalition forces before they arrived in [the] country. Therefore, we'd spend a lot of time talking about all the good we were doing for the Iraqi people. Some Iraqi people were great. They'd come in from the village to visit their loved ones at the hospital. We'd give them whatever supplies we had, such as toothbrushes, coloring books, and things like that. They'd go back to the village to tell everyone what great care we'd be giving their sons or husbands. You could tell they were very grateful. It was just very hard because we were getting mortared several times a night. It was at 12 a.m., 2 a.m., 4 a.m., and you'd just have to grab your weapon and helmet and run out to the nearest bunker."

Robert continued, "When we were reassigned to Al Asad, we opened the first combat support hospital for injured troops in Anbar province. They had to fly too far to Baghdad to get care. We would be their stopover point. It was great to leave the danger of Mosul, but it was also scary because after 6 months in Mosul, we knew exactly what we were doing. We finally got into a rhythm, and then we had to pack up and move. Our entire hospital of over 300 personnel moved. Another smaller hospital came to take our place. We literally built a brand-new trailer hospital in Anbar province. It was different now because we were in the desert. You could see for miles and miles. It was harder to get mortared because the enemy didn't have any place to hide. If they wanted to come in close enough to mortar you, you could see them coming from miles away because it was flat desert. We had an airfield on Al Asad. It was an entirely different tempo. You definitely felt safer because you didn't have the mortars coming in every other night. It was also harder for the enemy to get on the base. We saw more injured Americans there, such as bilateral amputees, gunshot wounds, burns, and polytrauma injuries. We also saw a lot more Iraqi children that got injured on the outskirts of town. I'd come in to work, and there would be four little bodies in ICU beds. We didn't get as many children at our hospital in Mosul. Therefore, our clientele changed, our tempo changed, and the pace wasn't as hectic as in Mosul. It was more dangerous in Mosul because there were both mortars and more injured people to deal with."

Robert related, "In Anbar province, our patients were coalition forces, local civilians, and sometimes, defense contractors. If we had a 'mass cal' [mass casualty situation], and we had several, the overflow of casualties from the ER would come to our ward. We had mass cal packets that we would break out and use. We would set up beds to triage patients. We would get casualties with gunshot wounds, blast injuries, burns from explosions, head injuries, blunt trauma, and you name it. The ER had 10 beds, the ICU had 12 beds, and we had an intermediate care ward with more beds. Therefore, in a mass cal, we could handle about 42 incoming casualties. We never got that many at once, thank God!"

Captain Trudi

Trudi was an Army reservist from the Cape Cod area. She had worked as an enlisted LPN (licensed practical nurse) before getting her commission as a registered nurse. She was one of a large number of reserve personnel transferred from the Army hospital in Mosul to Al Asad in Anbar Province, Iraq. Trudi remarked, "Mosul is the second-largest city in Iraq with a population of 4 million. The city was all around us. Our medevac helicopters would fly in and take off to transport the wounded. There were all these back roads in Mosul. The insurgents would put a mortar or two in the back of a little Toyota pickup and just pop them over the walls of our compound. So we got mortared a lot right into our hospital compound. Later in our tour, we did our last 6 months in Al Asad before coming home. I got a taste of the rough life in Mosul and a taste of a little-less-rough life in Al Asad. We realized we were safer after the move out of Mosul, if there is such a thing as feeling safe in a war zone. In Al Asad, we had a large ICU, an intermediate care ward, a large triage area, CAT scanners, pharmacy, radiology, laboratory, power plant, and various offices. The only thing we didn't have was MRI capability. Otherwise, we were like a stateside trauma center, and we could handle just about anything. We had generators all around because we had to make our own power. There was no power grid in most of Iraq."

Lieutenant Colonel Judd

Judd, an Army Reserve nurse practitioner, reported, "When we moved from Mosul to Al Asad, I thought I was going to be back doing routine sick call every day since I was a nurse practitioner. However, they needed me in surgery as first assistant in the operating room. I said, 'I don't do ORs. I don't know what an OR even looks like!' They said, 'Don't worry, we'll teach you.' So they taught me, and I did first assist in surgery. With all the amputations that were coming in, I was very busy. The equipment we have today is great for soldiers. The helmets are made of Kevlar. The body armor is great. However, when it comes to limbs, limbs are still exposed and vulnerable. Therefore, I was doing a lot of amputations in Iraq. I was cleaning up the limbs and doing some very gross reconstruction. We stabilized many amputees so they could fly on the medevac to Germany. Many would have more definitive surgery there."

Major Fran

Fran was assigned as a mental health nurse and combat stress team leader in Iraq. She spent most of her tour of duty in the area around Tallil, Iraq. Fran summarized her feelings about casualty trauma. "Mass cal situations were always very tough for me. They always made me sick in my stomach. Every time we got the call for a mass cal, I got that sick feeling in the pit of my stomach. You never knew what you were going to get. We'd have some mass cals when only two or three living patients showed up, and the rest were dead. Other times, we had 20 wounded people. Sometimes, everyone was dead by the time they arrived. Some casualties came by helicopter, and others were driven through the main gate to the FOB, and some were 'walking wounded.' The triage area just dripped in blood with people moaning and screaming."

Captain Tina

Tina, an active-duty Air Force nurse, was assigned to Balad Air Base, Iraq, shortly after the war in Iraq began. Later in 2007, she was assigned at the coalition forces hospital on FOB Salerno in Afghanistan. She described her schedule and routine working in this small hospital in Afghanistan. "Well, I worked the night shift. I would get report, and then I'd go see all my patients. We had translators, who were great to help us communicate. I also tried to learn a little bit of the language. I would introduce myself, tell them I was their nurse and that I would be giving them medications and changing their dressings. I would be responsible for all the medications on my patients. My medics and I would do the dressing changes together. We would bring chai to the patients, which was a tea. For my American soldier patients, I would also try to get to know them, talk with them about their care, and listen to their stories. I would remind them to call their family to let them know how they were progressing."

Tina continued, "Once all the patients were asleep, I remember a lot of good times talking with other nurses. We'd share bits of information about our homes and families. We also shared different stories we heard about things that had been happening. There were always surgeons around or sleeping in the on-call room. If there were any problems, we could alert the surgeons quickly. It was a small hospital, so you really got to know everyone. It was like a family. I worked nights the whole time I was deployed. We would have 3 days on, then 1 day off, for 12-hour shifts. I liked working night shift. It was usually a little slower paced, and we had good people. I got to meet people deployed from Germany, Japan, and other Air Force bases in the States. We also had a lot of Air Force reservists there. The hospital had primarily Air Force people, but the base had more Army people."

DETAINEE HOSPITALS

The coalition forces have maintained three primary detainee encampments in Iraq, all of which contain hospitals to support the detainee population. The three main detainee care facilities include Camp Bucca, Abu Ghraib Prison Hospital, and Camp Cropper. Camp Bucca is the largest, spanning 1 square mile and located at the southern border of Iraq. Camp Bucca encompasses 29 independent compounds that can hold as many as 15,000 detainees at once. Since the beginning of Operation Iraqi Freedom, more than 100,000 detainees have been held at this location. Camp Bucca houses a state-of-the-art medical facility, the 115th Combat Support Hospital, which provides the highest level of care on a nonstop basis to a diverse detainee population. Local area casualties are also provided emergency care at Camp Bucca.

Camp Cropper is a smaller detainee center established near Baghdad, Iraq, in April 2003. In August 2006, a new hospital was opened on Camp Cropper to treat both coalition soldiers and detainees. The hospital was originally staffed by members of the 21st Combat Support Hospital from Fort Hood, Texas. This is the only facility to hold some female detainees.

Abu Ghraib prison was known as Central Baghdad Prison during the reign of Saddam Hussein. Since the beginning of the current war in Iraq, Abu Ghraib has served as both a forward operating base (FOB) and a detention facility. When the United States was using Abu Ghraib prison as a detention facility, it housed approximately 7,500 detainees in March 2004. The prison hospital operated as a 60-bed CSH with triage, ER, ICU, and operating room capabilities. The Abu Ghraib prison hospital was closed in 2006 with the opening of the new detainee medical facility at Camp Cropper.

Lieutenant Colonel Victoria

Most of the nurses responsible for detainee care were assigned to either the Abu Ghraib Prison outside of Baghdad or Camp Bucca in southern Iraq. Victoria, a seasoned Army nurse, described her assignment in detainee care. "I had a very unique assignment. I did my first 12 months in Camp Bucca, Iraq, with detainee operations. I was the assistant chief nurse of the largest detainee prison hospital in Iraq. I was there during the troop surge. We were extremely busy and short staffed, but we made it. We lived in tents and trailers. We provided care to detainees in a combination of tent and trailer medical facilities. Some detainees had wounds from the fighting. Others had medical-surgical conditions, such as diabetes, renal disease, nutritional disorders, cellulitis, appendicitis, hernias, and gastrointestinal complaints."

Victoria further reported, "The detainees would frequently fight among themselves, so there were many injuries to take care of. Sometimes, they would gang up on a prisoner and beat him or rape him. Prisoner-on-prisoner trauma was common. We never took care of any women detainees at Camp Bucca, only men."

LOCAL HOSPITALS

The U.S. military sent nursing and medical specialists to teach and mentor Afghan medical military personnel at regional ANA hospitals. There are five regional ANA hospitals located in Kabul, Kandahar, Herat, Paktya, and Mazer-e-Sharif. Coalition forces have sent 12- to 20-person medical mentoring teams to help the Afghan medical personnel to learn western medical techniques and practices. The coalition forces also took over local hospitals in Mosul, Tikrit, and Baghdad, Iraq, as well as the prison hospitals at Camp Bucca and Abu Ghraib, to provide care for coalition forces, local civilians, and detainees.

Major Michelle

Michelle was an active-duty Air Force nurse anesthetist on a medical mentoring team.

Michelle described her assignment at the ANA hospital. "The U.S. government built a military hospital for the Afghan army in Kandahar. I was sent there to train the local military personnel in anesthesia care. It was called a 'mentor program,' but I ended up doing about 300 anesthesia cases myself, as well as teaching anesthesia care. We built four hospitals for the Afghan national army, and the grand plan was to assign medical mentoring pools to those hospitals to mentor the Afghan medics who worked there. I was the anesthesia mentor and the only anesthesia provider on my 16-person team."

Michelle recalled, "My job was to teach them to give anesthesia care the right way. My definition of the right way and their definition were at polar opposites when I first arrived. When I got there, I was horrified at what they considered an anesthetic. It was torture. They never used narcotics. They didn't even have any narcotics in the hospital. That was very ironic because Afghanistan is the world capital of illegal opium and heroin production. However, they didn't have medical-grade narcotics for their own patients. Luckily, I was able to get a hold of some narcotics, such as fentanyl, diazepam, delaudid, morphine, and ketamine. You won't believe where this cache of drugs was found. It was found further north next to an incinerator by some Marines. It was left by a unit that was redeploying. All the drugs were still good and had not expired. Thankfully, the guy that was operating the incinerator got in touch with us to see if we needed any of these drugs. We drove up there to the trash bin to pick up the narcotics and other drugs. I was able to get these medications for our patients, and that was a big positive for me! We began to be able to provide painkillers for our patients that came to the ER. Culturally, a lot of the Afghanis were taught to ignore pain."

Michelle went on to describe the local people and the surgery caseload. "A lot of the local people were addicted to opium and heroin. They would roll it up and smoke it. We did everything from tonsillectomies to appendectomies to massive trauma cases. The only cases we didn't do were thoracic and neurosurgery, since we didn't have surgeons on our team with those skills. We did a lot of belly and limb trauma cases. We did the best we could with any head traumas or chest traumas. We'd try to stabilize them and ship them out to the nearby NATO [North American Treaty Organization] hospital. All my surgical cases were Afghanis. We didn't take care of American troops. They went to the Air Force hospital at Bagram or the NATO hospital down the road. My patients were Afghan army, Afghan police, and local civilians. Word got out that an American surgical team was at the hospital, so the locals flocked to us for care. They knew we would provide better care than anything they had available locally. They came in droves to our hospital. About 80% of what we saw was trauma injuries. We saw injuries from IEDs, gunshot wounds, and burns. You name it, and we got it. I was also able to teach them in surgery what good anesthesia was. They had never seen good anesthesia support in surgery before. I taught them what they should try to achieve for their patients. You want the patient to wake up but not be in agony. I taught them to give a local anesthetic before they sew up a hand or finger. Before this, they would literally smack a patient if the patient moved. I taught them to do anesthesia blocks to numb up areas before suturing."

Michelle related, "Once we got some training done and lots of learning squared away, I'd come in the morning and look at the board where all the cases were listed. We'd note any add-ons, make any changes, go to the 07:30 briefing, and then on to the operating room. We worked until we got all our cases done. On a good day, that was 4 or 5 p.m. On a not-so-good day, it would be 11 o'clock at night. We saved a lot of Afghan lives over there. We added to the quality of life for many people with combat and noncombat surgical diagnoses. We even operated on kids with congenital birth defects. Some days were long but amazingly gratifying."

Commander Josie

Josie, an active-duty Navy nurse, reported on her unique assignment mentoring Afghan nurses at an ANA hospital in Mazer-e-Sharif. "I would get up, have breakfast, go to the office, and check email if the computer was working. Then I'd go over to the hospital by 8 a.m. for the morning report. After morning report, the doctors would make rounds. Twice a week, there would be grand rounds where the entire physician staff and several nurses would go room to room to visit each individual patient. Many mornings, we had a nursing education session following morning report. Then I would start doing bedside training with the nursing staff. It took me months to get them to add an I & O [intake and output] sheet to the patient record and to calculate it correctly. We had a lot of renal patients. I used these patients to try to help the nursing staff understand the importance of I & O. They needed instruction in very basic nursing care."

Josie recalled, "My Navy hospital administrator and I would walk back to Camp Mike Spann for lunch. It was a mile walk. It was the American camp inside the Afghan army base. Later, we would walk back in the afternoon after lunch. We always had a class in the afternoon. One day, it was an English class. The next day, it would be a nursing class. A computer class would follow. The hospital staff would get classes that we felt they needed. The hospital shift for the Afghans was over at 3 o'clock in the afternoon. Most of our patients were Afghan national police or Afghan national army troops. The police in that country were the ones who were engaged in knocking doors down, fighting the Taliban, and keeping the nation secure. The Afghan national police did search, seizure, and urban warfare, not the national army. This Afghan national army hospital was built by the U.S. in 2006. It was one of only a handful of buildings in Afghanistan that had air-conditioning, and hot and cold running water. There was an X-ray technician, Nazir, who lived in the hospital. I once asked him, 'Nazir, why do you live in the hospital?' He answered, 'Air-conditioning, beds, toilets, running water; why would I go anywhere else?' After I learned that most people lived in mud huts with no plumbing, it certainly made sense to me."

Major Yvonne

Yvonne was an active-duty Army nurse assigned in Afghanistan to an airborne infantry brigade as the brigade training nurse. Yvonne usually augmented the staff at the CSH at Bagram Air Base at least 1 day a week to keep her clinical skills current. Yvonne recalled, "One of my primary jobs augmenting the nurses at Bagram was to go down to the local Afghan hospital to do burn care. I'd go down there with a supply of pain meds, dressings, and other supplies. I would accompany a physician's assistant and couple of medics to take care of the burn patients. The local hospital didn't have running water or screens on the windows. It was amazing how you'd load somebody up on pain meds back in the States, and you'd have to fill out 20 pages of paperwork. Here, I'd just put a pulse ox [oximeter] on a finger. Most of us are lucky enough to be able to say that we have changed people's lives. That's one of the great things about nursing—to change people's lives whether they are soldiers, Afghanis, or Iraqis. It's made me a better nurse."

FLIGHT NURSING AND AEROMEDICAL EVACUATION

Air Force flight nurses and critical care air transport team (CCATT) members flew missions inside Iraq and Afghanistan as well as air evacuation missions from Iraq and Afghanistan to Ramstein Air Base, Germany, where nearby Landsthul Military Medical Center is located. From Ramstein, these nurses crewed medical evacuation flights to the Washington, DC area, transporting casualties to the National Naval Medical Center in Bethesda, Maryland, the Walter Reed Army Medical Center in Washington, DC, and the Malcolm Grow U.S. Air Force Medical Center in Camp Springs, Maryland. Some of the flights carrying burned patients would occasionally fly to San Antonio, Texas, to Brooke Army Burn Center at Fort Sam Houston.

The "workhorse" of in-country aeromedical evacuation in Iraq and Afghanistan is the C-130 Hercules aircraft. The "heavy lifter" for moving casualties from Iraq and Afghanistan to Germany and on to the United States is the C-17 Globemaster. The C-17 is a long-range multirole jet aircraft. The C-17 can be reconfigured very quickly to accommodate pulmonary ventilators; cardiac monitors; intravenous fluid pumps; litter stanchions to support patients confined to litters (stretchers); and a team of flight nurses, air evacuation technicians, and CCATT personnel if they are needed. This aircraft has a built-in oxygen system for therapeutic patient oxygen and extra electrical hookups for medical equipment. The interior fuselage is well lit to facilitate patient care and assessment.

Major Christina

Christina, a flight nurse, described herself and her job. "I am active-duty Air Force, and I've been in the Air Force for 11 years. I am a nurse and a major. I was deployed to Balad Air Base, Iraq as a flight nurse. My job was to serve the Iraq area and some parts of Saudi Arabia, to transport patients by air in and out. I dealt with all levels of acuity. Some may just need evaluation, and some were in an area of Iraq where they didn't have all the medical specialties. At Balad Air Base, they had a lot of specialties. Sometimes, if we didn't have the specialty, then we would transport the casualties to Germany or maybe directly to the States. For the most part, we would air evac patients from remote locations, where they didn't have a lot of medical equipment to sustain life, or for further treatment to Balad or Germany. We would go into these austere areas and transport patients out. Sometimes, we'd only have 1 patient, and other times, we'd have 50 patients. We'd bring them back to Balad Air Base. Sometimes, we'd fly out on an alert mission [urgent air evacuation] where there would be life-threatening injuries from an explosion or gunshot wounds. We'd bypass Balad and go right to Germany with these severe trauma patients."

Christina continued, "I flew on the C-130 and the C-17. The C-17 is the 'Cadillac of wartime aeromedical evacuation.' It is larger and nicer than the C-130. It is environmentally controlled. We use the C-130 throughout Iraq. Then, if the patient [needed] to go to Germany, we'd often transfer them to a C-17 for the flight to Germany. We used the C-130 primarily within Iraq because it can land on a barren dirt strip, but the C-17 needs a real aircraft runway."

Captain Liz

Liz was from Pittsburgh, Pennsylvania. She joined the Air Force about 2 years after graduating from a large university in the Pittsburgh area. Before being deployed as a flight nurse, she had two assignments at large Air Force medical centers in California and Ohio. Liz had worked as a medical-surgical nurse and critical care nurse in the Air Force. She attended the Air Force Flight Nurse Course during her ICU assignment in Ohio. The mission of her unit was aeromedical evacuation, and Liz deployed to Iraq in 2006 and to Afghanistan in 2008.

Liz described her typical day. "A typical day was actually boring. It was a lot of waiting around for something to happen. We'd sit on alert depending upon where we were. We [were] usually attached to a cell phone or a pager. We also [had] routine scheduled missions where you['d] pick patients up and fly them to the bigger hospitals for more surgery. When we [got] called for a mission, we'd have to pick up all our medical equipment and make sure it

[was] in serviceable condition. When we [had] everything we need[ed], we'd go out to preflight the plane. We'd take off and go to the location that has patients for us. We['d] bring them back to either Balad Air Base in Iraq or Bagram Air Base in Afghanistan since that is where the biggest U.S. hospitals are located. Both hospitals had most of the specialists. They had neurosurgeons, eye surgeons, maxillofacial surgeons, [and] plastic surgeons, so a lot of in-country air evac missions ended up there."

Liz recalled, "Each day on alert duty, you never know what the day [would] bring or where you [would] be that night. It was an exciting job, but it was dangerous, too. We'd come back and count the bullet holes in the plane from landings in hot areas where we rushed to get the patients onboard, spending minimal time on the ground."

Captain Alice

Alice was an active-duty Air Force nurse deployed to Afghanistan as a CCATT nurse. Although she was not a flight nurse, she frequently accompanied the most critical patients on their air evacuation flight. She cared only for patients requiring one-to-one or one-to-two nursing care. Alice described urgent care in flight. "We'd fly out on an alert mission where we picked up people with life-threatening injuries. These people were fresh trauma from the fighting who had usually been temporarily stabilized in the field by a fast-forward surgical team. We'd sometimes bypass in-country military hospitals and go straight to Germany. I flew on both the C-130 and C-17 aircraft. We would have patients stacked in litter tiers in both types of planes. We had cardiac monitors and ventilators for use, if we needed them. Some patients were so critical, we'd bring a critical care nurse, physician, and a respiratory therapist just for that one patient, while the two flight nurses and air evac technicians took care of the rest of the casualties."

Captain Meaghan

Meaghan, an active-duty Air Force nurse, described her role as a CCATT nurse. "It was my first deployment. I was gone from June 2003 till Nov 2003. I was assigned to take care of the most critical patient on air evac flights. We spent most of our time in Iraq and Kuwait. I am not a flight nurse, but I am assigned to air evac flights that have one or more very critical patients that need pretty much one-to-one care. The two flight nurses on a flight may be responsible for 50 other patients. Some of our missions took us back to the U.S. with patients for Walter Reed Army Medical Center or the National Naval Medical Center in Bethesda, Maryland. We only use a CCAT team of a critical care nurse, an ICU physician, and a respiratory therapist when the patient is very critical, on life support."

Captain Tina

Tina, an active-duty Air Force nurse, was assigned to Iraq early in the war. In 2007, Tina was deployed again to Afghanistan. Although she was not a flight nurse, she was sometimes called upon to accompany critically wounded patients on Army Blackhawk helicopters in Afghanistan. Tina explained, "Sometimes, when casualties arrived at our small FOB, there was no time to call in an aeromedical evacuation aircraft with its flight nurses and maybe a CCAT team. I had been an Air Force nurse for over 10 years. I was assigned to a forward operating base manned by the Army. I was there to work as an ICU nurse. The FOB has about a 6-mile radius, and there are probably about a thousand people coming in and out each day. Most are Army with various assignments in Afghanistan. I was serving mostly as an ICU nurse on the ground, but sometimes, I had to do air evacuation when patients were critical and needed to be transported by helicopter. Most of the time, the Army had their own medical technicians on the helicopters. When the patients have surgeries, are very unstable, and are on ventilators, a nurse had to go with them. The Air Force also has what is called CCATT, critical care air transport teams. They come in to pick up very critical patients and bring their own crew. However, sometimes, they can't come because of the time frame. They have to come within 6 to 8 hours. Therefore, if the patient needs to be transported right away, we used the helicopter because it was faster and available to go at any time. I was at FOB Salerno in Afghanistan for 4 months."

AEROMEDICAL STAGING FACILITY (ASF)

An aeromedical staging facility is a medical unit operating with transient patient beds located on or in the vicinity of an air base or airstrip. An ASF provides reception, administration, processing, ground transportation, feeding and limited medical care for patients entering or leaving the aeromedical evacuation system (*Dictionary*, 2005.)

In Iraq and Afghanistan, the ASFs are located on air bases that house a hospital and an active runway. Most of the ASFs are separate from the hospital but located near the hospital and flight line. Air Force nurses and medical technicians provide staffing for the ASF.

Major Diana

Diana, an Air Force Reserve nurse from Dayton, Ohio, was assigned to the ASF at Balad Air Base, Iraq. She described the flow of casualties from Baghdad to Balad. "Once they came from the Baghdad facility, they came to the U.S. Air Force theater hospital in Balad. At our hospital, they had surgery or other treatments. When they were deemed stable enough to fly, we got them at our staging facility. Once they came to us, we knew that a flight was en route to get them within 12 hours. We would provide for them and give them whatever they needed. It might be a pain medication injection or one dose of antibiotics prior to flight. We made sure they had a good IV port. If they were ambulatory, they might be given enough medication to self-medicate themselves during the flight. We tried to make sure that they had all those needs met for flight. We just made sure everything was ready for flight, such as fresh dressing changes and medications. Some patients came from very small sites. We never had anybody come straight from the field. They had all received care at some sort of hospital before they came to the aeromedical staging facility. I was at the ASF for 5 months."

Captain Suzanne

Suzanne was an active-duty Air Force nurse deployed to Balad Air Base, Iraq. She was assigned to the ASF at Balad Air Base. Suzanne described a typical shift. "We worked 12-hour shifts. I would go in around 7 p.m. to get report about our patients from the previous shift. We ran a computer program called 'TRAC2ES' [Transcom Regulating Aeromedical Command and Control Evacuation System], which captures data on all the patients entered into the air evac system. When a physician wrote an order to air evac a patient from one hospital to another, the nurse or physician entered the patient data in TRAC2ES. Then, that data was automatically sent to the flight surgeon's office. The flight surgeon would review the patient's clinical data and either validates that patient for flight or rejects that patient for flight, pending more clinical data or improved clinical data over time. This provided a clinical picture of the patient. The flight surgeon could get a summary of clinical data and assess how stable the patient was. They all had to be stable enough to fly. These would be mostly air evac flights to the big military medical center in Landsthul, Germany. They had to be stable enough for the long flight to Germany."

Suzanne recalled, "We also had helicopters coming in every night with casualties. They would land on the helipad. We would move them to the emergency room for triage. The walking wounded would come straight to our tent. We would evaluate and triage them and then send them over to the hospital. Later, in the emergency room, we would assess them again with a flight surgeon and get all their information into TRAC2ES. If the patients needed to have surgery, they would be admitted to an inpatient unit and go straight to surgery. We would then get their information into TRAC2ES so the next shift would have that info and, if they were stable enough after surgery, the next shift could get them out on an air evac flight to Germany. The aeromedical evacuation system is dynamic. For it to run optimally, it involves the close coordination of the forward mobile surgical units in the field, combat support hospitals in country, the medical center in Germany, and the aircraft flight crews and flight nursing personnel who actually pick up and transport the patients. It requires all the military services to provide administrative and operational input even though operational control for all fixed-wing air evac falls under the U.S. Air Force. We could say air evac is really a team effort."

COMBAT STRESS NURSING

Combat stress teams are small mobile teams composed of a mix of mental health professionals including psychiatrists, psychologists, mental health nurses, psychiatric social workers, and occupational therapists. These teams have their own vehicles to move forward to augment the combat support units, military medical facilities, and chaplains over a wide area.

Major Fran

Fran, an active-duty Air Force mental health nurse, described her assignment in Iraq. "I was assigned to a combat stress unit. We also had a medical facility nearby with an ER and a small ICU. I was the combat stress outreach coordinator. I taught a 2-day seminar for the soldiers in an effort to reduce the effects of posttraumatic stress disorder [PTSD]. It involved five phases: talking, sleeping, eating, exercising, and stress management activities. I also coordinated the schedule of the remaining members of the combat stress management team in providing additional services to the rest of the base. There were 11,000 troops on the base."

Fran continued, "When I was doing the training, it was 2 days of 4-hour sessions working with the soldiers. If I wasn't doing that, I was visiting one of the units. I assigned all of the units on base to the members of the combat stress control team. We would go out and visit the units. It would be on-site visits to bring the services to the members instead of them always having to come to us. I would also get to know the folks in the unit, so they wouldn't be so fearful of mental health personnel. In effect, we built relationships with them so that when something happened to their personnel, we were not strangers to them. For example, we received fatal rocket fire, and three soldiers were killed. We were able to go into the units of the dead soldiers because they knew us as they were processing the loss of these soldiers. It gave us an opportunity to help them. If we hadn't built those relationships, there would be that stigma of 'The mental health people are coming.' We had the relationships built, we were already known in the units, and we were accepted as helping people. We weren't so scary because they already knew us. We knew the commanders, and we knew their troops."

REFERENCE

Dictionary of military and associated terms. (2005). Washington, DC: U.S. Department of Defense.

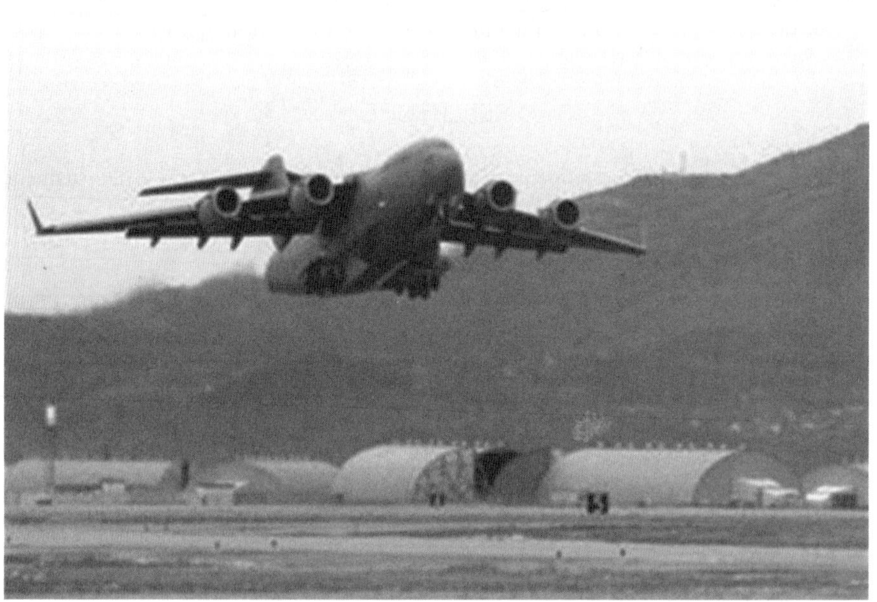

Photo Courtesy of U.S. Air Force.

C-17 aeromedical evacuation mission, Bagram Air Base, Afghanistan.

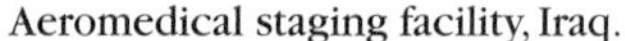

Aeromedical staging facility, Iraq.

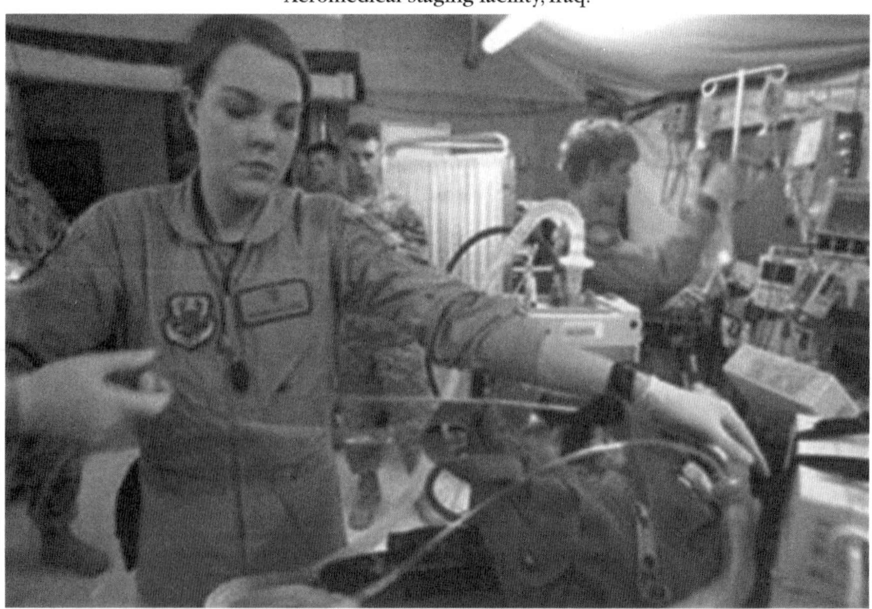

Photo Courtesy of U.S. Air Force.

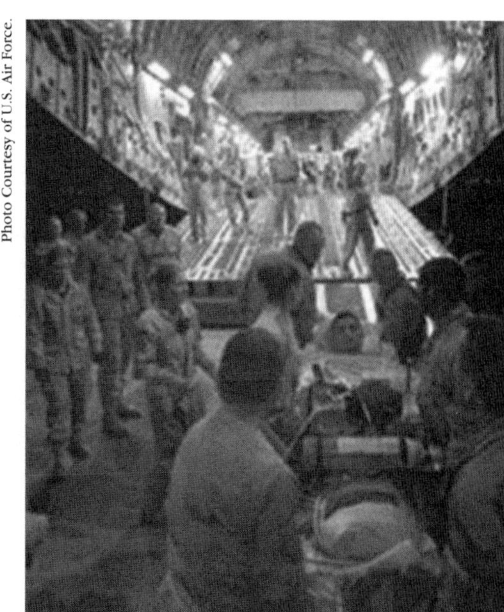

Photo Courtesy of U.S. Air Force.

Loading C-17 air evacuation patients.

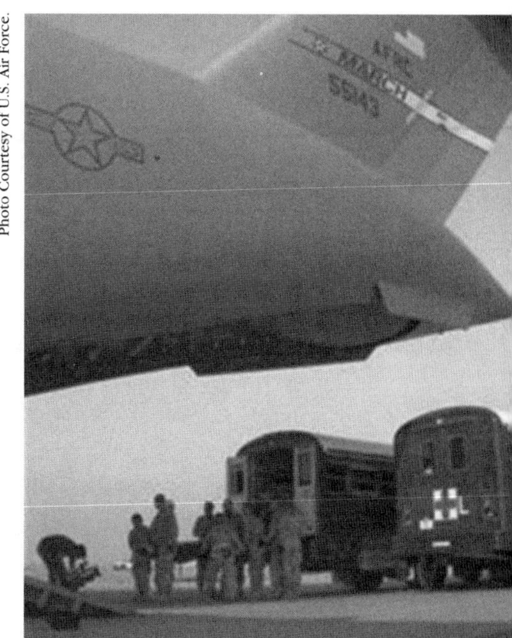

Photo Courtesy of U.S. Air Force.

Loading patients.

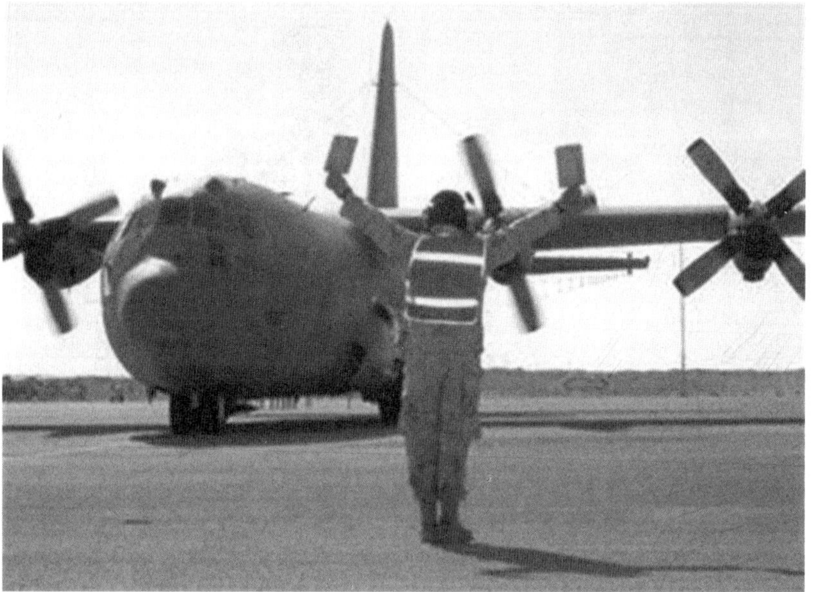
Photo Courtesy of U.S. Air Force.

C-130 air evacuation aircraft landing at Balad Air Base, Iraq.

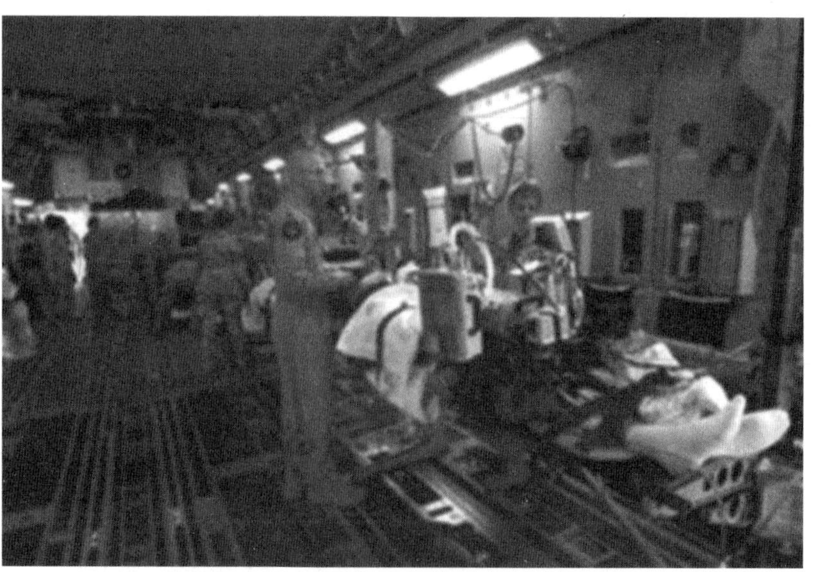
Photo Courtesy of U.S. Air Force.

Interior of C-17 aeromedical evacuation aircraft.

Photo Courtesy of U.S. Air Force.

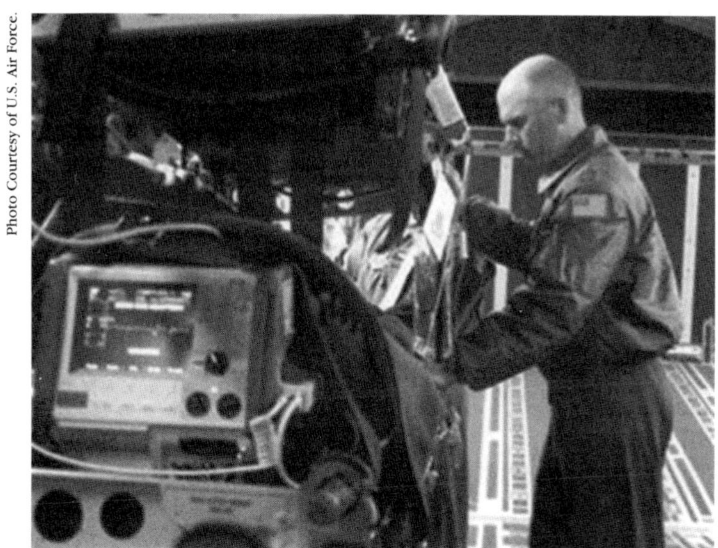

Critically injured soldier on C-130 air evacuation.

Photo Courtesy of U.S. Air Force.

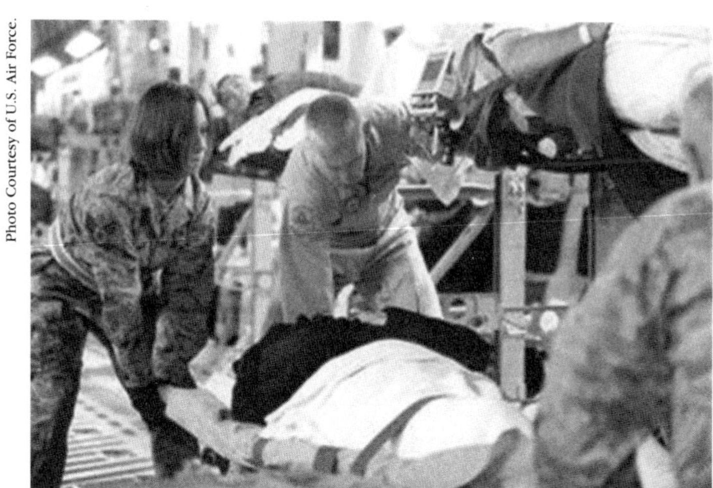

Loading patient in litter tier on C-17 aircraft.

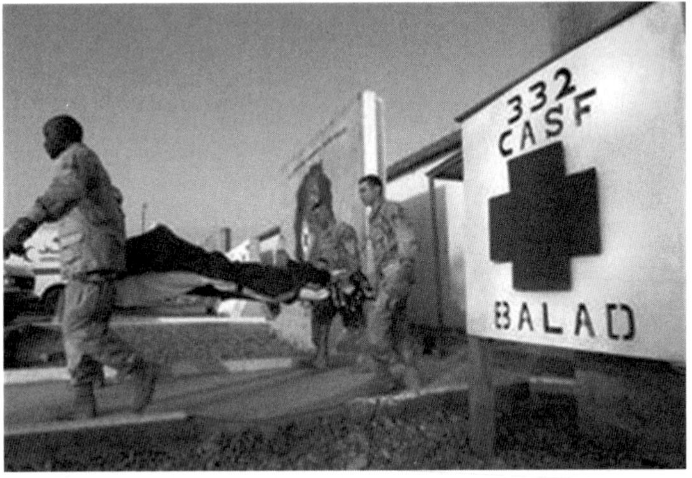

Photo Courtesy of U.S. Air Force.

Combat aeromedical staging facility, Balad Air Base, Iraq.

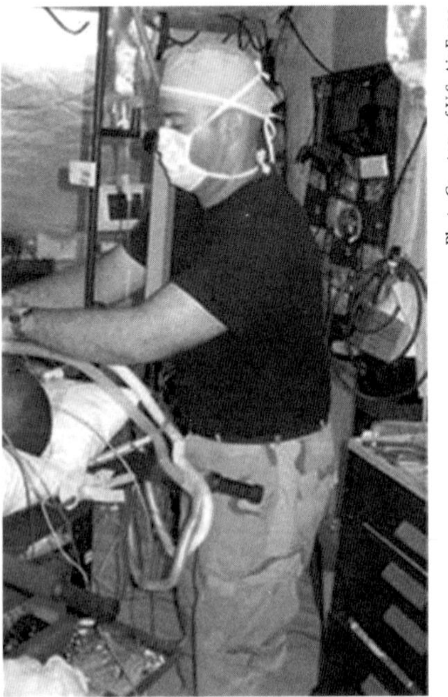

Photo Courtesy of U.S. Air Force.

Nurse anesthetist, Iraq.

Photo Courtesy of U.S. Air Force.

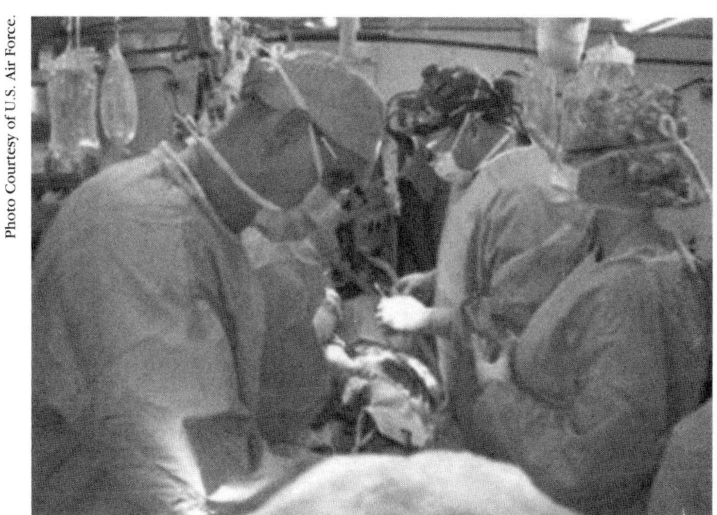

Operating room, Bagram Air Base, Afghanistan.

Photo Courtesy of U.S. Air Force.

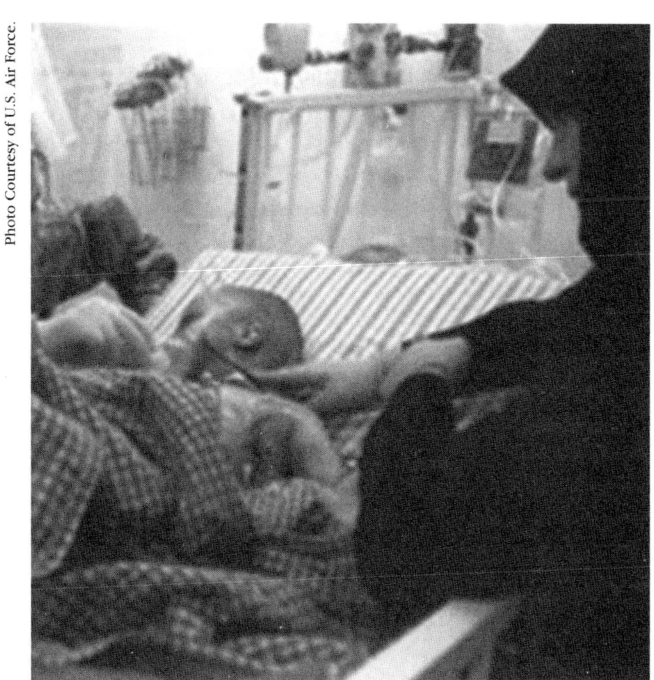

Mother and injured child, Afghanistan.

6

Diversions From War: A Piece of Home

Nurses tried to instill a piece of home into their wartime duty. Some nurses became involved in church activities, such as bible study groups, book review groups, and choirs, and even social activities like line dancing. Others used their time off duty to improve their physical fitness. Even most of the smallest bases had a makeshift gym or workout room. Jogging and biking around the guarded base perimeters became popular. On some bases, sports leagues were set up and thrived in an atmosphere of healthy competition, including traditional interservice rivalries. Some nurses enrolled in academic online courses, mostly pursuing a master's degree in nursing education or business administration. Others volunteered or were tasked to provide humanitarian services to the local population. All agreed that having activities outside their assigned clinical duties was crucial to balancing the stresses inherent in war nursing and family separation.

Major Michelle

Michelle, an active-duty Air Force nurse anesthetist who served at an Afghan national army hospital, stated, "When you are deployed, you have to find something that is an outlet for you. Either sewing, reading, exercising in the gym, writing in a journal, or playing sports with others, whatever you like and have available in your environment can serve as diversions and outlets. Without an outlet away from the work we do in the hospital, the carnage, danger, and stress will get to you."

Captain Vanessa

Vanessa, an Army reservist, remarked, "I would tell anyone who was deploying to make sure you have some type of outlet so you get a break, and your work is not all-consuming. Outlets make the time go faster, help you meet people, and relieve a lot of the stress. Luckily, sports provided a big outlet for me. Our volleyball team was an awesome support for me."

Major Vivian

Vivian, an Air Force reservist, remarked, "I was able to talk to my husband almost every day. He wasn't active duty at the time, but he worked on a military base, so we were able to communicate because of phone cards, and we also had email access."

Vivian remembered helping her patients by doing extra things for them. She recalled, "Another thing I liked to do was doing errands for my patients, especially the soldiers that we had for a while at the hospital. The dining facility did an outstanding job and made sure we had everything we could possibly want. What was neat, too, was we'd come over on our days off and pick up hot meals for our patients, so we were able to give them a good meal before they flew out or returned to duty. I must say that some of those guys and gals hadn't had a hot meal in a very long time. Some had been eating MREs [meals ready to eat] for quite a while. We felt good that we were able to get them a decent hot meal. Some nurses also did the soldiers' laundry if they needed a clean uniform or sweatshirt. We also let them watch TV, play video games, watch videos, and provided computer access to them. When we had time, we'd play cards or video games with them. They were able to communicate with their families back home using the Internet or free phone cards. These things were big for them, and it made us feel good, too."

Major Millie

Millie, an Army operating room nurse, recalled, "I am thankful for the opportunities around the base. I tried to get out of the hospital to do things during my off-duty time. The chapel office offered activities that were such an important outlet. They had church services, discussion groups, and social activities. It was such an important outlet from work. They had country line dancing, game night, and other recreational activities. We had a bible study group and a fellowship group led by a young soldier. We all read *Purpose Driven Life*, too. We would meet to redirect some of the emotion about being away from home. It helped if you had faith and believed in God. It just made you stronger and more positive about life."

Millie further reported, "As far as I'm concerned, life was pretty good at my base. Sometimes we had 14-hour days in the OR nonstop and some sad outcomes. However, we were doing what we were there for, and we saw some miracles as well. We changed some lives by giving injured people a second chance at life. The bible study and fellowship members were just tremendous. These were good outlets for me. The group members were mostly Army and Air Force folks of all ranks and many career fields, so it wasn't just medical people. I also learned a lot about what other occupations do in the military. These folks became a support group for each other."

Lieutenant Colonel Judd

Judd, an Army Reserve nurse practitioner, stated, "I had a good time going to chapel. We had a little choir. We would get together and sing. I played keyboard at Mass in the chapel on Sundays. It helped my mental health. Whenever I could, I was at the gym working out. I would work out with one of the, I won't say older, but 'more mature' officers in charge of the operating room. She needed a workout partner, so we worked out together. We were almost the same age, so it worked out well for us."

Judd told of some nurses becoming involved in charity projects for the local populace. Judd elaborated, "There was a school in Mosul that our Army chaplain was working with. The children needed clothes for the winter. They didn't have the money to buy fuel oil to heat the school in wintertime. Our hospital people got wind of it and wanted to help. The hospital people made out-of-pocket donations of $5,000 to buy heating oil for this school. In addition, we all called home for the clothes. They had airplane after airplane come in with clothing. We got 1,500 boxes of clothes for these kids. This was a civil affairs operation. We couldn't go in and even see these kids. We also started a library for the people in the hospital and for the people on the base. Later, we started a music library for everyone."

Judd also told of the satisfaction he received working with the younger troops in Iraq. Judd recalled, "Working with the kids, the younger people, was incredible. I was like a dad to some of them. After I treated them in sick call for minor ailments, sometimes, I would close the door and they would cry on my shoulder. After you got to know these young troops, they would pour their hearts out to you. They'd confide in me about relationship problems with their special person back home or just decompress about the horrors they were seeing out in the field. Many of these young people had never seen a dead body before. They were very young to see the level of carnage a war brings. Most had lost at least one person from their unit. I had been in Vietnam as a young soldier before I became a nurse, so I could really appreciate the perspective of the young grunt."

Major Derek

Derek, an Army reservist, was assigned to Camp Bucca Detainee Hospital early in his assignment to Iraq. Later, he was transferred to Abu Ghraib Prison Hospital. Derek stated, "We really enjoyed going to the gym when we were off at both detainee compounds. Everyone tried to stay healthy. The gym was a good outlet, and we tried to stay in shape. There were not a lot of things to do when you were off. They had good equipment in both of the gyms. It was a good distraction, and the gym facilities were very good."

Lieutenant Donna

Donna grew up in Virginia. Donna recalled, "I didn't have the money for college without taking out student loans. I didn't want to start my career as a registered nurse with thousands of dollars of debt. I got some literature in the mail about Navy ROTC at the college I was planning to attend. I filled out all the application paperwork, sent in the application, passed the physical, went for an interview, and then got a letter offering me the scholarship. It was a lot of hard work doing all the ROTC classes and training, plus all my nursing courses, but it was worth it in the end. I got my bachelor's degree in nursing without going into any debt. Other people in my class had to work while going to school, and I had everything paid for by the Navy. I even got a subsistence stipend to live on." *Donna graduated from college and entered active duty shortly thereafter. Donna was assigned to a large Navy medical center in Southern California for 4 years. At the end of her fourth year, she was deployed to a hospital in Kandahar, Afghanistan.*

Donna described how she used her spare time during her deployment to work on a master's degree. "I used my off-duty time to take courses. I worked on my master's in nursing education. There were two of us taking the same program, so we cheered each other on and formed a study group. It was an online program, so all we needed was Internet access. Luckily, we weren't at a real remote location. The Internet was available to us 9 out of 10 days. We both felt we were accomplishing something important to our careers. We didn't have the distractions of our families, so it was a useful way to spend our time."

Donna told of some volunteer work that she became involved with. "There was a group of us that volunteered to work in free clinics for the local villagers. I volunteered there on my days off. I spent time in the pediatric clinics because I wanted to do something very different from my usual work. It was important for me to get time to interact with the local people in a bit more of their environment. I would see the women with their burkas [head scarves] come in with their children. I got to see a glimpse of their more 'normal' life."

Commander Josie

Not all nurses who intended to take Internet courses fared as well as the aforementioned Navy nurse. Josie, an active-duty Navy nurse, remarked, "Many of us had planned to take courses over the Internet, but access was so poor that it was a problem for us at the Afghan national army hospital where I was assigned. We could get Internet access, but it was sporadic. After about a month, we gave up and got a refund of our money from the university. We were just too remote for regular consistent Internet connectivity. I was taking health care administration courses with one of our hospital administration officers."

Some nurses became involved in activities on their bases that they probably would have never had an interest in at their stateside bases before deployment. Josie described an unusual extracurricular activity she volunteered for while in Afghanistan. She stated, "Friday night was boxing night. I usually volunteered to be the boxing nurse. It was fun to watch these kids. It was good stuff and a morale builder. It was entertainment. They didn't fight that many rounds, and they wore protective gear. It was a great source of entertainment, and the kids loved it. Even one of our doctors, who was 58 years old, signed up to box. He boxed a 23-year-old kid. The doc didn't win, but he went the whole three-round match. It was just amazing. The doc had boxed in college, and he held his own against this kid. It was good fun. Everyone found ways to help support each other. Sporting events were a big morale boost for everyone. You couldn't drink. There was no alcohol over there. We did have the 'mousey beer,' which is the nonalcoholic beer. Therefore, we had happy hour on Friday nights with nonalcoholic beer and boxing matches. We kind of made the best of a bad situation."

Captain Tina

Tina, an active-duty Air Force nurse assigned in Iraq and Afghanistan, recalled her volunteer work in Iraq, "We volunteered to do weekly humanitarian missions in the villages. We found a little girl with a tumor on her tongue and referred her to the surgeons. We saw quite a few Iraqi families. We treated them for a variety of ailments. Many people had old injuries that had gone untreated. People had old wound infections. Some children had congenital anomalies, such as clubfoot and cleft palate. I was there for about 7 months. We did a lot to improve the health of the locals. It was a very rewarding aspect of my deployment. We made life better for a lot of people."

Captain Robert

Robert, an Army Reserve nurse, related how U.S. soldiers on patrol in the villages of Iraq looked out for the health and welfare of the local population. "Besides taking care of soldiers and marines, we did humanitarian missions, too. If the marines or the soldiers were out in a neighborhood and saw something wrong, like injured children who were being tended to by the families and not getting better or getting progressively worse, they called us in, and we would provide care for them. I really got to love the children. When we had them in the hospital or clinic, we would play with them. Kids everywhere are so resilient. They just like to be kids."

Major Samantha

Although most nurses who performed humanitarian missions in Iraq and Afghanistan felt a sense of accomplishment that they were making a positive difference in the lives of poor people who did not have access to good health care, some nurses encountered frustrating culturally induced situations in these local villages. Samantha, an Army nurse assigned to Bagram Air Base, Afghanistan, explained, "One of the things my husband told me not to do when I left was to volunteer for anything outside of the wire. My husband is a retired marine, and he truly feared for my safety. I had an opportunity to do this humanitarian mission in a village where we set up a clinic for the day to care for the Afghani people in the village. With the help of an interpreter, we let the people tell us what was wrong with them. We handed out a lot of Tylenol and Motrin for their aches and pains that they probably had for 15 years. In one of the mud huts, I got to see a woman who was 9 months pregnant, who had taken a fall. The baby was dead inside of her for a few days. I have thought of her so often inside my head because the men would not let her go with us where we could get her some treatment. I just wonder what happened to her. Did her body finally expel the dead baby, or did she die?"

Samantha continued, "There were several other women who needed our help as well, but the men would not let them go back with us. This one woman had gangrene on her arm and needed an amputation, but they would not let her go. The men would accompany some of the children back with us, but not the women. The whole situation with the women was, at times, very sad. It makes us appreciate what we have back in the U.S."

Captain Marie

Nurses who arrived in Iraq and Afghanistan after 2006 reported improved base infrastructure, which usually translated into better and more diverse activities and venues on the U.S. military bases. Marie, an Army reservist assigned to three bases in Iraq, reported, "MWR [morale, welfare, and recreation] at Balad Air Base was awesome in 2006. They had a theater in Balad and an ice cream place. That's the Air Force! They really take care of their people. The Air Force people always have nicer barracks and facilities."

Major Yvonne

Yvonne, who was an active-duty Army nurse assigned to an airborne infantry brigade near Bagram Air Base, Afghanistan, recalled, "Your deployment experience was often tied to where you were in country. I was near the big Air Force hospital in Bagram. I was lucky in Bagram. We had a coffee shop, a Dairy Queen, and a great fitness facility. They had just added a theater. Rumors were circulating that they might add a bowling alley. I had no complaints with how to spend my off-duty time. I felt sorry for the nurses and other troops at remote sites who didn't even have the Internet."

Major Olga

Nurses at remote sites used their ingenuity to find outlets for the stress of living and working in a combat zone. Olga was an Army nurse assigned to a fast-forward mobile surgical team that deployed to remote sites and FOBs in Iraq. Olga remarked, "We played board games and cards just like we did at home. Even though we were a small unit usually traveling to isolated FOBs, I spent my personal down time reading, exercising, doing needlepoint, and writing almost every day in my journal. I tried to stay busy because then the time passed quicker."

Olga continued, "Stress management was also very important because there wasn't a lot to do. Physical fitness took on a new value for me. I did very well in my physical fitness training, and I see where I used it as a motivator. For example, if I was feeling kind of down or depressed, I knew it was time to go running. I also helped form a coed volleyball team. For many of us at these tiny remote bases, sports activities were a way to pass the time, interact with others outside of our unit, and stay in good physical shape."

Lieutenant Colonel Victoria

Victoria, a career Army nurse, stated, "I was running 6 days a week. It really helped me cope and got me in great shape. At 5 o'clock in the morning, I was out there with our commander, a family practice doctor, running in gravel and sand. We started a running club and got other people to come out and run with us during the 15 months we were in Iraq."

Many of the nurses said that the high point of their day was getting mail from home. Victoria recalled, "Mail from home was a positive thing, and the majority of it was email from my family. I emailed them about my experiences. They wrote back with supportive messages. They also sent packages of cookies, nuts, deodorant, and toothpaste. I got emails and packages from my extended family, too. People readily shared the goodies from home with their coworkers and even their patients. Most people over there were such giving people."

Major Alene

Alene was an Army reservist assigned to the coalition hospital in Mosul, Iraq. Later in her career, she served a second deployment to Afghanistan. Alene had joined the Army Reserve in 1991 as an enlisted member before attending college. Four years later, she completed her baccalaureate degree in nursing from a large university in the northeastern United States. Her first civilian job was in medical-surgical nursing at a Boston-area medical center. Later, she moved to the emergency room to gain experience that was more varied.

Alene described how some nurses took the initiative to expand their relationships with other coalition forces. Alene related, "We had about 10 Romanian nurses and doctors with us. We had some fun times. We'd do things at the recreation center together. They liked to challenge us to games of billiards, air hockey, and ping-pong. We taught them more English words, and they taught us some Romanian words."

Alene also reported, "We were also located near a German hospital unit and a Canadian communications unit. We'd have parties and sports matches and invite these guys over to our compound. We'd drink nonalcoholic beer and eat snacks from the mess hall. It was fun meeting people from other countries and listening to their music instead of just hip-hop and country music from the U.S. We had a Halloween party at our hospital, and everyone got dressed up. It took a lot of creativity to put a costume together. Some of the men dressed up with makeup and girly clothes. They formed a chorus line of dancers. They were a riot! Our commander, a surgeon, came as a vampire, and the chief nurse came as a baby doll in pajamas. These types of fun activities built morale and drew us closer together as a unit."

Captain Meaghan

Meaghan, an active-duty Air Force CCATT nurse, described how Thanksgiving was celebrated at Bagram Air Base, Afghanistan. "The mess hall put on a great Thanksgiving dinner with all the trimmings. After dinner, we sang Christmas carols before they served the pumpkin pie. Then people got in line to use the free phones to call home. I took lots of pictures, so I will always be able to look back and remember my Thanksgiving and Christmas in Afghanistan."

Major Diana

Diana was an Air Force reservist who worked at the aeromedical staging facility in Balad, Iraq. She reported, "My shift team kept our sense of humor for the most part. A couple of them had the same night off as me. We would work four nights on and one night off for 12-hour shifts. We'd stay up all night keeping each other company and telling stories. We told a lot of stories and talked a lot, when we were not extremely busy with patients. We'd play music, listen to the radio, and had Internet access. We'd always find something to laugh about. We would do stupid things to make others laugh and break the tension of our jobs and environment."

Captain Trudi

Trudi, an Army reservist in her 40s, reflected, "When you are there, you really don't have time off. At a combat support hospital, you work your shift, go to the gym, maybe watch a movie, and go to bed. Life is so simple when you are there. You don't have to cook, and you don't have to grocery shop. You just show up and do your job. It's like the movie *Groundhog Day*. The simplicity of a deployed life was good for me. It gave me time to read, journal, and reflect; to sort out what is really important in my life and what is not."

First Lieutenant Lisa

Lisa grew up outside of Providence, Rhode Island. She attended college at a large New England university. After her graduation, she was employed in a large medical center in Boston. She joined an Army Reserve unit for some adventure and to help pay off student loans. She was deployed to the coalition forces hospital in Mosul, Iraq, where she worked in the emergency room and intensive care unit.

Lisa shared, "One thing I did to escape the war zone environment at Mosul was to read romance novels and the autobiographies of famous people. I read the autobiographies of Madeline Albright and Colin Powell. I won't tell you which romance novels I read because they were quite racy but fun. We passed around books, and you could take whichever ones caught your interest. Reading was a good way to escape."

7

Remembrance of War: Most Chaotic Scene

As traumatized soldiers, civilians, and insurgents moved through triage areas and emergency rooms, nurses learned about the chaos of war each and every day. Quickly, they became adept at treating injuries that were so devastating and brutal that you would not even find them in an urban trauma center in the United States.

The severity of the injuries along with the youth of the patients also made the nurses' jobs that much harder. Ordinance wounds are rarely simple. Bullets and other projectiles pierce the flesh and explode. A wound taken in the stomach would also tear up the intestines, pancreas, gallbladder, lower esophagus, and liver.

Sometimes, the enemy used women and children as suicide bombers. It was difficult to determine whether a family driving up to a military checkpoint was a family needing help for their injured child or a pack of suicide bombers posing as a family. Other times, women and children might be used as human shields hiding an insurgent within the car. These circumstances added to the chaos and complexity of serving in a war zone.

Major Vivian

Vivian was an Air Force reservist who served in both Iraq and Afghanistan. Vivian commented, "War injuries are terrible. People with their legs blown off, bloody flesh that looks like chunks of meat hanging off missing legs or feet, blood splattering everywhere, and people crying. It is the most chaotic scene one could imagine. I think with all the hard things that we saw, it was tough. The rooms and rooms full of injured people were hard to deal with emotionally. Most were so young. Many were so terribly injured. You sometimes ask yourself, 'How can this happen?' I think getting to know my patients as people made it easier to handle, but it was surely the most chaotic scene."

Commander Rita

Rita, an active-duty Navy nurse anesthetist assigned to a fast-forward surgical unit, reported, "When the war started, we took on heavy casualties. The first seven days were some of the worst casualties. We never came out of the original gear we started the war with. I went without a shower for 11 days when the war started. We had two beds in each of our operating rooms for a total of four beds. We worked head to head in providing anesthesia, so the two anesthesia providers were back to back. We did this so if one of us had to leave the OR [operating room] to pee, the other could briefly manage both patients. It also allowed us to move patients in and out of the tents quite easily. We worked 24 hours 'round the clock when we had a steady stream of casualties. You were on an adrenaline high. No one came in with a single wound. Everyone had multiple wounds. Most of the bullets blew up on impact, so there was usually a lot of structural damage within each wound. What went in as a shoulder hit might also take out part of a lung. What went in as a low colon hit might also take out part of the stomach, the pancreas, and the gallbladder. The bullets sort of pierced and exploded. Our tent did the head, chest, and abdominal cases, and the other tent took on the orthopedic and extremity surgeries. This way, the surgeons, anesthesia providers, and OR nurses were assigned to one tent or the other. After the first month of the war, the stream of casualties slowed a bit."

Major Olga

Olga was an active-duty Army nurse assigned to a fast-forward surgical team. She recalled, "We saw a lot of truly horrible injuries. We saw faces blown away, soldiers with multiple traumatic amputations, people with massive head trauma exposing what was left of their brains, gaping holes where eyes used to be, jaws blown away from facial structures, open abdomens with intestines ripped to shreds, and macerated genitals that looked like hamburger. Rocket-propelled grenades (RPGs) just ripped away bone, muscle, organs, and skin. Convoys were slow moving and regularly attacked with IEDs [improvised explosive devices] and RPGs. Many of the 'mass cals' resulted from an ambush on troop or supply convoys. That's when we'd receive 10 or

20 casualties, and they were usually bad injuries with many deaths. They would arrive by chopper. You could see blood pouring off the floor and skids of the chopper as it landed on the helipad outside the ER. Honest to God, some of these troops just looked like they were slaughtered."

Captain Penny

Penny was an Army nurse assigned to a fast-forward surgical team in Afghanistan. She recalled, "Communication, you know, can make problems. There is no one to point a finger at. We were the guinea pigs. What we did as a forward team had not been done before. This concept of operations was new."

Penny went on to relate, "Communication was sometimes a problem because what the leaders in Washington saw on paper was not really the way it happened over there. We have been in Afghanistan a long time, and many of us have done multiple tours of duty over there. Some days we were just overwhelmed with casualties. We had abdomens busted open, faces blasted and burned beyond recognition, young bodies just about sliced in half by explosive devices, eyeballs and limbs hanging by a thread of tissue. You name it and it came to us in the field, and not much has changed over these few years."

Penny recalled a particularly trying day. "We had four airmen brought in from a convoy that had been attacked by rocket-propelled grenades. Two came in DOA (dead on arrival), and two others were critically wounded. One airman had half his face gone. His jaw was completely gone, with only a few upper back teeth left intact. It looked like hamburger where his mouth had been. There was sand and dirt where his mouth had been. One of his arms was gone, with bands of tendons and ligaments hanging out of where his shoulder joint used to be. He was unconscious and bleeding to death when we got him at our forward surgical unit. The other airman had a traumatic amputation of one leg all the way up in his groin, and the other leg was mangled below the knee. He was semiconscious and disoriented. We worked like crazy in the OR to save these guys. We used all the blood we had on hand. When we shipped them out, they were both still alive. I often wonder whether they made it or not."

Captain Robert

Robert was an Army reservist assigned to Tikrit, Mosul, and Al Asad, Iraq, during his 1-year tour of duty in the war zone. He commented, "War is chaotic. One thing that really pissed me off was that some of our guys are being tried for alleged war crimes, like shooting civilians, but the generals basically told all of us, 'If you tell them to get back and they don't get back, you shoot them. Then you put another bullet in them just to make sure they are dead.' If you don't kill them, they will certainly kill you. People would come up to our compound in civilian cars, and you would swear to God they looked innocent, but the woman would have a bomb under her skirt. They just wanted to get close enough so they could kill everybody around them as well as themselves. You lived in fear. Is this just a child that wants candy, or is he rigged up with a bomb? This is one of the things I struggled with the most. Trying to understand why, sometimes, our troops are charged with things like killing civilians when most people don't know what it is like over there and how truly dangerous it is."

Major Christina

Christina was an active-duty Air Force flight nurse who served in Iraq and Afghanistan. Christina recalled, "There is a lot of learning taking place, too. You are dealing with a lot of different injuries. I was a med–surg nurse before doing air evac. We saw a lot of children with mainly burns from explosions and gunshot wounds. There were a lot of Iraqis who would like to slice our throats. As a nurse, you are helping this person, and they'd like to kill you. It takes you through a lot of different emotions. You are angry. You are sad. One minute you don't want to be in the military, and the next minute you do. Working with Iraqi patients was sometimes scary. You don't want to let your guard down. They have a flat demeanor. They stare at you with their eyes. They have this look. They are dark and dreary."

Christina reported, "I was deployed to both Iraq and Afghanistan. There's a big difference between Iraq and Afghanistan. In Iraq, we were considered occupiers, and in Afghanistan we were consider liberators. Therefore, in Afghanistan, any local national who came to our gate who was at risk of losing life, limb, or eyesight had to be taken in and provided with medical care. Therefore, we saw a very large number of injured local nationals. In Iraq, our soldiers were suspicious of any nationals approaching the base. Too many soldiers and Marines got blown up at the gates from insurgents posing as families or innocent locals needing medical assistance."

Lieutenant Colonel Victoria

Victoria, an active-duty career Army officer, was assigned to Camp Bucca Detainee Hospital for her second deployment in Iraq. She remembered, "One time, we had a couple of RPGs that came into the compound right next to the hospital. They were meant for the hospital. They launched them right into the hospital compound, and they did it right at the change of shift. Within about five minutes, we had about eighty traumas in our little ER. Keep in mind that we are only a 44-bed hospital, but we could expand using hallways. However, we did it! We pulled it together and made it happen.

However, you want to talk about chaos? We had chaos! Many of the detainees came in without guards and those types of things. We had to calm down a lot of people. We knew that the RPGs were meant for us. We did very well, but it was hard. It happened at the beginning of the deployment in June. We had another year to go, taking care of these 'little gentlemen.' It was very hard. Imagine having to take care of people you despise and fear at the same time. Most of them just wanted us dead."

Victoria's first deployment in Iraq was at the small hospital in Mosul. She described this assignment in Mosul at the beginning of the war. "I was in Iraq for four months in 2003. We were the first hospital to set up in the middle of the desert. We were actually set up without any security at all. That was scary. It wasn't planned that way. It was due to other circumstances. We got hit with the worst sandstorm in 100 years. That was probably good because, otherwise, we would have got[ten] overrun. Because the weather was so bad, the bad guys weren't moving around on us. Everyone had to do his or her part. Once Baghdad fell, they moved another hospital up there. Our jobs were very important. We got the first casualties of the war, along with a few mobile surgical hospitals that moved across the border at the same time we did. It was a very scary environment the whole time I was there, but especially the first few weeks of the war."

Commander Josie

Josie was an active-duty Navy nurse assigned with a 16-person mentoring team to an Afghan National Army Hospital in Mazer-e-Sharif, Afghanistan. Josie described how her roommate was killed in an ambush attack on their Afghan Army base. "I loved my roommate. Even though I was twenty years her senior, we got along great. We were both married. We had left husbands and kids back in the States. We ate together. We went to the latrine together. We worked together at the hospital, and we ran together. We went to the gym together, and we were 'battle buddies,' meaning we were security partners. We didn't venture out alone after dark. She cut my hair. I built stuff for her cubicle. I would go to the woodworking shop. She would want something, and I would build it for her. We had the best breakfasts together. We had a tray with peeled sliced kiwi somebody spent hours doing. We counted our blessings, even though we had none of the amenities that other bases had. We had no salons. No Mickey D's or Burger King, and no Starbucks. We had our MWR (morale, welfare, and recreation) shack, a home theater box where you could watch movies. The 'D-Fac' was the only restaurant in town, and it was open 24/7."

Josie continued, "When she was cold, I caulked the entire B-hut so she would not be cold. She was my baby. She was almost like my child.

My oldest daughter will be 30 soon, and my roommate was 35. We both had birthdays in November, and we celebrated them together. We served Thanksgiving lunch together for a group of U.S. and Afghan medics. We went shooting with the German soldiers together. She talked me into it. We shot their weapons for target practice. It was a competition, and she got an expert gold medal. I got a bronze. She was just that good. There was nothing she touched that wasn't gold. She was a hospital administrator, a Medical Service Corps officer. She was killed in an ambush on our Afghan base. She was shot in the leg and then finished off with two shots in the back."

Captain Olivia

Olivia was sent with a large cadre of people from her reserve unit to the coalition forces hospital in Mosul, Iraq. Olivia remarked, "I went out on a fair number of helicopter missions to pick up wounded troops or civilians. I felt that sometimes I had to play God out in the field. If I was out on a mission, sometimes I had two patients that were critically wounded. I felt like sometimes I had to flip a coin and say 'heads, you get the care, or tails, he gets the care.' I hated that, particularly when the patients were kids. I lost a lot of friends over there. I was friends with a lot of soldiers. I not only went out on missions to pick up the wounded, but I also went out on 'angel flights' where we would pick up those killed in action. We believed in leaving no soldiers behind. The dead come in pieces sometimes."

Olivia recalled losing a friend in Iraq: "There is one time that I will always remember. There was this Marine that I became friends with, but we were just friends. If I would see him at lunch, I would go sit with him and have lunch. We would sometimes go to the gym together. Whenever we could meet up, we would just chitchat over coffee. Then one time, he said he wouldn't be around for a while because he was going out on a mission. Three days later, I get a call that it's my turn to go out on an angel flight to pick up bodies. Well, it was him. The only way I found out was we found his dog tag attached to his boot. They were hit with an IED, and there were no bodies, just pieces. There were three of them together. Apparently, one of them stepped on an IED."

Olivia went on to describe another situation she will never forget, "One day, I had to pick up three little kids. It was two little twin girls and their brother. I had to do my best, and there was just a medic and me. We lost all three of them. There is only so much you can do in a helicopter. They all had head injuries. I was trying to stop the bleeding on all of them, and it was horrible. I got in trouble when we landed back at the hospital. I had put the twins on the same stretcher because they were small. I caught flak because of that. That was not the SOP (standard operating procedure) we were supposed to follow. I felt they needed to be together. They were twins. They came into the world together, and I felt they should go out of the world together. The grandfather was the primary caretaker for these three kids. He came to the hospital on another helicopter. He got upset with me because all three of them died. He hit me in the shoulder. He was grief-stricken. Females do not have a predominant role in the society there. I had become the caretaker for his three kids and they all died."

Captain Tina

Tina was an Air Force nurse assigned to FOB Salerno in Afghanistan. This was her second deployment. She served at Balad Air Base, Iraq, earlier in her career. Tina recalled her experiences in Afghanistan. "I was shocked at the emotions that I felt over there. I felt emotions that I never felt before. The number one emotion was anger. I was so angry. I haven't ever been that angry. I could never really put my finger on what it was that made me so angry. It was just a combination of everything. There was so much death over there. There was tragedy and injured children. There was such a sense of hopelessness and helplessness. There were sleep interruptions from nightly mortar attacks. There was constant noise from planes and choppers. I'm trained as a flight nurse, even though I was assigned to a field hospital. They have a term called 'stressors of flight.' It is the things that you experience in an aircraft. It's heat, altitude, noise, vibration, and turbulence. I was experiencing all these things on the ground."

Major Samantha

Samantha was an active-duty Army nurse assigned to the hospital at Bagram Air Base, Afghanistan. Samantha recalled, "I had very little experience with pediatric patients prior to this deployment. Now, I could resuscitate a burned child if I had to. Things that you just look at, and in your mind you say, 'That's not right,' this person does not have any legs. It's just not right. It doesn't make sense in my brain. I can't wrap my head around what I'm seeing. It's not right. It's like seeing someone with two heads. I think a lot of the nurses got involved, and it may have led to compassion fatigue. I did the complete opposite. I didn't get involved. I didn't talk to patients, and I didn't even look at their faces, because I couldn't. My way of coping was looking at the equipment, focusing on the task at hand, and waiting for the midnight meal because then I'd know the shift was half over."

Lieutenant Donna

Donna was an active-duty Navy nurse assigned to a combat support hospital in Kandahar, Afghanistan. She described the usual flow of injured troops and locals. "At our hospital, if we got in American troops, we would transfer them right away to Bagram if they were seriously injured. However, if the patient was a local Afghani, we would try to manage them. If they were seriously injured, we would transport them to Bagram, too. There was at least one flight a week to take Americans who were not seriously injured to Germany. Patients need to be stable to fly unless there is a Critical Care Air Transport Team (CCATT) where they can do intensive care in the sky. Most of the time, they do the first surgery in a forward surgical unit on an FOB close to where the troops were injured. Then the doctors will do another surgery here or at Bagram, where the specialists are located."

Captain Marie

Marie, an Army reservist, preferred working in the intensive care unit (ICU) or on the medical-surgical units at the large Air Force Hospital at Balad Air Base, Iraq. However, sometimes, she was reassigned to the emergency room when they were very busy there or short on staff. Marie recalled, "I worked in the ER when they needed me. It was an open-door policy for the troops. We worked 12-hour shifts. Therefore, if there was a soldier whose feet were bothering him at 2 a.m., he would come in. People get sick no matter where they are, so we would have emergency appendectomies that would come in. You had your trauma patients that came in by chopper or truck, or whatever. We had Marines who would come zooming in with their trucks or Humvees. We had insurgents who were brought in when an IED blew up while they were planting it. We had more and bigger trauma than you would see here in the States. However, we would also see routine things like strep throat and earaches. We saw the full gamut. Sometimes, it was so crazy in the ER, with all levels of injuries and illnesses."

Captain Erin

Erin was a new Air Force flight nurse from the Pacific Northwest. She was assigned to an air evacuation squadron based in North Carolina. She had been on active duty for about five years. Erin described how her work was physically and emotionally exhausting. The demands of providing nursing care contributed significantly to her stress. She added that she was not alone in this, because it was a recurrent theme in her conversations with her nurse colleagues. She shared that ongoing "venting," as she called it, was therapeutic for the nurses, and she felt close to the other nurses. She recalled, "Flight nursing was physically demanding. We carried a lot of gear onto our C-130 or C-17. Some of the gear was patient care equipment, and some was personal safety equipment. We had to reconfigure these cargo planes to accommodate patients. We had to string oxygen and electrical lines. We had to set up litter stations to support patients lying on litters."

Erin continued, "Our patient population varied depending on what was going on. We cared for a lot of patients from truck convoys. Convoys would get blown up by IEDs, resulting in polytrauma injuries for many of the troops. You'd have the gunner up in the turret that got thrown out, and he was unconscious with a head injury and broken bones. Others would have blast injuries from IEDs. Small-arms fire and IED explosions resulted in many traumatic amputations. Gunshot wounds hit major arteries in the legs or neck. There were also knife wounds, suicides and attempted suicides, and burns. Sometimes, depression made up our days."

Lieutenant Colonel Heidi

Heidi, an active-duty Army nurse researcher, described how her perspective on deployment changed after she deployed to Iraq and returned. "I was at Walter Reed Army Medical Center when the first Gulf War started. I felt horrible about not going. I felt I should be over there since I was a senior Captain with a lot of critical care experience. More recently in my career, I learned that nursing is easier in a combat zone. Using the general term for soldier, Joe, all Joe worries about when he gets shot up is, where's my weapon, when can I go back, are my buddies okay, and is my 'junk' (meaning private parts) alright. That's all they care about there. It's not until people get back to places like Walter Reed (Walter Reed Army Medical Center) and they go through this long-term convalescence that reality takes hold. You have people that are incredibly disfigured or injured for life, and that is incredibly difficult. Nursing in places like Walter Reed is much more difficult. You have to help someone get better and learn to live again. I have tons of respect for people who work in places like that and have not deployed, and what they are dealing with on a daily basis. We all have our roles to play. It's a lot more emotionally draining to do long-term care. However, I didn't have this perspective until I deployed to Iraq and realized that my two years caring for war casualties at Walter Reed was much more taxing on me than my year in Iraq. Nurses back home also have to be there for the injured soldiers' families as well as the soldiers needing long-term care."

Photo Courtesy of U.S. Air Force.

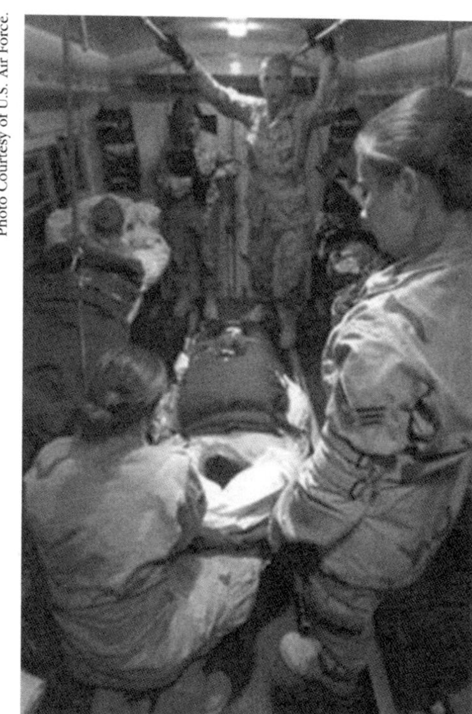

Air Force medics on Ambus with air evacuation patients.

Photo Courtesy of U.S. Air Force.

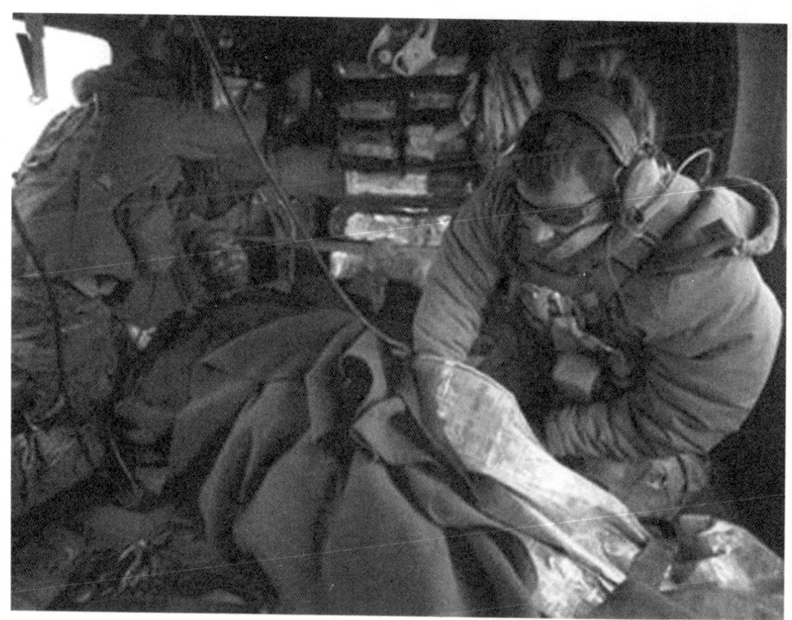

Army medics with Afghan patient on Blackhawk helicopter.

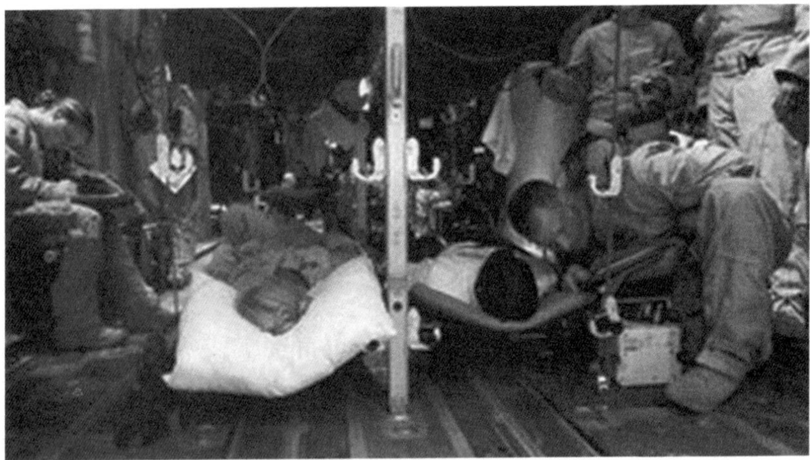
Photo Courtesy of U.S. Air Force.

C-130 air evacuation flight, Iraq.

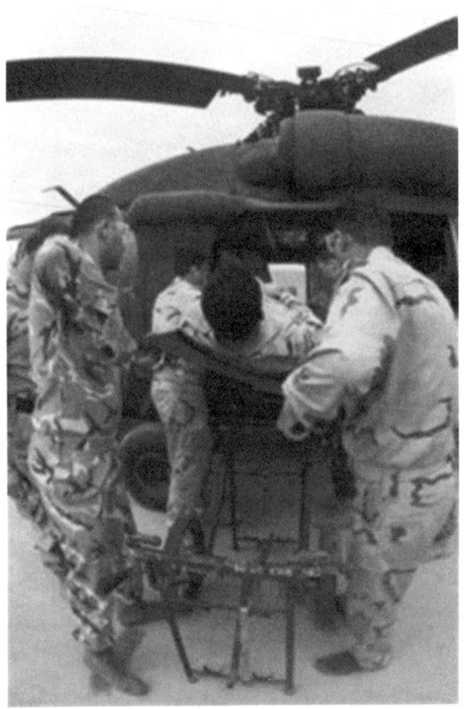
Photo Courtesy of U.S. Air Force.

Patient loaded on Army Blackhawk helicopter.

Photo Courtesy of U.S. Navy.

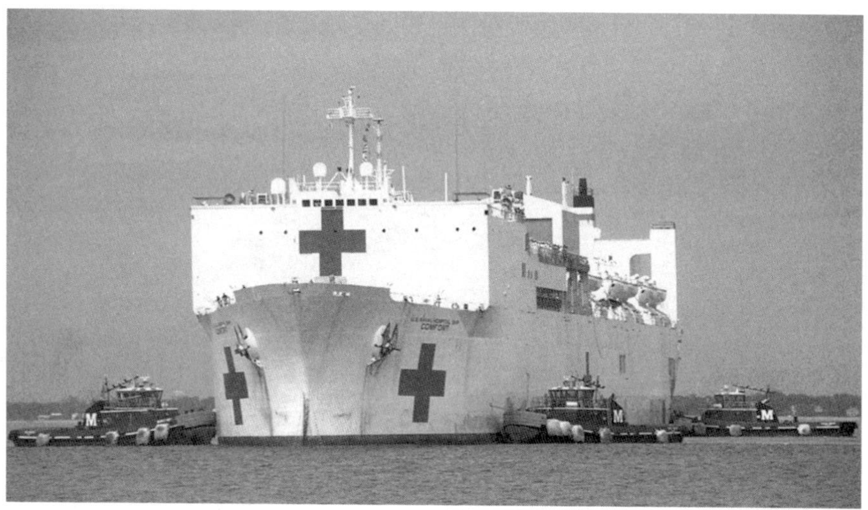

U.S. Navy Hospital Ship Comfort.

Photo Courtesy of U.S. Navy.

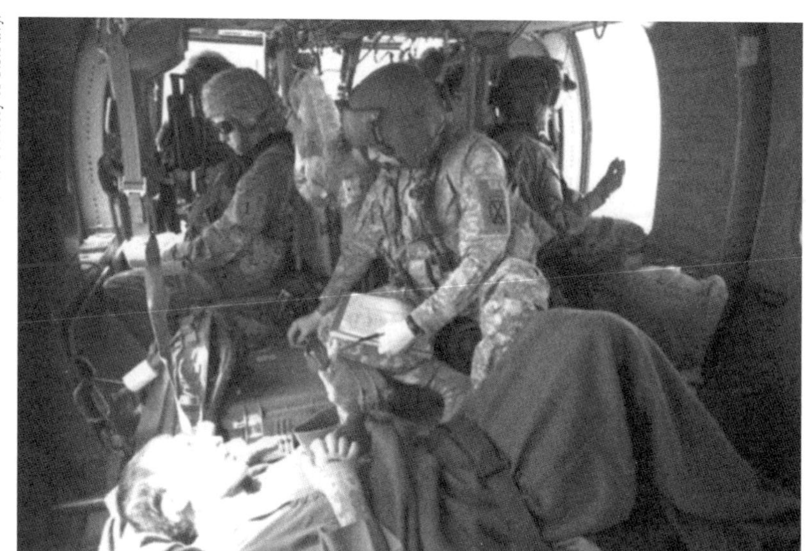

Army medics care for injured Afghan civilians on Army Blackhawk helicopter.

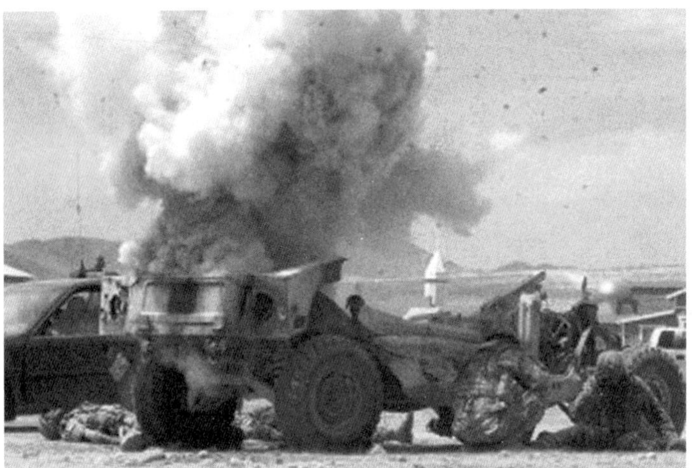

Photo Courtesy of U.S. Army.

Soldiers injured from car bomb at Army checkpoint.

8

War Memories: Sensations Etched in My Mind

Nurses recalled the sounds, smells, images, and thoughts of the war zone that defined their experiences in Iraq or Afghanistan. Many stated that these sensory elements would be etched in their minds forever. Most nurses described Iraq and Afghanistan as noisy, smelly, and dangerous places they would never forget. War is not quiet. Machine guns, mortars, rockets, fighter jets, grenades, IED (improvised explosive device) explosions, and helicopters reverberate. Electrical generators, ventilators, medical device alarm systems, and suction machines add to the noise within a combat support hospital or mobile field hospital. In the hospital compound, at high volume and with a sense of urgency, the public address system blares the warning, "Incoming, incoming, incoming, take cover, take cover." Here, the noise level and sense of chaos were sustained.

War has an odor indigenous to where it is being fought. For Iraq, it was the raw sewage, the military base burn pits, or the burning oil fields. For Afghanistan, some nurses recalled a pervasive smell of body odor, curry cooking scents, and jet fuel.

Sights of the desert sands dominated the rather austere vision of Iraq. For many nurses, Afghanistan was a contrast of views. Some nurses focused on the picturesque snow-capped mountain landscapes, whereas others recalled burned and maimed soldiers and children. Through it all were the soldiers fighting outside the wire and the casualties the nurses cared for inside the wire in their combat hospitals.

SOUNDS OF WAR

Major Diana

Diana was an Air Force reservist assigned to the aeromedical staging facility in Balad, Iraq. She described the sounds of her experience. "The sound of Iraq was the roar of Air Force C-130 and C-17 airplanes that we used for air evac. I hear the sound of helicopters and jet engines, too. Our living area was close to the runway, so the jets taking off and landing were loud. Our hospital was right next to the helipad, so helicopters would be coming in and taking off all the time. Another primary sound was the generator next to our tent. I was sure I was going to come home with hearing loss because the generator was so loud. It was probably 50 feet from the front of my tent to the front of the hospital. You could hear that generator all the time."

Lieutenant Colonel Judd

Judd was a nurse practitioner in the Army Reserve. His first assignment in Iraq was in Mosul. He described the noises of that environment. "Our base was in the middle of the city of Mosul. I could hear mortars going off almost every night. They would shoot mortars into our compound from pickup trucks. They were very loud, with a characteristic dull thud or thump sound followed by a loud explosion. I would also hear helicopters coming into the hospital helipad and airplanes in the distance. I can hear the alarm system going off, saying, 'Incoming, incoming, incoming,' when we were under mortar attack. Mosul was a very loud place compared to my next assignment in Anbar Province."

Captain Tina

Tina, an active-duty Air Force nurse, described FOB Salerno, Afghanistan. "Our base had a perimeter of landmines for security to keep insurgents and other people out. I remember hearing the 'click' and then the explosion of the landmines if someone tried to breach the perimeter. Usually, a stray animal would set them off. Once a landmine exploded, the alarm sirens would sound to warn us that someone or something tried to break through our lines. The siren would alert us to put our 'battle rattle' [helmet and body armor] on and be prepared for an attack."

Captain Marie

Marie was an Army reservist assigned to Balad, then Mosul, and then Anbar Province, Iraq. Marie recalled, "The other day, we were on vacation camping. I heard about five fighter jets in a very short period. I said to my husband, 'Put the radio on, something is going on. There are jets all over; something is going on today.' I spent my first 3 months in Iraq at Balad Air Base, and every morning, I heard the fighter jets take off. This sound that morning took my mind right back to Balad. The other noises for me were the alarms, explosions, helicopters, and cargo aircraft. Sometimes, you had to run and get down and take cover. You might be eating dinner, and all of a sudden, an alarm goes off, and you get on the floor for your own safety."

Major Alene

Alene was an Army reservist assigned to the coalition forces hospital in Mosul, Iraq, and later in her career, to Bagram Air Base, Afghanistan. She reported, "Iraq is really loud. Even if there weren't a war going on, I think it would still be very loud. The place had generators instead of regular electricity. The generators were terribly loud. The generator noise was like your worst OSHA [occupational health and safety association] violation. It was the worst OSHA violation in the world! You could get killed accidently on almost anything over there. I can hear the sound of the mortars. You hear it through the air, and you don't know where it's going to land. I can also hear the hustle-bustle sound of the intensive care unit with all the suction machines and beeping monitors. I can also hear the call to prayer in the city of Mosul since our hospital compound was in the middle of the city and right near a mosque."

SMELLS OF THE WAR ZONE

Lieutenant Colonel Judd

Along with the sounds in their wartime environment, nurses identified some odors unique to their deployment location. Judd, an Army Reserve nurse practitioner, remarked, "When I was in Mosul, Iraq, there was a lot of open sewage. It literally smelled like a sewer. The smell of raw sewage was so strong for the first month, I walked around nauseated. It was really pretty awful. Mosul is a city, so the smell permeated the whole city, not just our hospital compound."

Captain Suzanne

Suzanne, an active-duty Air Force nurse assigned to the aeromedical staging unit at Balad Air Base, Iraq, recalled, "I smell the acrid smell of the burn pit. All waste from the base went into this huge burn pit, so you smelled hospital waste, plastics and leftover food from the mess tent, garbage, and sewage from the latrines, and who knows what else. A cloud of smoke from the burn pit always hung over the base and seemed to burn the back of your throat as you breathed. I hear they have gotten better about the burning pits by not doing it every day and using different locations on the base now. If I smell burning trash 20 years from now, it will take me right back to Iraq."

Major Fran

Fran was an Air Force mental health nurse and combat stress team leader. She spent most of her tour of duty in the area around Tallil, Iraq. Fran commented, "Iraq always had a musty smell. The hospital always smelled like dead tissue, charred tissue, and infected flesh. When the oil fields were burning, you could smell that, too. I would also say that the whole country had a lingering musty smell. Like a moderate body odor smell. Kuwait was even worse because it was much hotter and windy."

Captain Richard

Richard had served 7 years on active duty in the Army after graduating from college on an ROTC scholarship. Prior to deploying, he had worked in medical-surgical nursing, the emergency room, and in critical care areas at two hospitals in Texas. Richard spent much of his deployment tour of duty in the detainee compound at Camp Bucca, Iraq. Richard recalled, "The people stunk to high heaven when I first got there. When they came in, they would take their shoes off, and we would move the shoes outside the building because they smelled so bad. These people don't bathe because they don't have much water. If water is scarce, you are not going to use it for bathing; you are going to drink it. So, the body odor of the detainees was pretty ripe, as was their rotting teeth and bad breath."

Lieutenant Donna

Donna, an active-duty Navy nurse assigned at the coalition forces hospital in Kandahar, Afghanistan, remarked, "The characteristic smells from Afghanistan included body odor, jet fuel, hydraulic fluid, and burning trash. Most Afghan people do not bathe, so most reeked of body odor. You just can't forget that odor. In addition, I remember the smell of curry because they put it on everything. I can't stand the smell of curry now. Afghanistan smelled like burning feces. We had to burn everything, including waste products from the latrines and hospital."

Major Michelle

Michelle, an active-duty Air Force nurse anesthetist assigned to mentoring duty at an Afghan national army hospital, recalled, "I can smell diesel fuel, jet fuel, and burning trash. The smell of things burning seemed to always be in the air. Burning trash was the smell that I will always remember. One of the first things I noticed when I came home was the lack of a smell in the air. Afghanistan, on the other hand, always smelled like something was burning."

Major Millie

Millie, an active-duty Army operating room nurse, recalled, "In Iraq, the raw sewage would come up from the latrines if the contractor hadn't pumped them out in a timely manner. When that happened, raw sewage would back up all over the place. Sometimes, I had to walk through a field of raw sewage to get to the hospital if there was a backup. It didn't happen that often, but when it did, it was just awful. The smells of hydraulic fluid from the C-130 aircraft and burning trash were Iraq for me. I can also smell infected wounds and burned flesh from my hospital."

First Lieutenant Lisa

Lisa was an Army Reserve nurse assigned to the coalition forces hospital in Mosul, Iraq. Lisa recalled, "When I think of Mosul, I smell cooking smells since our compound was surrounded by the city. I can also remember a musty or damp smell in the early morning before the sun got so hot. The hospital smelled from the antiseptic spray that we used."

SIGHTS OF THE WAR ZONE

Lieutenant Colonel Judd

These nurses associated many sights with Iraq or Afghanistan during their wartime deployment. Judd, an Army Reserve nurse practitioner, described his environment. "I see sand. I see a total desert of sand. It was very fine sand. The sand was permeating everything. You just couldn't get clean. You could vacuum the floor in your little CHU [containerized housing unit], you could wash the floor in your little CHU, but in 24 hours, you would run your hand over it, and there was sand dust in there again all the time. It is like confectionary sugar. It is the consistency of powdered sugar."

Lieutenant Colonel Victoria

Victoria, a career active-duty Army officer, remarked, "On my first deployment to Mosul, we had a lot of sand storms. You would see a big orange cloud coming toward you. Sandstorms are just awful. You would have to go outside and hold down the sides of the tent in a sandstorm. I also see a swarm of sand flies flying around my head. They were just awful. They were everywhere, and they totally grossed me out. I would be sweating in the 130-degree heat and fighting off the sand flies. It was just miserable."

Victoria continued, "Iraq is a huge sandbox. I see no trees. It was very isolated. Maybe I see a couple of straggly palm trees near the prison. I had the opportunity to do a couple of medevacs during the rainy season. I'm looking out of the helicopter, and all I see is just a giant mud pit. It goes from being a giant sandbox to being a giant mud pit. I didn't think there was anything attractive about the country at all. Everything was always coated in a fine layer of sand. Everything always felt dirty, but you get used to that, too. I see the waves of heat coming off the desert. I see dust and dirt everywhere. I see my canvas tent where I lived with a horde of my best friends. I see my cot that is so close to the women on both sides of me that I can hold their hands. It added new meaning to the word *cozy*. I see the matlike weave floors and the mice scurrying about at night."

Major Christina

Christina served tours of duty as an active-duty Air Force flight nurse in Iraq and Afghanistan. She reported, "I can see the flares going off outside the plane, [regardless of] whether we are being shot at or not. The flares will go off when our plane is taking fire. They go off to distract or divert heat-seeking missiles away from the plane. I can see tracer rounds coming up from the ground toward our air evac plane. All of this is kind of unnerving when it happens. However, you learn to deal with it. It goes with the job of being a flight nurse flying in a war zone."

Lieutenant Colonel Heidi

Heidi, an active-duty Army nurse researcher, recalled, "I see cars driving by with bullet holes in them. Being shot at or blown up was a way of life over there. I see wrecked convoy vehicles scattered on the side of the road. I see burned-out cars and military trucks. I see children blown up and dead soldiers. I see lines of body bags. I hated zipping up body bags, and trying to scoop up the brains of the babies and stick them in body bags so that all parts of the 'biologicals' were together. I see lots of death and destruction, a landscape of the injured, the dying, and the dead."

Commander Josie

Some nurses described the terrain in Afghanistan to be beautiful. Josie, an active-duty Navy nurse assigned to mentoring duty at the Afghan national army hospital in Mazer-e-Sharif, remarked, "The first things I see are the snowcapped mountains surrounding our base. I see the Afghan local women with the burka [women's scarf], white hat, and their weather-worn but beautiful faces. I see the destitute but grateful children. I see children happy to see Americans taking care of their people. Most of my sights are associated with the Mazer-e-Sharif area. I see the plywood B-huts we lived in and the hospital we worked in. I also see the smiling faces of the Afghan people we worked with at the Afghan hospital. I see the pharmacist, the X-ray technician, the housekeepers, and the doctors."

Major Michelle

Michelle was an active-duty Air Force nurse anesthetist assigned to an Afghan army national hospital. She recalled, "I see the faces of the injured, but not all are sad. I see injured kids smiling when they are feeling better and getting ready to go on the helicopter back to where they came from. I see the hopeful faces of some injured soldiers getting ready to fly out to Germany. I also see dirt. Everything was just dirty in Afghanistan. Even in the hospital, everything was dirty. Hygiene for them was not a priority. Even decontaminating our surgical instruments was not a priority for them."

Lieutenant Commander Clare

The sights of human misery were paramount in many nurses' visual memories. Clare, an active-duty Navy critical care trauma nurse, shared her visual memories. "I see blood everywhere. Blood is all over the trauma area, on the floors, on the walls, on the medics, and on the patients. I see the helicopter doors open, and a red river of blood gushes out. I see a convoy of vehicles approach the trauma area and casualties being quickly off-loaded. I see marines frantically running around in the triage area as they off-load their wounded and dead. Later, I see some marines crying and trying to console each other outside the triage area. I see big 6-foot-tall marines crying and hugging each other."

Captain Olivia

Olivia, an Army reservist, remarked, "I just see uniform after uniform after uniform. I see weapons and soldiers carrying weapons. I see convoys mounting up and heading out of our compound. I see greenish brown tents, plywood huts, and tan-colored trailers everywhere. I see Blackhawks [helicopters] landing in Mosul and the injured being carried to the triage area outside the emergency room."

THOUGHTS OF THE WAR ZONE

Major Diana

Nurses described a plethora of thoughts about Iraq and Afghanistan. Most thoughts centered on the people of these two foreign lands and the wars. Diana, an Air Force reservist, stated, "When I hear the word *Iraq*, that brings me right back to the time I was there caring for patients and moving them to the planes bound for Germany. I think of all the patients I've cared for over there. I think about our guys and gals being out in Humvees and convoys on the roads, dodging the threat of IEDs and insurgent attacks with small-arms fire. I think about our people outside the wire and the danger out there. I've seen firsthand what devastation the weapons can do."

Major Derek

Derek, an Army reservist assigned to the Camp Bucca hospital and Abu Ghraib Detainee Hospital, remarked, "I think about the danger. I think about the near misses from mortar and rocket attacks and some hard landings in our medevac helicopter. I think about the time we landed and then got hit with an RPG [rocket-propelled grenade]. I think about all my safety concerns. It was not safe there. I think about the detainee compounds. The staff was angry, and the detainees were angry. No one wanted to be there, not the nursing staff, not the medical staff, not the military guards, and not the detainees. The words *angry* and *unsafe* come to mind for me. It was such a dirty and emotionally toxic place. Of course, we were at the world's largest prison, so it wasn't exactly a spa. We had 28,000 detainees at Camp Bucca. We had grown from 11,000 to about 28,000 by the end of the troop surge. The hospital was in the middle of the prison compound. Therefore, you were in it, around it, you lived a half mile from it, and you had to walk through the prison to get to the hospital every day. We never got away from it, and a year there was just too long."

Lieutenant Colonel Heidi

Heidi, an active-duty Army nurse researcher assigned to Baghdad, recalled, "Fear is the first thought that comes to mind. Fear because it was a dangerous place. I had to jump over my cot because we were receiving incoming rocket fire on several occasions. Seeing explosions outside the window of my trailer was a fearful experience."

First Lieutenant Leah

Several nurses reported that when they think of their experiences in Iraq or Afghanistan, their thoughts focus on the feelings of frustration and futility. Leah was an Army reservist. Her combat assignment was working in the intensive care unit at the coalition hospital in Mosul, Iraq. She recalled, "I think about the frustration we experienced in Iraq. Every time I hear Iraq being mentioned or talked about, it reminds me of unfinished business. Nothing seemed to get finished over there. As a medical person, I truly thought a lot of the seriously injured Iraqi people we treated would end up dying once we sent them back to their villages. There would be no follow-up for these people once they got home. Back in the States, if someone needs to follow up in a week or a month from now, you won't have a second thought about that. In Iraq, everything you do, you almost feel like you need to frontload the rest of that kid's life with all the care he needs today because he might not be able to get it once he gets home. Of course, that is just impossible. I think a lot about the frustration and futility of the situation in Iraq."

Lieutenant Colonel Judd

Judd, an Army reservist and nurse practitioner, was assigned to three bases in Iraq. He shared his thoughts, "As far as my thoughts, *frustration* is a word that comes to mind. Also, *futility*, because of a lot of what we did is like putting a Band-Aid on a much bigger wound. It is going to take years and years of rebuilding and a lot of time and effort and resources to help them rebuild. It is so backwards. I tell my wife it is like going back 150 years in time and trying to work with people with that mentality to move forward into the 21st century. It's frustrating. The culture is frustrating, especially the way they treat women. They didn't let the women come into the hospital unless they were escorted by their husband or a male elder from the family. It's frustrating working with that type of culture."

Captain Erin

Erin was an active-duty Air Force flight nurse assigned to Bagram Air Base, Afghanistan. She recalled, "I think of the frustration and the futility of what we were trying to do in Afghanistan. Working with Americans was very rewarding. You'd patch them up and get them better. We would expend a lot of time and energy into saving injured Afghan nationals, and then you have to send them back out to what. You didn't know what you were sending them back to."

Erin continued, "I remember one case. I was not flying that day, so I was helping at the hospital. We had a baby who came in. It was obvious child abuse. They had dunked the kid in hot boiling water. Their abuse to the women and children over there is rampant. Of course, Dad said it was an accident, and the mother wasn't allowed to come in. The child was about 2 1/2 years old. It was obvious what caused the burns. She was dunked in hot water. We called her 'Baby Gracie.' She went through 4 months of rehabilitation and skin grafting. At the end of all that, you have to send her back to her family. You have no idea what becomes of these children. You wonder if it will happen again. It's very frustrating."

Major Michelle

Michelle was an active-duty Air Force nurse anesthetist assigned at an Afghan national army hospital to mentor and teach anesthesia care to Afghan medical teams. She stated, "The first thought or word that comes to mind for me is *frustration*. As mentors, we were sent there with really no guidelines from our headquarters. It was, 'Just go over there and teach them what they need to know.' We gave them a new facility. It was a state-of-the-art facility by their standards. They were in mud huts before we built this place. We gave them all the equipment, but they had no idea how to use it. Most of them had no training. They were self-declared medical personnel. They could not prove or validate any of their training. Many of them were illiterate. We didn't have any goals or end point or any direction from our headquarters. We were just told to make this hospital work. There were so many hurdles for every little thing that we did."

Michelle continued, "We made strides, but they came at a high cost. For example, the Afghan army had no money. They had no way of supplying their own hospital. The logistics system was just so antiquated that we just couldn't get supplies. We had mentors in supply up in Kabul. They couldn't even help us because they had nothing. Therefore, our own supply people couldn't help us. We were faced with massive traumas coming in, and we didn't even have simple supplies. We had to deal with no supplies, a lack of education, cultural differences, and their work ethic was horrible. The Afghan workers at the hospital would find every excuse not to work. They would work hard at not working. Their excuses to not work were crazy. They'd say, 'I have to go have some tea, or I have to go take care of my brother-in-law's cousin's uncle.' They would take leave, and they would stay away for months. There just weren't any repercussions for poor performance."

Major Millie

Millie was a seasoned active-duty Army operating room nurse. She described how she kept her feelings to herself while deployed. Millie explained, "I often think about how we never talked about what was bothering us over there. I might see three young soldiers die in the OR today. I'd go back to my tent and not say a word about what I just saw and experienced to anyone. My best friend was a mental health nurse over there, but I wouldn't say anything to her. I thought I couldn't let it out. I couldn't talk about how I felt. Maybe I was afraid to let it out. My feeling was that I've got this stuff I feel, but I can't talk about it. I have to hold it together. I think everyone there had similar thoughts and feelings. I didn't talk about what bothered me till I got home. Luckily, I could talk to my husband because he was a retired military member. He understood. He was in Iraq in 2003, shortly after the war began."

Captain Richard

Other nurses had a variety of mixed thoughts about their Iraq or Afghanistan deployment experience. Richard, an active-duty Army nurse assigned in Iraq, commented, "When I think of Iraq, I think if it weren't for the oil, I don't see why anyone would ever want to live there. There is nothing about the country that had any type of charm or any type of attraction. I just heard the Iraqi government is starting a tourism bureau. How ludicrous is that! I know if you look at it from a historical point of view, it is the cradle of civilization. From an archeological perspective, there is probably a lot there. However, there isn't anything attractive about the country."

Captain Tina

Tina, an active-duty Air Force nurse, reflected on her thoughts about living in Iraq. "I think about the primitive conditions we lived and worked in. The hospital had air-conditioning. We had a couple of generators, but just about every other afternoon, one of the generators would go out. We'd have to move the patients to an area that still had air-conditioning because we had patients with serious injuries, fluid problems, and they couldn't withstand the temperatures up around 120 degrees in the afternoon."

Commander Josie

Josie was a senior active-duty Navy nurse assigned to mentor Afghan medical personnel at the Afghan national army hospital in Mazer-e-Sharif. She remarked, "When I think of Afghanistan, I think about how women were treated over there. Women in the south of Afghanistan, where we were, are very sheltered. They were covered from head to toe when they left their homes. After puberty, many girls never left the house. They stayed tucked away. There were 5,000 Afghan soldiers on our base. Many never saw a woman not covered from head to toe. Most were very young single men. It got to the point where I was just disgusted. They stared at us all the time. I didn't understand what they were saying, but the innuendos were nonverbally communicated. It was like walking through a construction site every day. They would just stare and say things I couldn't hear or understand. They would ask us women for pictures. They asked for more pictures every day. I was just disgusted and felt harassed. My roommate and I were the youngest of the 4 women in our group of 16 Americans, and we got it more than the other 2 older women."

Major Vivian

Vivian was an Air Force reservist from Delaware. She reflected on the camaraderie as one of her primary thoughts about her experience. "I might be at the mall, and someone says the word *Iraq*, and it might take me back. There were 60 of us who deployed from my reserve unit. We all left from the same place. When I think of Iraq, I think of the camaraderie we had prior to leaving that even grew stronger in Iraq. We all left together and we all came home together. For me, that was the best part of the time in Iraq. Of course, taking care of the patients was so important to all of us. However, it was nice to have each other. It helped us get through it."

Lieutenant Donna

Donna, an active-duty Navy nurse assigned to the coalition forces hospital in Kandahar, Afghanistan, summarized the thoughts of many. "When I think about our deployment, I think about the pride, honor, and privilege to have served my country and taken care of our wounded military personnel. There is no more noble a deed for a military nurse. The hard work, long days, and other sacrifices were worth it for us medics because our troops in the field were making an even bigger sacrifice. We had a job to do, and we did it to the best of our ability. It is the price of freedom."

9

My Warrior Patients

Many nurses had a patient or two that they will never forget—a marine or airman who was severely injured or a soldier who died too young and too far from home. The nurse could tell you what this patient looked like, what injuries he or she sustained, the patient's rank and branch of service, and the circumstances surrounding the injury. If the patient was conscious, the nurse would remember what he or she had to say. The nurse would remember if this special patient wore a Star of David, or a cross, or a crucifix around the neck, as well as any tattoos that were present. The nurse would remember the patient's buddies and what his or her buddies had to say about the patient. The nurse would carry memories of this patient far after these wars end. Perhaps these memories would leave an indelible imprint for this nurse of a life cut short, a life forever changed by battle injuries, and questions about this soldier's or airman's sacrifice.

Lieutenant Commander Clare

Clare, a seasoned active-duty Navy critical care trauma nurse, remarked, "I think every nurse had one or two patients that he or she will never forget. The circumstances of the encounter will remain vividly etched in one's mind forever, as will the injuries this patient sustained and whether this patient lived or died."

Clare worked at a large Navy medical center in Virginia before being deployed to a mobile field surgical unit in Anbar Province, Iraq. "Most of the casualties we cared for in Anbar province were marines because that area was heavy with Marine units. I was a shock-trauma nurse in our hospital. We had an intensive care unit (ICU), three inpatient units, and a medevac holding area. Most of our medevacs went out by helicopter, but we did have a flight line for C-130 Air Force transport aircraft to land. Sometimes, these big planes would bring in supplies such as ammunition, food, bandages, intravenous fluids, blankets, portable generators, and refrigeration units. Then the aircrew would reconfigure the back of the plane with litter stanchions, oxygen, and electrical lines to support several tiers of three or four patients for the medevac flight to Balad Air Base, Iraq, or Ramstein Air Base, Germany."

Clare enjoyed the challenge of taking care of injured marines right from the battlefield, but she admitted that the sheer volume of patients with catastrophic injuries was difficult to deal with. She remembers the first war casualty she ever cared for. "My patient was a marine sergeant. He was my first Iraq casualty. We got a radio call that they were bringing in a 'tourniquet injury,' which means his limbs were blown off. He was a typical marine, and marines 'take it.' His corpsman had tourniqueted his extremities, and he was dusky gray. He lost a lot of blood, but he was still conscious and talking. He leaned up close to me and said, 'Ma'am, please tell my mother and my sister I'm sorry.' Then the doc said, 'Okay, we're taking the tourniquets down now,' and within about 7 seconds, he was gone."

After 6 months in Iraq, Clare looked forward to returning to the United States and seeing family and friends. She counted the days till she was going to return to California for a new assignment in San Diego. "Right before I came home, I took care of a young gal from California. We got a horrible call from the Marines.We couldn't really make out what they were saying on the radio, except that they were very upset. Anytime marines get hurt, they are upset. However, this was different. We couldn't hear anything they were saying because there was so much screaming. The Humvees came around the corner. We could see the patient's head was all wrapped and bleeding profusely. Finally, we get this patient on the table, we cut through the uniform, and we see breasts. This is a woman marine. She was the only woman in this unit and had just gotten promoted to sergeant. A sniper got her and blew off half of her head. There was not much we could do. She was a very pretty girl, what was left of her. The back of her head was completely gone."

Clare summarized her experience and feelings. "There were many patients I took care of in Iraq. We had some detainee [prisoner] patients, little kids caught in firefights, local villagers, and many soldiers from the U.S. and other coalition countries. The two that I will never forget are the first and last casualties I cared for. They both died. They were both marines. They were two of the most severely injured to ever enter my trauma unit. Neither marine could have been more than 25 years old. They had their whole lives ahead of them. It is sad to see anyone die, but seeing young troops die is the saddest for me. I wondered about their families back home getting the word that they were dead. I wondered if their fellow marines would be haunted by their deaths. I wondered what their lives would have been like if they were not ever sent to Iraq. These two losses were the hardest for me."

Major Lee

Major Lee had been a nurse for almost 30 years. She had worked in a large city emergency room (ER) in Philadelphia for nearly 20 years. Lee joined the Air Force Reserve after her son and daughter were in high school. She joined because of two friends who were in the reserves. They had told her about how much they learned as military nurses, the strong sense of purpose and pride that they felt, and the continuing education opportunities available.

Lee remarked, "I was at a point in my life where the kids were old enough to be more autonomous, my husband's business was well established, and I wanted something more out of life. Joining the reserves seemed like the perfect way to expand my professional practice as a nurse while doing something important for our country."

After several years in the reserves, Lee had never deployed to a war zone before but had participated in two humanitarian deployments to South America with the Air Force. Lee deployed with her reserve unit in January 2005 for 6 months. Their mission was to augment the active-duty Air Force staff at the hospital in Balad, Iraq. Balad Air Base hosts the largest military hospital in Iraq. All severe medical or trauma-related emergencies are routed through the 332nd Expeditionary Medical Operations Squadron ICU at Balad Air Base. The mission of the ICU is to take care of the patients brought in from throughout Iraq, whether they are U.S. military personnel, coalition forces, defense contractors, local villagers, or wounded insurgents.

Lee vividly described two experiences in Iraq that were especially painful to think about. "One of my worse nights was when we had an 18-year-old soldier who got pinned down behind a truck. His platoon leader, a lieutenant, went after him to try to save him, and the lieutenant got shot in the process. They put them on a helicopter. When they landed, they brought the lieutenant off the helicopter while doing CPR on him, and he died. It was Easter Sunday, and he died right there in the emergency room. The young soldier died, too. It was a bad night. I will remember the lieutenant and the young soldier for the rest of my life."

Although that was a difficult day for Lee as an ER nurse, she recalled, "I will never forget my worst day in the ER and the soldiers I cared for on that day. We had three young soldiers; an RPG [rocket-propelled grenade] had ripped through their Humvee a little below sitting height, and it traumatically amputated every one of their six legs. One of them was on a ventilator when they brought them into the triage area. Another was doing okay, and he was awake and alert. The third one was like a squirrel set out in the middle of the road and didn't know which way to go. He was panic-stricken. He sat up on that gurney and looked down where his legs should have been and just screamed bloody murder. 'Oh my God, I don't have any legs!' He threw himself back on the gurney and continued to scream and cry out. I actually had to leave and go outside and throw up. It just made me physically sick to see this poor child the way he was. I think it was the first time he realized that he actually didn't have any legs anymore. It took hours to try to get this child calmed down so we could get him on an airplane to Germany that morning."

Lee described the anguish and frustration soldiers experienced when they lost buddies. "I took care of a soldier who survived an IED explosion but lost all his comrades in the attack. This soldier was driving a vehicle that ran over a bomb. Four other American troops were killed. They are now being flown out on what is known as an 'Angel flight.' This poor guy felt so terrible, so guilty about what happened. I really felt for him. I wonder if he will ever be normal again after such a tragedy in his life, or will this event define the rest of his life? Our ASF staff used to go to the flight line and stand there in formation when an Angel Flight was departing. These C-17 flights contained the flag-draped metal caskets of our fallen comrades. These were some of the toughest days."

Captain Olivia

Olivia, an Army reservist, described some tough experiences. "One time, we were supposed to get four troops from the first cav [first cavalry of the U.S. Army], and we didn't get anybody because they were all killed. We were waiting for them, we got everything ready, and then we were told they were all dead. It was very hard for us.We knew the first cav guys. If they are breathing and have a heartbeat, we could pretty much ensure that they would get to Germany alive. Most of the time, if they have a heartbeat, they are going to live. You know, we all ate our meals in the same dining hall, we lived on the same base, and it was just that we had so much in common with the first cav. The first cav was one of the most famous and most decorated combat divisions in the Army. They were based out of Fort Hood in Killeen, Texas. They were our friends, and some were our boyfriends. It was so tough for us nurses to see this unit get hit so hard."

Although Olivia took care of many critically injured patients, she recalled the man she calls her "miracle soldier." "I took care of soldiers with lots of blast injuries, gunshot wounds, and traumatic amputations. I had this one guy have a bullet go through his neck and come out the other side. He only had soft tissue injuries. The bullet missed all the vital structures. It was truly an amazing wound. He got a bandage on it and left that same afternoon to return to his unit. This was the most miraculous injury I saw the entire time I was over there. The doctors and I had never cared for a luckier soldier. I call this guy my 'miracle soldier,' and I will never forget him or what we saw that day."

Olivia related, "I always provided the best care I could for my patients. I would tell a wounded soldier that he was in American hands, and we were going to take care of him. I would never tell them that they would be 'okay' because that is never something you should tell a severely injured patient, but I would try to allay as much anxiety as possible. I let them know that we were here for them, and we were going to take good care of them. With people who were catastrophically injured, sometimes you get an injury that will blind you, not because of an eye injury but because you are in so much pain that you will lose sight. It is comforting for the dying soldier to know he is not alone and he is being cared for by other Americans who care about him. Even though it was hard, I got some measure of satisfaction being with our troops in their last moments. They would have peace that they knew they died in American hands, and they did not die alone."

Captain Alice

Alice was an active-duty Air Force critical care air transport team (CCATT) nurse. She was assigned to Iraq to care for critically injured patients while being transported aboard aeromedical evacuation aircraft. Alice reported, "More of the air evac missions occurred at night, so I mostly slept during the day and worked at night. We would go check in at the air evac command post to see if anything was going on. Sometimes, critical care patients were added to a flight at the very last moment, and sometimes, you knew about them for a while before you took off to go get them. I flew many missions with lots of stable injured soldiers as well as with CCATT patients onboard. The CCATT patients were so critical, they needed an ICU physician, critical care nurse, and a respiratory therapist just for their care alone. I remember taking care of a soldier who lost three limbs and had other serious chest and abdominal injuries. He was probably the most critical patient I cared for in flight. He was ventilator dependent and receiving lots of antibiotics because his wounds were imbedded with debris from the soil and the IED. We heard his Humvee ran over an IED, and everyone else was killed.

He was in his early 20s and had a strong heart. If he was not in such good physical shape before the blast, he probably wouldn't have survived. I was the CCATT nurse assigned to take care of him. I often think about him and wonder what his life is like now."

Later in 2007, Alice was deployed to Afghanistan as a CCATT nurse. She remarked, "I have some patients that I will never forget. In Afghanistan, we went to Camp Bastion down south near Kandahar, which is a big Marine base. We were picking up some injured marines. We had one marine that was intubated, but he wasn't quite sedated enough. He was not knocked out. He kept asking me where his weapon was, how were his buddies, and how [his squad was] doing. He told me I needed to pull the tube out so he could go back to the firefight. He was actually missing a limb, but he wanted to go back to the fight. The attitude of so many of these injured guys was, 'You['ve] got to let me go back for my troops, I['ve] got to go back to my guys, they need me there.' There was such a strong show of camaraderie with these injured troops that I will never forget. You have to be firm and tell them they can't go back and that they are injured and they are going home. They are defiant because home for them is with their troops. Some cried when told they could not go back. I will always remember their faces and their spirit."

Lieutenant Donna

Donna was an active-duty Navy nurse assigned to the coalition forces hospital in Kandahar, Afghanistan. She described a patient she will never forget. She remembered, "I had a lot of trauma and ICU training. Probably my weakest area was burn care since I just never got the opportunity to care for a lot of burn patients. The services sent the most badly burned soldiers, sailors, airmen, and marines to the Army burn units. The Army always took the lead in burn care. When I was in Iraq, the patient that stands out in my mind the most is a soldier who we responded to in the ER. He looked like he was burnt to a crisp. It was the worst thing I had ever seen. He was still alive when we first started to work on him. We had to crack his chest in the ER and try to revive him, but it didn't work. He was the victim of a blast injury, probably from an IED. To this day, I can close my eyes and remember what he looked like."

Donna recalled another patient care situation etched in her memory. "Another patient I will never forget was an Army captain. He had gone out on his first convoy. It was not something he usually did. It was not his normal job, but he was sent out on this convoy. His truck got hit by an RPG, and the truck rolled down an embankment. None of their injuries was too bad, but they were shaken up. Once they were stabilized, I spent some time talking with them and listening to their stories. We put them all in the same room so they could check on each other and kind of debrief what they had just gone through. We tried to do this with people from the same unit who were not real seriously injured. It helped them to recover. You could see how much they really cared about each other. This group made a big impact on me. The soldier bonding was an incredible thing. They knew they had come very close to losing their lives together. They were a good group. They were appreciative of everything we did for them. It just felt like they were our brothers."

Donna recalled caring for a patient who, with the extent of his injuries, should not have survived. "I had this one patient in pulmonary edema. I could push down on his chest like giving chest compressions, and lots of fluid came out through the ET [endotracheal] tube. It wasn't just foam; it was gushing out. He got wounded while sitting in his Humvee. He had a through-and-through that got him in the ribs then tunneled through his liver and then out the other side. He was very lucky to recover. We lost him about three times but always got him back. He is so lucky to have completely recovered now. He has no deficits whatsoever. He is very lucky because he was so critical. I cared for him for 4 days. I couldn't even leave the bedside because he was so critical. Our chief doctor said I was the primary nurse for this guy. I could take a couple of short naps, but I was to remain at his bedside. I'd have people relieve me so I could take a half-hour or 2-hour nap, but I pretty much was there for 4 days. Today, he is home with his wife. I tracked him through the military evacuation system. I was still in Iraq when he left, but I tracked him to Bethesda Naval Medical Center. I would email the nurses that were caring for him there. I can tell you someone was watching over him on that day, the day he got shot."

Major Alene

Alene was an Army reservist assigned in Mosul, Iraq, during her first deployment and to Bagram, Afghanistan on her second deployment. Alene related, "I joined the Army Reserve during peacetime. I was single at the time and just really wanted to meet people and do something different. I knew it would be extra money, which was good, but I didn't really join because of the money. I really wanted to meet people and expand my social network while at the same time doing something different from the average person. I guess I just wanted another dimension in my life. I guess I felt the Army Reserve would fill a professional and personal void. The thought of deploying to a war never entered my mind back in 1996."

Alene stated, "I'd been a nurse for a long time and thought I had seen just about everything I could see in terms of trauma. I'd cared for lots of gunshot wounds, stabbing victims, car accidents, diving accidents, near drowning, a helicopter crash, house fire victims, and head injuries. When my reserve unit got activated and mobilized for Afghanistan in 2007, I truly believed I was prepared for whatever came to our hospital. I believed that I learned a lot on my earlier deployment to Iraq. Now, I was assigned to the Air Force hospital in Bagram, Afghanistan, augmenting the Air Force critical care nursing staff. There were four other Army Reserve nurses assigned there to help out."

Alene recalled some of the patients she cared for while in Afghanistan. "We had some Afghanis who were in some terrible explosions. This one 20-year-old Afghan national army soldier had lost both his legs, was blind, had both eardrums blown, and severely burned hands, and nobody knew his name. He was not even identifiable, and there was no way to communicate with him. Here we were trying to take care of him. Every time we'd do nursing care, he would just struggle and wrestle because it hurt so much, and he didn't know where he was. I just remember my technician and I, after doing all the dressing changes, trying to think of a way we could communicate care to him. We just started to massage his arms where he was not burned, and he settled down and started crying. We realized there is still a way, and we found one, to communicate love and caring to another human being. He was stable after a while, but then he was transferred back to the Afghan national army hospital. The care there was not very good. They didn't even have trained nurses there, so I didn't offer much hope for him in the long run. Maybe they could find his family, and then maybe they would care for him. However, I just don't know. He was so young."

Major Diana

Diana was an Air Force reservist assigned to the Aeromedical Staging Facility at Balad Air Base, Iraq. She recalled, "Although we weren't flight nurses, we worked in aeromedical staging and also in the ER. Aeromedical staging is when you take care of patients awaiting an aeromedical evacuation flight to another hospital in Iraq or to Landsthul Military Medical Center near Ramstein Air Base, Germany. Occasionally, we had some flights go right from Iraq to the Washington, DC, area and then on to the Brooke Army Burn Center in San Antonio, but that was not a common occurrence. That happened only when there were a lot of severely burned patients at once."

Diana continued, "The scariest thing for me was not knowing what was going to come off the helicopters every night. We never knew what we were going to see as far as injuries, the psychological state the young folks would be in, and most were young boys 18, 19, and 20 years old. You didn't know what they were going to be feeling and how they would be responding to their injuries. It was real[ly] scary for about the first month, until you really got used to what to expect when those helicopters landed. Still, you never really knew if something tragic was going to happen that day. You didn't know if you were going to get a pile of dead bodies coming off that helicopter."

Diana recalled, "Seeing the young kids come in was hard for me. These young troops had gunshot wounds, burns, traumatic amputations, and IED blast injuries. I have a 19-year-old son back home, and these guys were his age. It just tore me up to have to see these kids all mangled, comatose, or missing limbs. I would think about their parents, girlfriends, and what the future would bring these guys."

Diana remembers a special soldier and the psychological and physical toll he endured. "I took care of a soldier who was haunted by guilt feelings from a previous deployment. One night, when he was having trouble sleeping, he confided in me that he felt he was being punished for killing an Iraqi during his last deployment. He said the Iraqi was reaching for something in his knapsack. In a split second, the soldier shot him because he feared the Iraqi was reaching for a weapon. It turned out that the Iraqi was reaching for a card in his knapsack with English phrases on it. He had no weapon. My patient lost both of his legs in a crazy rollover truck accident in southern Iraq. He felt this was his punishment for the shooting."

Diana also recalled the positive attitude expressed by some of the casualties she cared for. "Some injuries were horrible, but some people really lucked out. Some patients, even those seriously injured, had a great attitude, and they appreciated what we did for them. There was this young marine who lost a leg from an IED blast. His name was Ted, and he was 23 years old. When he woke up, all he asked about was his squad of men. He looked down and saw his leg was missing but was only concerned about the fate of his squad. I remember how happy he was a few hours later when three squad members came to visit. It struck me just how these men cared for each other. Ted told me before he was flown out to Germany, 'I'll be fine. None of my guys were killed, and I have six younger brothers and sisters back home that are waiting for me.'I will remember him and his reddish-blonde hair and big blue eyes for the rest of my life. For me, he put a face and a voice on this war."

Amid the carnage of war, Diana could still recount humorous situations in caring for injured soldiers."We got a chance to listen to the soldiers', marines', and airmen's stories. We did whatever little things we could do to try to make a difference in their lives. We got to know some of them really well, and we took pictures of them. One marine comes to mind in particular; his name was Robbie. He had a bad infection in his finger and was on intravenous antibiotics. We called him 'Robbie Finger.' It happened to be his middle finger, too. One time, a general was visiting the hospital, asking all the troops why they were there. Robbie said, 'Sir, I have an infection in my finger' and proceeded to hold up his middle finger for the general. The rest of us just instantly doubled over in laughter. Luckily, the general laughed, too! Some of these guys were really comic relief. Robbie was with us for more than 3 weeks. He helped run errands for us between the ASF and the hospital. He would help us by stocking shelves, mopping floors, and taking patients to X-ray. He would hand out meal trays for other patients and would interact with the other troops. He was a sweet guy and a big help to the nurses at the ASF and hospital. Sometimes, the mood on the unit would be lighter depending on the patients and the severity of injuries. Sometimes, we would have time to joke around with the patients. Robbie would play cards with other patients and had everyone listening to country-western music. He was special."

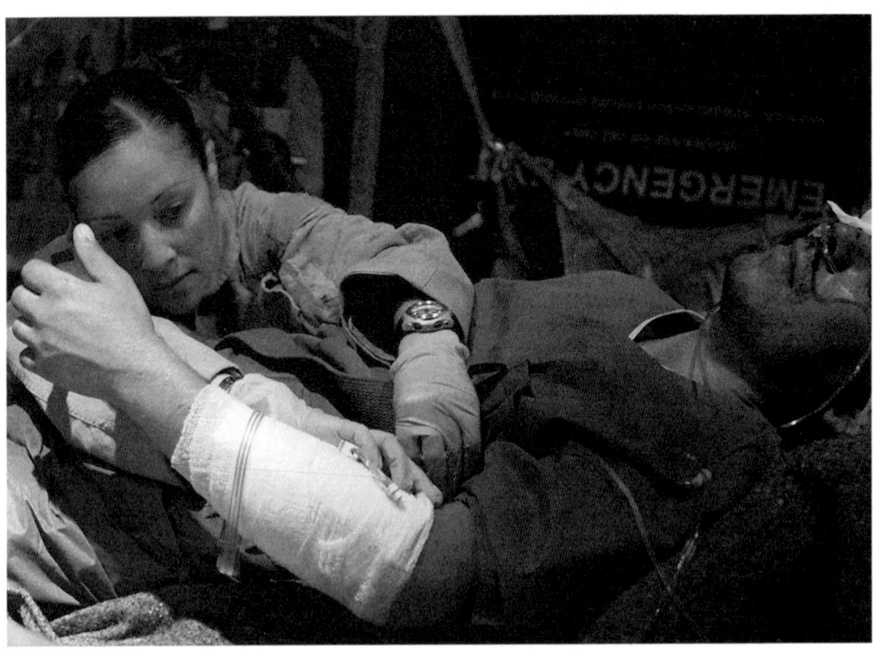

Photo Courtesy of U.S. Air Force.

Injured soldier and nurse on an aeromedical evacuation flight to Germany.

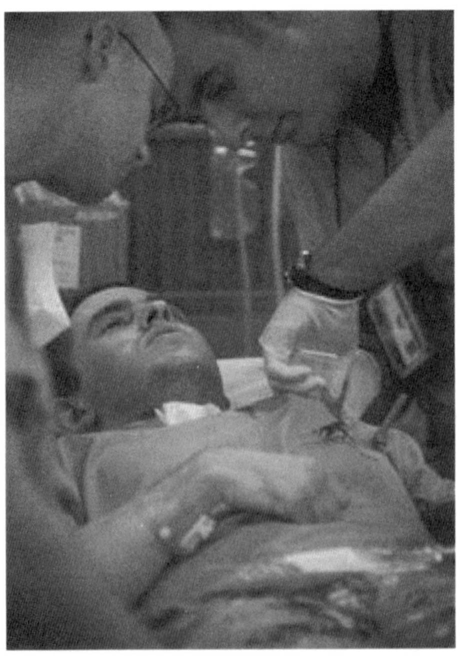

Photo Courtesy of U.S. Air Force.

Injured airmen, Balad Air Base Hospital, Iraq.

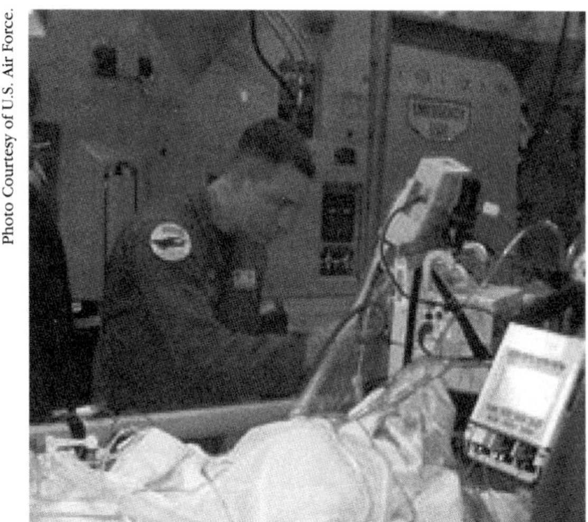

Photo Courtesy of U.S. Air Force.

Flight nurse and critically wounded patient aboard C-17 air evacuation flight.

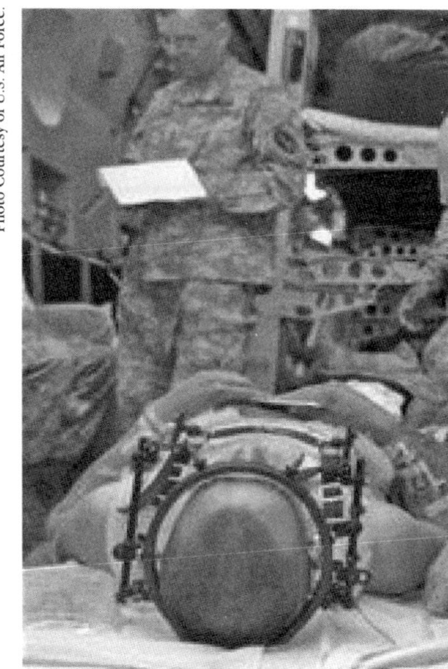

Photo Courtesy of U.S. Air Force.

Injured soldier awaiting air evacuation.

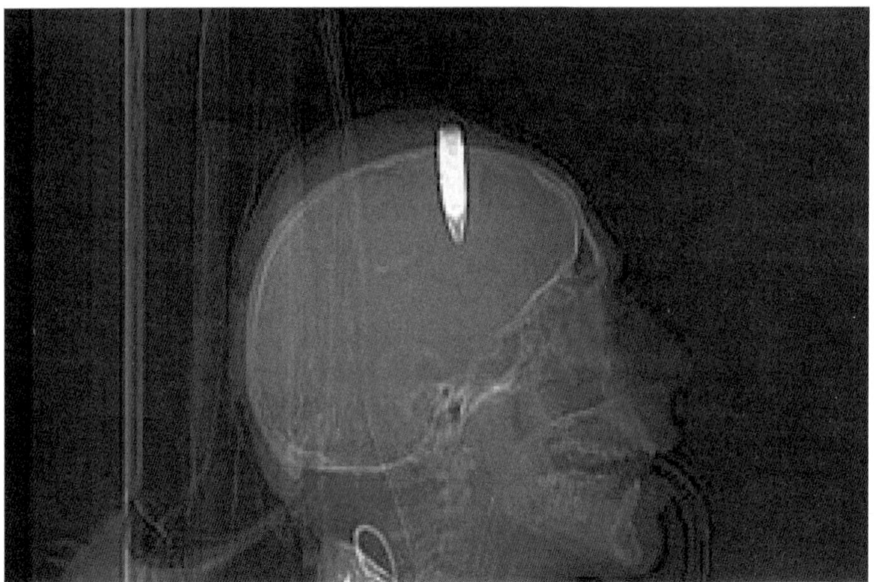

Photo Courtesy of U.S. Air Force.

Unexploded shell penetrating soldier's skull, Iraq.

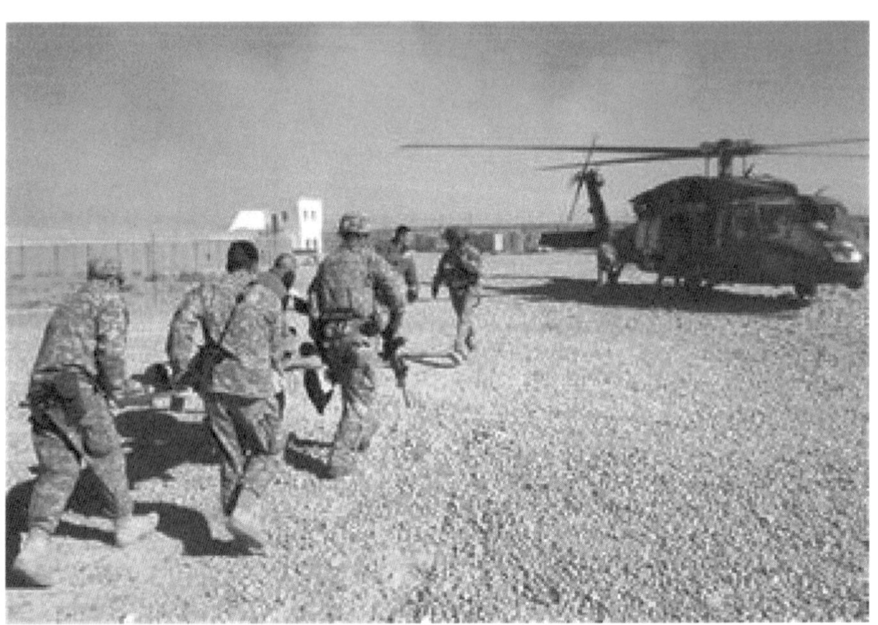

Photo Courtesy of U.S. Air Force.

Wounded soldier moved to Army Blackhawk medical evacuation.

10

Caring for the Enemy

Nurses addressed many issues surrounding the mission of detainee care. Some of these issues included that most medical personnel did not want to do this mission; some feared for their own safety; there were moral and ethical dilemmas surrounding care of the enemy; and detainee-on-detainee violence was commonplace. All of the interviewees who performed detainee care at the Camp Bucca, Camp Cropper, and Abu Ghraib prison hospitals were either active-duty Army or Army reserve nurses. Within Iraq, the Army was tasked with the detainee care mission. Army, Navy, and Air Force nurses all cared for enemy prisoners of war (EPWs) admitted to their hospitals for emergency care, but this was before the EPWs had been moved to detainee care centers. Nurses assigned to the detainee care mission vividly described their environment and situation. It is estimated that less than 5% of the Army reservists and 1% to 2% of active-duty Army nurses were tasked to provide nursing care at the three main detention centers.

Major Derek

Derek, an Army reservist who had assignments at Camp Bucca and Abu Ghraib prison, recalled, "When the terrorist attacks of 9/11/2001 occurred, I had been in the Army Reserve for many years. I was working in a large hospital in New York State. I had always volunteered for special assignments and deployments within my reserve unit but had never been chosen before to deploy. My unit was a very large combat support hospital based in the New York City area. For the Iraq deployment, they needed a large number of people to deploy."

Derek reported, "I didn't learn until I got to the training FOB in Wisconsin what our mission would be in Iraq. I have to admit I was a little surprised and a little disappointed when I learned that we were going to do detainee care. We were the first hospital mobilized, and that was going to be our whole mission. We were trained to take care of coalition troops but were tagged to be taking care of detainees. As I said, I was a little shocked by that and a little disappointed, but it was what it was, and it was no big deal. I was assigned to Camp Bucca, Iraq. The camp was named after one of the New York City firefighters killed on 9/11, and he was an Army reservist. Camp Bucca is the largest detention center in Iraq. It is not that far from Kuwait. About 200 personnel from our unit went to Abu Ghraib prison, and about 100 of us went to Camp Bucca. I was the head nurse on the largest inpatient detainee intermediate care ward of 34 beds. I was there during the troop surge. We were extremely busy. We did not always have enough staff, but overall, I think we did well in view of the circumstances."

Derek related, "One thing about this mission suited my unit well. Many people in my unit were from the New York City area, and we were used to dealing with foreigners. It was not too much of a difference. Working with translators, working with hand signals, having people around from different cultures, we were used to that in New York City hospitals. Our unit was made up of so many immigrants, people of different religions, and different cultures. People in our unit speak many languages. We were well suited for the mission of working so closely with the Iraqi detainees."

None of the nurses was assigned to care for women detainees. Derek explained, "We did not take care of any women detainees. If there were female detainees, they went to Camp Cropper. If they came to us, they would have to be flown in at night, under cover, and we would have to section off a separate area for their care. Culturally and religionwise, having any women was an issue. We would get women in the ER, such as if women were in a vehicle that got blown up or shot up in close proximity to Camp Bucca. However, we would transfer them as soon as we could. We would stabilize them and then try to get them moved out. We would transfer them to a combat support hospital in the green zone. Coalition forces had taken over a private hospital that had been just for Saddam and his soldiers. It had separate floors now for men and women."

Derek stated, "Since we were [providing] detainee care, we also had the opportunity to take care of patients with medical emergencies. We took care of folks with heart attacks. One guy that was a particularly interesting case had renal failure, and we actually did peritoneal dialysis on him. When I was transferred to Abu Ghraib prison from Camp Bucca, we had a very busy intensive care unit (ICU) up there. We had an 8-bed ICU that could expand to 12 beds. About 90% of the time, our ICU beds were full. We took care of a lot of acute trauma patients with blast injuries, gunshot wounds, traumatic amputations, and burns."

Derek further commented, "We had one burn patient when I arrived at Abu Ghraib. He was still there 10 months later when I left. He had burns over 50% of his body. In a combat zone, usually, anything over 40% burns, you are not going to make it. We kept him alive the whole time we were there, but I understand from nurses who were there after us that he died after we left. Every night I was on, he was one of my patients. I'd spend about an hour debriding his burns every night. I'd medicate him because he was in a lot of pain, and then I'd clip his dead skin off his burns."

Captain Vanessa

Vanessa, an Army reservist, was assigned to detainee care. She reported, "We were sent to Abu Ghraib detainee hospital in Iraq. When I knew where we were going, the reports about Abu Ghraib had previously not been good. I thought, 'What was I going to do if I saw evidence of torture? What was I going to do in a war zone if I saw people being hurt? Moreover, what was my responsibility? Was my responsibility to my license, my ethics, or to my Army peers?' I almost went to the commander and said, 'You don't want me on this mission'. I'm a nurse, and if anyone gets in the way of my job, there is going to be a problem. I'm not going to back off of my ethics. No one is going to change that. It is the one thing I have in my life that I have always adhered to. The Army has core values: honor, integrity, self-sacrifice, and courage. Therefore, I decided not to say anything, and I went over there. I actually wrote an article about my worries, and it was published. It was called 'A Letter from Iraq.' I tried to talk about my worries of discovering torture and how you are supposed to handle it. I had discussed this with my chief nurse in a meeting with other people. The Army says if you see it, you are supposed to report it, and that is very clear."

Vanessa further reported, "When I went to Abu Ghraib, we had a very busy ICU. We took care of acute blast injuries, gunshot wounds, traumatic amputations, and burns. Since we were providing detainee care, we also had detainees with heart attacks, renal failure, and the like. No one wanted to do the detainee care mission. We were afraid of them, and I think if we had a choice ahead of time, we would have all left."

Vanessa went on to report that she encountered a few instances or situations where she felt appreciated by some detainees. She recalled, "There were small moments with the detainees that were heartwarming, things that I'll always remember. We had patients who were there for months. You got to know them. They laughed with us. They would try to teach us songs. One medic was a barber. One night, he brought in his buzzer and clippers and gave all the patients haircuts. The war was going on, but we were singing and smiling in our little hospital. We were a mix of nationalities, but we were all part of humanity. I played my recorder for the patients, and they really liked it."

Vanessa related, "Many of these young guys were so badly injured, it was like their lives were over or at least drastically changed. Dressing change time was a big deal. We had so many wound dressings to change every day. Some of the detainees were quadriplegics and paraplegics. We had many amputees. We had one young man who had both arms and both legs amputated. He was with us for a long time. He was driving a truck that rode over a bomb and went up. When we first got him, he had one leg left, but it had to be amputated later. We tried to save his last leg. He was failing due to infection, so we had to take the leg off. He got healthier as the infection subsided."

Vanessa described how the military police (MP) and the hospital staff worked together. "In the prison ICU, we had all these ventilators, and the patients were tied down. We had no potable water. At the end of the hallway is an MP with a weapon to protect us. The MPs sometimes helped us at the bedside to turn patients and lift patients who could not help themselves. You'd see the MPs every day, and we got to know them. Together with the MPs and our hospital staff, I think we did the best we could to make sure that the detainees got the care they needed."

Lieutenant Colonel Victoria

Victoria, a seasoned Army nurse assigned to detainee care, remarked, "I was an experienced Army nurse serving my second tour in Iraq. Having had a little detainee care experience on my first deployment, I think the second time around allowed me to have more empathy for my staff. Detainee care is a very difficult mission. My staff at Camp Bucca was very disheartened that they were assigned to do detainee care. I was the assistant chief nurse. I would bounce back and forth between the ER and the ICU. I was everywhere. I was the senior-ranking person there under the chief nurse, so if she went out to the field, I was the acting chief nurse at that site."

Victoria continued, "The hospital was surrounded by 34 compounds. This mobile trailer had been extended and extended and extended right in the middle of all these compounds. Each compound had 3,600 detainees, and they would move them around. We were not supposed to know why they were there. However, they would talk too much, or the guards would tell us, or somehow we would find out. Therefore, that was very unpleasant for us. Because of this and being far into the war, most of us knew someone who was injured or killed. It was very challenging for me and my staff to accomplish the detainee mission."

Victoria went on to report, "This was not the normal kind of nursing that we do at home. Even when I worked in the burn unit in Texas, I would get some kind of feedback from the patient or the family. It was a very challenging type of nursing, but feedback would motivate me to put in another 12 hours. With this type of patient population, there was no feedback. They hated our guts and wanted to kill us. Very few would say, 'Thank you, thank you, I want to move to America.' Most would act as if we owed it to them to take care of them. It was very challenging. I tried to reiterate to staff that we were not only there as nurses, but also, we were diplomats. This was a very different type of nursing than we will ever do. The culture over there is for men. Their mothers take care of them until they get married. Therefore, they thought we were there to take care of them and do everything for them. I was very glad the guards were there. They could keep us centered, and we would keep them centered. They would get frustrated, too. Most of these guys were SOBs. Before I left, we had started to take death row detainees. I was very proud of my staff and how professional they were."

Captain Holly

Holly was an Army reservist from New Jersey. She had worked in civilian hospitals in New Jersey, New York, and Connecticut for about 15 years. She joined an Army Reserve combat support hospital because several of her friends from work had joined. Holly wanted to be part of an organization that made a difference. She believed that the Army Reserve made a difference in people's lives during peacetime, natural and manmade disasters, and war. Holly belonged to a large combat support hospital from the greater New York City area. Her unit was mobilized to provide detainee care in Iraq.

Holly found the detainee care mission difficult. She recalled, "I found what we had to do was horrible because of having to feel like you are splitting yourself. You are taking care of people who are the enemy. I tried not to think about the person and what he may have done or didn't do. I tried to concentrate on procedures, the specific procedures we had to do on these patients. Put in the IV line, debride the burns, change the dressing, whatever. Do that procedure. Make sure they are taken care of medically. That way, I didn't have to get involved with their life. I would also have to go over to the ER and help with mass casualties."

Holly added, "We trained for 4 months before we went to Iraq. We were trained on how to handle detainee personnel and how to protect ourselves. However, once I was there, at no time did I feel threatened. Some were arrested and later cleared and let go. Others were arrested, and they were probably guilty, but I never felt threatened at all. Based on the training, we were prepared to be threatened by the prisoners. However, I never did feel in jeopardy. We were told we would never have to do body searches; the MPs would do that. We were very clear that our role was to provide medical care. There was still the scar of what military personnel had done at Abu Ghraib prison in 2003 and 2004. The Department of Defense had invested a lot of time and money to ensure that people assigned to detainee care were prepared going in. I think the military has done a good job with the training for folks taking care of detainees. The military also did a good job of making sure that detainees' rights were protected. They made sure that we, as medical personnel, did not have to cross that line as combatants. In the military, you are always a soldier first. The medical people always walk a fine line. We are going to take care of everybody who needs care. That is what we are trained to do. Even though, as medics, we still have soldier skills, we really are not there to use them unless we absolutely have to."

Nurses reported that detainee-on-detainee violence was commonplace in the prison compounds at Abu Ghraib and Camp Bucca, Iraq. Holly elaborated, "We would have mass casualty events from incidents that happened in the prison. A couple of times, there was a riot among the detainees. Sometimes, it was Sunni-Shiite. Other times, it was just that something upset someone and started a riot. Sometimes, the guards had to use rubber bullets. We actually had one detainee die from a head injury when he was hit over the head by another detainee. Another time, one older detainee, we used to call them 'hodgees' because they had gone on the hajj [the Islamic pilgrimage to Mecca], was attacked by a tribe of five guys while he was sleeping. They each took a limb, and they twisted him. He came in with fractures in all his limbs in several places. There was one leg that we could get a blood pressure on. He ended up losing the other leg. It was so sad. He was in such severe pain. They had tortured their own countryman.

Holly continued, "The detainees weren't always fighting each other. Most just prayed, did their laundry, read their prayer book, and stayed peaceful. The guys who weren't going along with the program and cooperating went to hut #6, which was like maximum security. The detainees would beat each other up all the time. They would sodomize each other all the time. It was disgusting, really disgusting, and the cultural stuff was really challenging. We would try to have an understanding and work with the guards and the interpreters. We would tell them, 'We'll respect your culture, but you also have to respect ours.' It was very hard on our staff. We felt like prisoners there, and nobody wanted to do this mission! For me, there wasn't any type of positive feedback mechanism with the patients. Number one, you didn't trust them, and number two, you didn't want to have any relationship with them. It was a very hard mission that we were asked to do."

Holly also reported that she believed some detainees appreciated the medical personnel. She stated, "Some of the detainees really appreciated us because we were medical. They saw a difference between the nonmedical forces and us. They didn't relate to us as enemies, and we didn't relate to them as enemies, because they were injured. We tried to help them get better, and they appreciated that. That part went very well. They were not only injured; some were sick. Some had diabetes, asthma, infections, renal failure, and anything you would see in medical patients."

Holly stated that even though detainee care was a tough mission, and even though most nurses were disappointed, upset, and stressed with the detainee mission, there were some special patients. Holly recalled a special patient she still wonders about. "There was this one 17-year-old who was a paraplegic. I took care of him for months. He was like my baby. He was not doing well physically, and he was very depressed. He didn't want to eat. He had a suprapubic catheter. He didn't want to believe the doctors that he would never walk again. He was getting thinner and thinner. He was beginning to waste away. He looked like he could go downhill and just die. When I worked the night shift, food would be brought to us because we couldn't leave the hospital. I would give him ice cream and chicken. I'd get him to eat fried chicken, and he liked it. I'd wake him up and give him the foods he liked. He started to gain weight."

Holly related that detainees got quality care given the circumstances. She exclaimed, "I think I did my best there for the detainees. We didn't know what they had done to get there. Most of them were just swept up in raids. They might have been in the wrong place at the wrong time. However, that didn't hold a lot of water. They were detainees, and you had to give them medical care without knowing their history. You didn't know their story. You had to ask questions through a translator, and everybody was tied down. These were not the best circumstances, but we didn't let it get in the way of providing quality care. I am proud of my unit for meeting the challenge of this very difficult mission. I know lives have been saved because of the care we provided."

Captain Olivia

Olivia was an Army reservist assigned to a coalition combat support hospital in Mosul, Iraq. She would receive critically injured EPWs in her

ICU. Olivia described the burden she felt in caring for EPWs during the beginning of the war. "In Iraq, our ICU had 36 ICU beds. We went there thinking we'd take care of injured kids and civilians as well as soldiers. However, one third of my ICU was designated to take care of Iraqi EPWs and local civilians. Most of the time, even if we shoot them up, we'll take care of them. Our staff was very angry about this, but we had the best staff of all. We embraced that role that no one else wanted. It allowed us to make the best of a bad situation. The more something sucked, the happier we were with it. That's what really brings out the best in people, when you challenge them and put them in unusual circumstances. We'd get these Iraqis in, and they thought we were going to kill them. They'd think they were going to be interrogated and then killed. By the time they left the hospital after we took care of them, they'd want to smoke a cigarette with us and would be joking with us. This was very early on in the war. They were still happy with us there. They left the hospital knowing we were the good guys and we were not going to hurt them. We honestly changed their lives."

Olivia further described the illnesses and injuries they encountered in caring for EPWs. "The Marines brought in some insurgents who were injured. They were treated the same as our forces who were injured. We treated even enemy patients with respect and gave them whatever care they needed. Our medical folks provide care to whoever needs it. If we had Iraqi troops on our wards or in our ICU, if an insurgent came in, the Iraqi troops got more upset than the Americans caring for them. What our translators would basically say to the Iraqi troops was that this was the American way and that the worse injured get taken care of first, even if it is the enemy."

Olivia shared a story about one of the EPWs. "I was taking care of two EPWs who were brothers. They were both shot at a security checkpoint. The less injured brother said to our translator, 'Look at the loving care she is showing my brother. I don't understand this. How can she do this? Her country is fighting with us. How can she do this?' That situation stuck with me because I educated him today. He learned something about Americans that day. The EPW put his hand on his heart and thanked me in Iraqi. He then understood that we are not there to try to hurt them; we are trying to help them. Yes, there was a moment he understood that we were not there to hurt him."

Olivia also wondered what the eventual fate of these EPW patients would be. Many of them were teenage boys or in their early 20s. Olivia recalled, "With the prisoners, we addressed every infection. When they were released, we wondered what they were going back to. What kind of care would they get? They would probably get no care. Many of them would probably die. I couldn't imagine when they went home that they would find adequate care in this war-torn country. It took three or four people to do the burn care three times a day. When they left, we believed many would get infected and die."

Captain Richard

Richard, an active-duty Army nurse assigned to the Detainee Center Hospital at Camp Bucca, Iraq, described measures MP guards had to take with detainees to provide security for everyone. Richard recalled, "We had insurgent patients. We had to keep them blindfolded in certain areas, and we had military police watching them all the time. They were always trying to take their blindfolds off. We had guards in every area. The detainees who were in the hospital, if they had four limbs, they had leather straps on one arm and on one leg. One day, I was working in the ICU. We had this one detainee who was a victim of detainee-on-detainee violence. He had two fractured elbows and two broken legs, and he couldn't feed himself. He couldn't do anything. He's strapped to the bed, and I'm trying to feed him. He is hollering at me. Finally, I put the plate down. Our orthopedic surgeon was standing behind me, observing my frustration. I turned to him and said, 'Nutrition is too highly overrated anyway!' Some of the detainees were so grateful for whatever we did for them, but not this guy in the ICU. I told the interpreter to tell this detainee that when he makes up his mind that he wants to eat, someone will be back to feed him. I knew what our junior staff was going through because I couldn't have any more patience for this guy and his antics."

First Lieutenant Lisa

Lisa was an Army reservist assigned in the ICU at the coalition hospital in Mosul, Iraq. She related, "We took care of insurgents occasionally in our ICU. We would partition them away from our coalition forces patients. We would have military police guards watching them, and they would usually have leather restraints on two extremities. If they were missing a limb, they would have at least one restraint. Some of these guys were in terrible shape. They usually didn't get to medical care as quick as the injured coalition forces. Many insurgents had burns, traumatic amputations, gunshot wounds, and some were peppered with shrapnel. A lot of them were young men in their late teens or early 20s. Most were too injured to give us any trouble. The guards ended up helping us lift and turn these guys during dressing changes."

Major Alene

Alene was an Army reservist assigned to the emergency room and medical-surgical units at the coalition forces hospital in Mosul, Iraq. Alene reported, "Whenever we got insurgents or suspected insurgents brought in to our ER, it made me very nervous. I would watch carefully as the military policemen conducted a body search because I always feared these guys had a hidden weapon when they were brought in. I saw more than one knife taken away right in our triage area outside the ER."

11

Children Caught in the Chaos of War

One of the elements of war that nurses reported as most troubling for them was the carnage inflicted on the children of Iraq and Afghanistan. Most reported caring for far more children than they expected. Some felt ill prepared for the volume and severity of pediatric injuries. Nurses reported empathy toward the children and outrage at the injuries inflicted on them.

Children were injured in these wars by accidentally stepping on land mines or by being shot at military checkpoints when they were traveling in a car that refused to stop, or simply because they were at the wrong place at the wrong time. Some children were injured at the hands of abusive fathers or by parental neglect. Parents were not always watchful when their children were playing near stoves or on building roofs when the houses became oppressively hot in the summertime. Some children were wounded when they picked up unexploded ordinance. Others became critically ill by accidentally drinking poisonous substances, like solvents or petroleum products stored in their homes.

Captain Olivia

Olivia was an Army reservist who was assigned to the intensive care unit (ICU) at the coalition forces hospital in Mosul, Iraq. Olivia recalled that she and her colleagues were initially surprised at the number of children who were injured in the chaos of the war.

Olivia told of two pediatric cases that particularly touched her heart. "We had one little boy for months. Apparently, his father had been painting and had a propane heater in the house. Somehow, the kid knocked over the heater, and it exploded. The boy had third-degree burns that just covered his body. The family was trying to care for him at home, and he was actively dying. He had no antibiotics. The Marines were doing a house-by-house search and found this little kid. They radioed back to us for permission to bring him in. We told them, 'absolutely.' Once we got him, he quickly became the most spoiled Iraqi child in the world. He got ice cream all the time once he came off hyperalimentation. The Marines who found him would bring him video games and toys."

Olivia described how an Iraqi orphan baby brightened the spirits of the nurses at Christmas. She recalled, "We had a child come to us. It was around Christmas time. There were a few of us who were moms with little babies at home in our group. Well, the story was that this little baby girl had been lost, and some Marines found her. They had hoped to find her parents. It was the strangest thing how this baby really made our Christmas for us. We were able to care for her, and at the same time, she filled a void for us. It was a positive experience. She had been injured, and they couldn't find anyone to take care of her. They didn't know who her guardians were. The Marines had brought her in, and we cared for her over the holidays. Her injuries were relatively minor compared to those we usually saw at our hospital. I'd love to know what happened to her and where she is now. It would be great to know. I'll always remember that precious little baby girl."

Captain Marie

Marie was an Army reservist with pediatric, emergency room (ER), and ICU experience. During her 12-month deployment, she was assigned to the hospital at Balad Air Base, then to the coalition hospital in Mosul, and finally, to the new combat support hospital in Anbar Province, Iraq. Marie reported being shocked at the violence, which was often directed toward children. She stated, "I remember we got seven children in at the same time because they were playing soccer and someone threw a mortar onto the soccer field. Our ER was filled with these children with blast injuries. I thought to myself, 'Who would do such a thing? It was obviously an angry, hateful, crazy person.' This action set me back a bit. It was hard for me. It made me sad and angry at the same time. When I was first deployed, I never thought that some of my patients would be children. Then the very next day, I took care of a little girl who was shot in the head when a bullet went through a window in her house. I remember thinking, 'Was this just a random bullet, or was it meant for the little girl just like the mortar that was thrown on the soccer field?' These incidents were a real wake-up call for me. They made me realize the brutality of war and the complete disregard for human life and the insanity of it all."

Captain Erin

An active-duty Air Force flight nurse assigned at Balad Air Base, Iraq, and later in her career at Bagram Air Base, Afghanistan, told of her pediatric experiences. "I took care of many burned children. Afghans used a kerosene type of kettle to heat up their rice. Children would catch themselves on fire. Some ended up 70% burned. I'll remember them for the rest of my life." *She added,* "Blood doesn't bother me, because I used to be an emergency room nurse. What bothered me was transporting injured children who had been shot or blown up or burned on our air evac plane. It really got to me, transporting 3-year olds to the combat support hospital to have exploratory surgery to find out where all the shrapnel was in their little bellies. This was the collateral damage of war. There was more than one of these kids whom I don't want to even think about. There were innocent women and children blown up in cars by roadside bombs and old people blown up and burned. The insurgents had no morals, no ethics. Soldier against soldier, I have no problem with. However, blowing up innocent people just for the sake of killing as many people as you can was horrendous, indiscriminate killing. The primitive living conditions added to the injuries and deaths of little children. Kids were injured by the kerosene stoves, the unexploded ordinance in the areas near their homes, and sometimes by abusive parents."

Captain Abby

Some nurses reported struggling with the moral dilemmas imposed by war nursing priorities. Abby was an active-duty Air Force nurse assigned to Bagram Air Base, Afghanistan. She shared, "I might be taking care of an injured child in one bed, and the guy who blew the child up was in the opposite bed. If an insurgent has more critical injuries than the U.S. Marine, or the injured child, the insurgent goes to the operating room first. That may not be what you want to do, but that's the way it is. That is triage priorities." *She added,* "It was very stressful for me in the first few days because not only was I working with ventilated patients, but my first patient was a pediatric burn patient. In terms of how prepared I was, I would say very poorly. Just because I had experience working with conscious sedation patients in my background did not prepare me as a good candidate to work in the ICU or with pediatric patients, but I learned quickly."

Abby continued, "I worked a lot with pediatric patients in Afghanistan. Most of these were head injuries because they had fallen off the roof of their homes. I understand that it gets very hot at nighttime, and they go up on top of their roofs. The kids aren't well supervised, so they fall off, giving way to head injuries and fractured arms and legs. It is a bad situation. I took care of a lot of them. I also took care of many burned children. They use a kerosene type of kettle. They heat up their rice in this contraption. I don't know what it is called, but it uses kerosene. The children would go light it, and they would catch themselves on fire. Even though the policy, I was told, was that we were not supposed to accept patients with greater than 30% of their body surface area burned, apparently, there were numerous cases where we took in children who had more than a 30% burn."

Abby went on to share information about one of her young patients. "I can give you the details of this one child, who was 3 years old, and he was hospitalized for the entire 4 months I was in Afghanistan. We took him to the operating room at least twice a week trying to graft his burns. They wouldn't take. Our resources were running slim, and at this point, the plastic surgeon determined that we should just discharge the patient after the fourth month. We sent him home with a feeding tube. The father ended up putting henna herb on this child's body, and he developed an infection. I heard he died about 2 weeks after being discharged from the hospital. I took care of this child numerous times. He had fallen into an oven. He was burned from the bottom of his feet to the top of his head. Every part of this child was completely burned. I couldn't believe he survived. It was one-on-one care. His care was mentally taxing, and I especially realized that after I came home. I remember all the hours we put into this child. We did not have all the resources in theater. If we were able to air evac this child to Germany, his chances for survival would have been a little higher. It was hard for me. You just pour your heart and soul into the care, hoping that he is going to come out okay, but it didn't work out that way. I'll remember him for the rest of my life."

Lieutenant Donna

Donna, a Navy nurse assigned to the combat support hospital in Kandahar, reported that safety measures were very lax in Afghanistan. "They don't use seat belts with their kids. They put kerosene in drinking water bottles. The kids accidently drink them. Stuff like that happens all the time. You have a brain-dead baby in the ICU, and you are trying to explain to the parents that it's really a bad idea to put kerosene in the drinking water bottles. The parents can't understand why you can't save the baby, because you're an American, and you can fix anything. Just multiply this by a thousand times, and that's their daily lives. It's just life for them."

Major Lee

Many nurses could not help but get attached to the children they cared for. Lee, an Air Force reservist assigned to Balad Air Base, Iraq, stated,

"The Iraqi children were absolutely gorgeous with their darkened skin, big brown eyes, and broad smiles," *She recalled,* "There was a little baby that had lost both of her parents. She kind of became our adopted child at the hospital for about 2 weeks till we could find out where her relatives were and we could send her back to them. We pretty much carried this baby around with us everywhere we went because she cried when we put her down. One of the civilian contractors wanted to adopt her so bad, but these children were not allowed to be adopted. He was brokenhearted because he sincerely wanted to take her home and adopt her. She would sit and play with him. You could tell she felt secure with him."

Major Samantha

Samantha was an active-duty Army nurse at the Joint Service Hospital at Bagram Air Base, Afghanistan. She stated, "I remember this little girl who we called 'Peanut.' Boiling water got poured on the anterior part of her abdomen and on her poor little hands. I don't even think she was 2 years old yet. Her hands were completely scorched. I mean, they were eschar tissue. That's how bad it was; her hands were gonna fall off on their own. The father came in, and he was with the Afghan police. You didn't see mothers around that often unless they were accompanied by a male elder. That's another thing that took me by surprise culturally. The fathers were Muslim and the authority figure. We pretty much had to say, 'Hey, listen, your child is going to die. You might want to tell your wife to come by and pay her last respects to her child before we withdraw the ventilator and care.' We had to have their permission, obviously, and we'd get the father's permission. Usually, the mothers would come in a day later and hold the child. The doctors would tell the parents what would happen in a few minutes. Just to see the mothers and their reactions was so sad. It was just so sad, just so horrible."

Captain Liz

Some nurses recounted how difficult it was for them to take care of injured children. Liz was an active-duty Air Force flight nurse who served tours of duty in Iraq and Afghanistan. Liz sometimes augmented the ICU staff for a day or two when she was not scheduled to fly a mission. She recalled, "It was tough with the children. I remember walking in my first day, and there was this little girl in the bed. I was getting my orientation to the ICU. Every time I walked by the bed, I wouldn't look at the little girl, because I had a little girl the same size back home. I said to myself, 'You've got to get over this and get a hold of yourself.' After a couple of hours, I asked about the little girl. The other nurses said she had been shot and she was doing well now. It was just unnerving for me, kids being shot."

Liz continued, "Another patient we got was a child who had the whole right side of his face blown off. He had picked up a grenade, and it had exploded. We were able to do surgery on him, but we had trouble finding further care for him. The civilian children's hospital in Kuwait wouldn't take him, because they wouldn't take any Iraqi patients. We finally got the patient accepted by a pediatric plastic surgeon who was only in Kuwait for a surgical conference. He convinced the Kuwait authorities to make an exception because it was a critically injured child. He was able to save this child's life."

Commander Josie

Some nurses, especially those assigned in Afghanistan, reported children and other locals being injured by mine blast explosions. Josie, a career Navy nurse assigned to mentoring duty at the National Afghan Army Hospital in Mazer-e-Sharif, explained, "In Afghanistan, when the Soviet Union pulled out in the early 1990s, they left a lot of minefields behind. They didn't clean things out on the air base. They actually planted mines so the Afghans couldn't use the airfield for their gain. You'd have these kids going out in these minefields collecting scrap metal to turn in for money. They'd step on a land mine or they'd be playing games in the field when it happened. We would actually end up dealing with quite a larger pediatric population in the trauma unit because of these land mines."

Captain Suzanne

Suzanne was an active-duty Air Force nurse assigned in Iraq. She shared some of the challenging and troubling situations she encountered. "We did lots of surgeries on local people and even children caught up in the gunfire and the bombings. One time, the Iraqis had taken two women and three children, strapped a propane tank to the front of a car, and put these people in the car. They had the car go toward the Marine checkpoint. The car did not stop, so the Marines opened fire on them. One woman and a child died right away. We worked on the others, but the baby also died. These kinds of casualties were especially tough to understand. They were innocent people killed by their own countrymen."

Suzanne further reported, "One patient experience stands out in my mind. It was about a young boy who comes in, and our guards didn't know whether to help this child. The guards were concerned about IEDs on suicide bombers, but it was a child begging for help, and the child was hurt. They decided at the time not to help the child because another child was involved similarly in killing their fellow soldier with an IED under his clothing. Situations like that are unforgettable."

Major Vivian

Nurses reported that getting acclimatized to cultural differences in Iraq and Afghanistan sometimes added to the stress. Major Vivian, an Air Force reservist and critical care nurse assigned to Iraq and later in Afghanistan, commented on her experience. "We had so many children come in with lice. We spent a great amount of time doing lice treatments on kids in the ICU. I felt this was not our job. There was no way we'd be doing this back in the States. It was a huge burden. One time, we had this family come in. I think we had bombed their village in a very remote area. It was probably in the Afghan mountains. I remember this one little girl. She did not know how to use a toilet. I saw her climb on top of the toilet. I had to call the custodian people to come in there and clean. I could not believe my eyes. I could not believe what I had seen. I guess she was used to a hole in the ground. I guess she had never seen a toilet before. It was sad, but it was one more thing you had to do in your day."

Vivian continued, "When I was assigned in Iraq, we had one little boy come in. He had gotten shot in the head with what I think was a stray bullet. He was shot straight down into the head. No one had heard the sound of the shot. The father didn't even realize that he had been shot until the son fell and they saw the blood coming from his head. He came into our ICU, but there was nothing we could do for him. They didn't even want to send him to the coalition forces hospital that had neurosurgeons. We just shut off the ventilator, gave him some morphine, and then he died. The family had been at some type of fair that evening. They were out on the streets in the village where they lived. Seeing the father cry for his son and pray for him was so tough. The father said this was okay. This was what Allah wanted. This was an example of the cultural differences and the violence that was happening over there. So often this happened to families who had nothing to do with the war fighting."

Vivian remembered, "As the weeks went on, we got more and more local people coming to us for care. One time, a woman brought us her 9-year-old son and tried to tell us that he had leukemia. Well, we were a surgical hospital. We had to tell her we couldn't help her."

Vivian went on further to describe nurse participation in humanitarian outreach missions in local villages as well as intervention when told about medical situations soldiers encountered when on patrol. She explained, "If the Marines or the soldiers were out in a neighborhood and saw something wrong, like injured children, who were being tended to by the families and not getting better or getting progressively worse, we would provide care for them." *She added,* "We made a difference over there. We helped a lot of people besides our own troops and coalition forces. We really cared about the little kids. They were special. You bring this little grubby kid in, and you give him a bath and wash his hair. You clean him up a bit and try to give him a quality of life he's never had. The interpreters came to our commander to tell him about a 2-month-old child who was dying. They had brought him to an Iraqi hospital, and the doctors there said there was nothing they could do for him. The interpreters said, 'Since you take care of so many people, can we bring the baby in?' It turned out he had Sprue; all we had to do was change the baby's formula, and he began thriving. The interpreters still get pictures from the parents of how big and beautiful this baby is. There is a Christmas card one of our surgeons used. It was a picture of him standing next to this baby after about a month of being with us and getting stronger and growing."

The nurses witnessed some terrible injuries inflicted on children, and some of those children died. Other children lived but faced an uncertain future as they returned with their families to live in primitive villages without the aid of modern medical care. Vivian summarized the sentiments of many in providing care to the children of Iraq and Afghanistan caught in the crossfire of war. "Sometimes, you have to be numb to it all. Just go to work, and do what you have to do."

Photo Courtesy of U.S. Air Force.

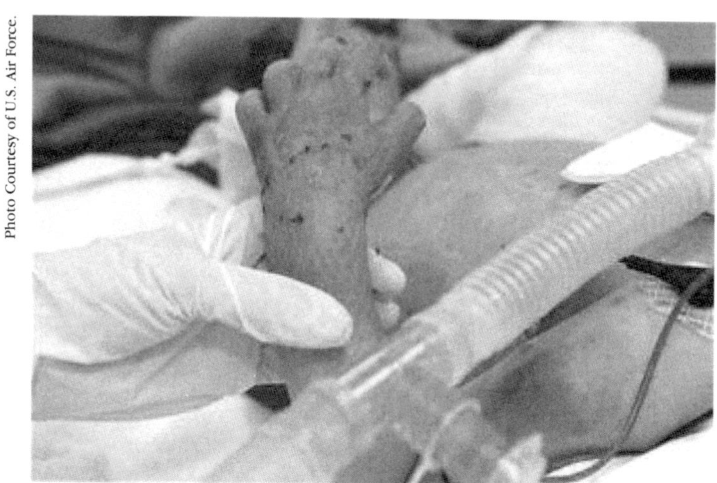

Iraqi child in Balad Air Base ICU.

Photo Courtesy of U.S. Air Force.

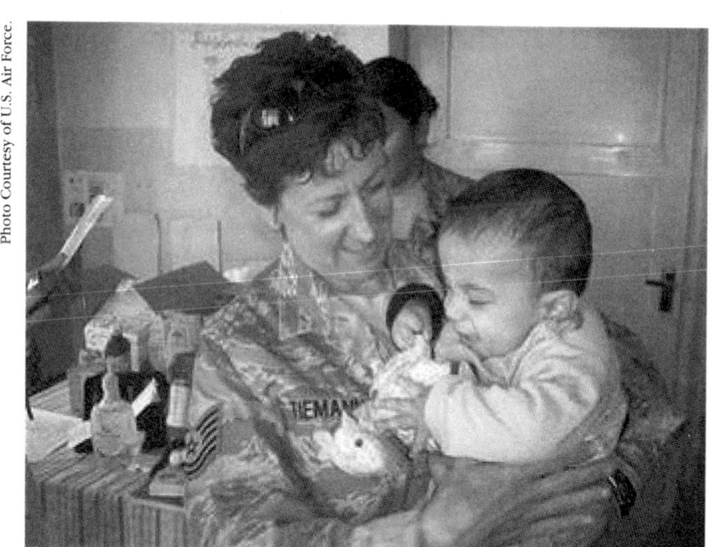

Afghan child with medical technician.

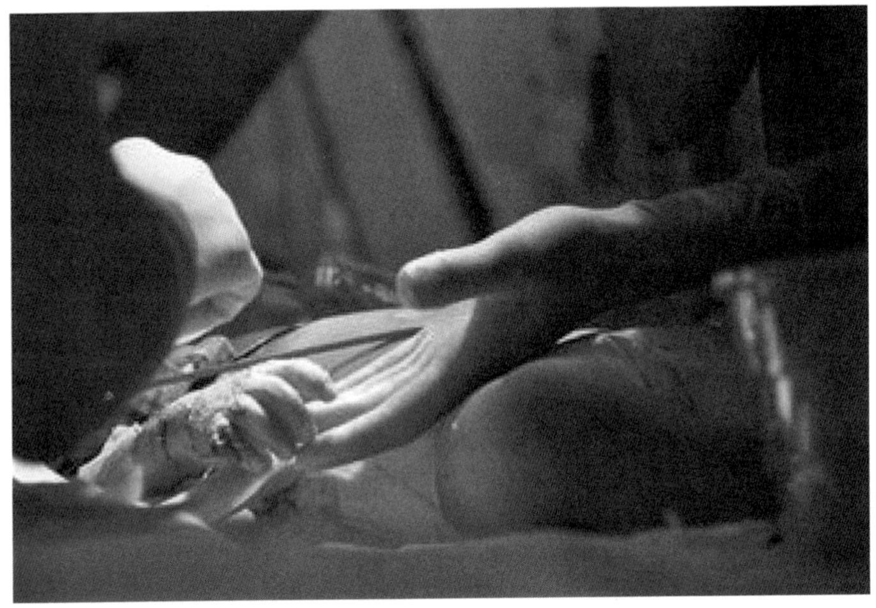

Photo Courtesy of U.S. Air Force.

Nurse holds hand of burned child in Iraq ICU.

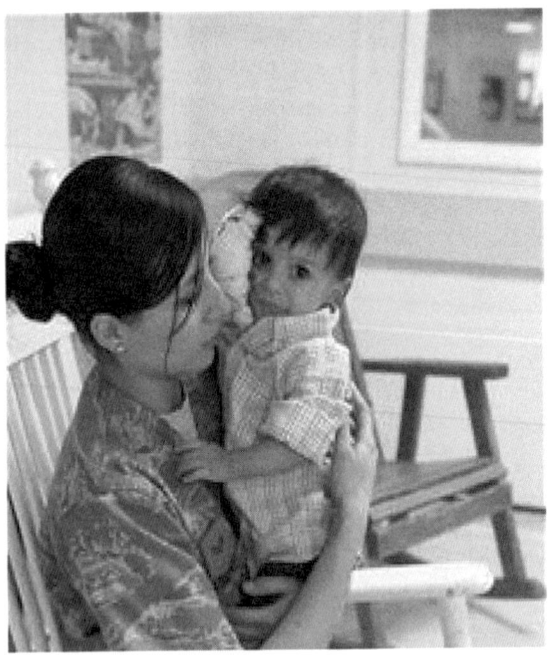

Photo Courtesy of U.S. Air Force.

Medical technician and injured Afghan child.

Photo Courtesy of U.S. Air Force.

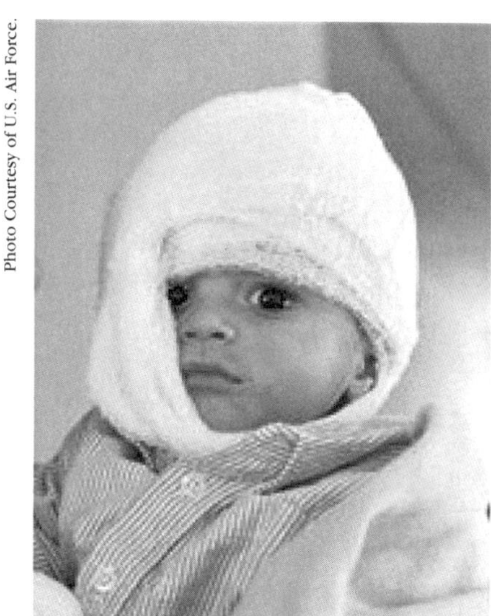

Injured boy, Balad Air Base hospital, Iraq.

Photo Courtesy of U.S. Air Force.

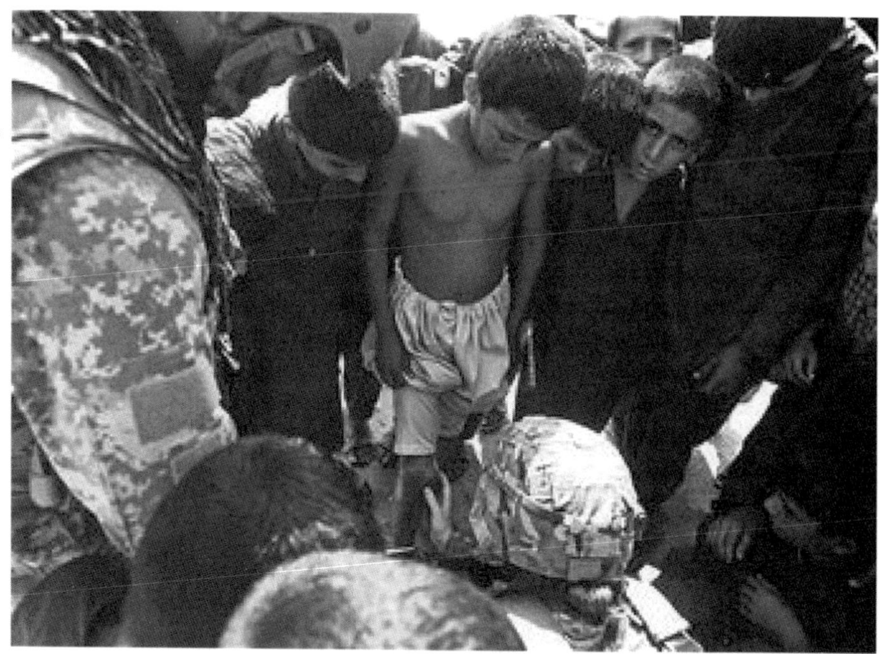

Injured boy examined by Air Force medic, Afghanistan.

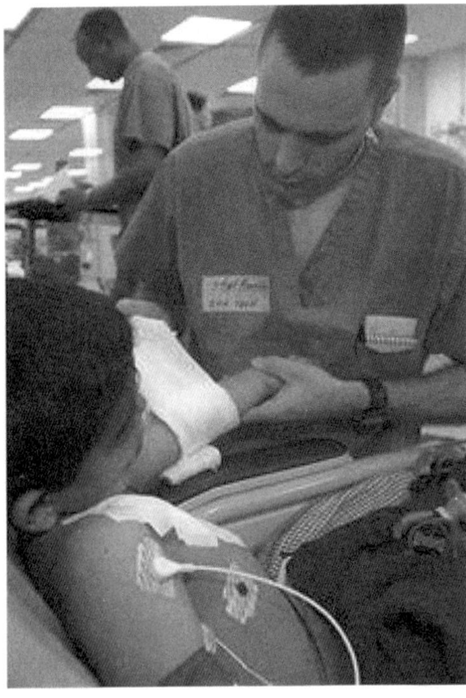

Photo Courtesy of U.S. Air Force.

Injured boy and Air Force medic, Afghanistan.

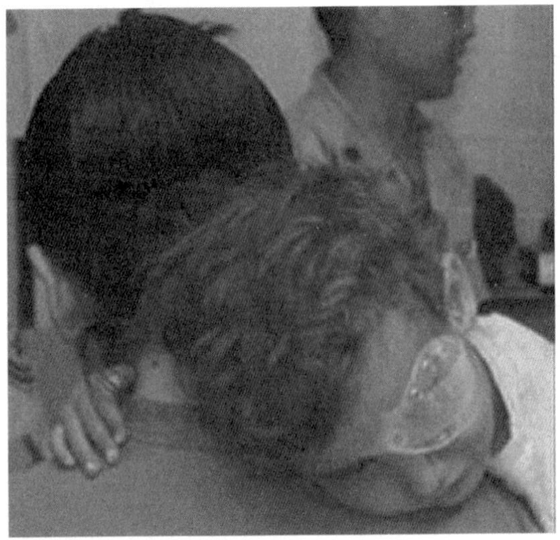

Photo Courtesy of U.S. Air Force.

Nurse holding injured boy, Afghanistan.

12

My Wartime Nursing Stress: I Am a Different Person Now

Nurses experienced multiple stressors in wartime nursing. The war changed them. Some of these stressors centered on the patients they cared for and the patient care environment. Nurses reported that not knowing the fate of the troops they cared for in hospitals or air evacuation planes was stressful. Another circumstance that was particularly stressful for the nurses was returning recovered patients to their combat units. Several of their former patients were injured a second time, and sometimes, the injuries were much worse or even fatal.

Attacks on the hospital compounds also took their toll on the nurses. Mortar and rocket attacks were terrifying, and most occurred in the darkness of night. These attacks as well as having to respond to mass casualty scenarios in the middle of the night contributed to sleep deprivation and increased stress.

Family illness and problems at home weighed heavily on some nurses while they were deployed. Other nurses were told their deployment would be for 12 months, and 2 months after deploying to Iraq, their deployment was extended to 15 months. Several nurses reported that the emotional stress of caring for so many terribly injured coalition troops, children, and local people contributed significantly to compassion fatigue. These nurses recalled feeling numb and spent, owing to the overwhelming burden of their nursing care duties. Some admitted to self-medication to help them sleep.

Major Lee

Lee, an Air Force reservist deployed to Balad Air Base, Iraq, aired her frustration. "We'd spend 2 days stabilizing these patients, debriding their wounds and burns, monitoring their fluids, changing their dressings, and sometimes listening to their stories. Then they would fly away on hospital planes to Germany or the U.S., and we never got any feedback regarding what happened to them. We never heard if they lived, how they adjusted to their injuries, or what happened to them after they left our care. It was rough. The not knowing was rough. We were without closure, and that was particularly stressful."

Lee shared the difficulty she had in readjusting to the practice of nursing in the United States. She reported, "I work in a civilian community hospital back home. The hospital back here is slower paced, and you have to follow doctors' orders. We all get caught up in trivial things. I found it hard to adjust to complaining patients who usually were having relatively minor procedures, such as gallbladder removal or hernia repair, and displayed an annoying sense of entitlement. I wanted to go back to Iraq, where our soldiers were so appreciative of the care they received and never complained about their serious injuries. I see things differently because of what I have seen in Iraq and the lives we saved there. We were doing what we wanted to do there, and it was important. I miss the excitement, the sense of teamwork and making a difference. When I came back, I was very impatient. You also question people's priorities. I look at people who are complaining, and I think, 'You need to go to Iraq.'"

Major Christina

Christina, an active-duty Air Force flight nurse who served in Iraq and Afghanistan, vented her frustration. "Some of the patients we cared for in aeromedical evacuation were really critically injured. Once we dropped them off, we usually never heard about what happened to them. We don't hear if they made it back to their families or not. We only have them for maybe 6 to 12 hours on the plane, and then you never hear what happened. That was hard on us. The lack of knowing and the wondering is tough. You never get to see that the loop gets closed. You never know if they made it home alive or not. We send them off to the hospital, and we hope for the best. That was very tough. The not knowing was very tough."

Along with the stress of not knowing the fate of their patients who were airlifted to Germany and the United States, nurses reported that it was stressful to care for patients who recovered from their illnesses or injuries in coalition hospitals in Iraq or Afghanistan and then returned to their combat units and the fighting. Many nurses expressed a feeling of "not wanting to let them go back" and some felt that their "maternal instincts" of protection and worry came to the forefront.

Captain Tina

Tina, an active-duty Air Force nurse assigned to tours of duty in Iraq and Afghanistan, reported experiencing an "internal tug of war" when she witnessed soldiers returning to battle. She related, "One kid was inside a building when a suicide bomber detonated an explosive. The soldier got glass shards in his eyes and a huge gash down his face. He was very lucky in the long run because he didn't lose his eyesight. We had taken care of him to heal and recover for about 10 days, and then he was sent back to his unit in Iraq. I used to visit him whenever I went to his FOB to run a clinic 1 day a week. He made a very good recovery and returned to the fighting. Later, he was killed in an attack on his unit. Returning recovered soldiers to the fighting is very stressful because they have "paid their dues" by being wounded, and now they return to the war and are killed. It took a lot out of me to see this happen again and again."

Tina continued, "I knew it was my job to help soldiers recover, but I felt really torn when I had to see them go back into harm's way. Sometimes, I felt enough was enough, and I literally wanted to take these young soldiers and put them in a protective bubble away from the fighting. I wanted to put them in a safe place and then send them home when the war was over. Of course, I had no idea when that time would come. I guess this was my fantasy, my dream. When I was feeling particularly down about sending these guys back into battle, I would share my thoughts and feelings with my colleagues. Many other nurses admitted to feeling the same way about protecting our patients against further harm. It was some consolation to me that other nurses felt the same way."

Tina also described dangers she encountered that were not expected occurrences of war. Tina exclaimed, "There was a nearby ammunition dump on base that caught fire. We had unexploded ordinance coming into the camp, and it was very scary and dangerous. We got holes blasted into the plywood hut that we lived in, and the hospital trailers got hit as well. I was at work, and we had to move patients to the floor and get down there with them. It was very frightening, and it was coming from our own base, not insurgents. This really stressed me out. I remember my body was shaking. Later, when I was giving out medications, my hands were trembling."

Captain Suzanne

Suzanne, an active-duty Air Force nurse assigned at Balad Air Base, Iraq, related, "We used to call patients who were treated at our hospital more than once 'frequent flyers' because of multiple admissions for care. These were usually simple injuries, such as a broken wrist, a flesh wound, or a piece of shrapnel to the buttocks or thigh. These conditions needed attention but did not require airlift out of the operational theater. We had these guys and gals on our wards for only a few days up to about 2 weeks. We would patch them up, give them a good rest, and then send them back to their combat units. Some would end up coming in several times over the year or 15-month tour with these rather self-limiting injuries. We got to know these people. Then, on their final visit to us, they would be critically or mortally wounded. This occurrence really took its toll on our staff. We felt so devastated when this happened, and it happened a lot! I know I will carry these memories with me for the rest of my life. These things haunt me now. I think they will still haunt me 10 years from now. For some reason, the happy memories don't stay with me with the same intensity as these dark ones, which literally burn in my gut and keep me lying awake at night."

Captain Alice

Nurses also found it stressful providing care and support for soldiers who survived bomb or mortar attacks while their comrades were killed or critically wounded. Alice reflected on her experiences as an active-duty Air Force nurse on a critical care air transport team. She recalled, "One guy was the lone survivor of an IED blast, who I took care of on a mission going back to the States. His driver was killed, and his teammates were killed. He really got to me because he kept asking the question, 'Why me? Why did I survive?' He really exemplified survivor guilt. I spent some time talking with him on the flight, and I just tried to help him cope with what was going on. His injuries were serious but not life threatening. He had shrapnel wounds all over and a leg badly broken in several places. I really felt for him. I wondered what his life would be like after he physically healed, and I questioned if he would ever psychologically heal."

Alice stated that many situations troubled her. "I feel we throw health care providers into completely ultratraumatic circumstances. We cared for not only the severely wounded or burned troops but also the guy who was sitting next to them in the vehicle that escaped with only minor injuries. This guy is also on your plane. He can see his buddy who is struggling to breathe and has burns all over and has three people taking care of him. I think we are going to suffer as a society for this ill-prepared situation for a long time to come. I think nurses who have done so much care have also been psychologically damaged and not as well prepared as they could have been. I am passionate about this because I found it disturbing. I was at a loss on so many occasions about how to talk to people and how to help them deal with the circumstances without simply giving them sedation or tranquilizing medications."

Captain Erin

Erin was an active-duty Air Force flight nurse. She stated, "When you fly air evac missions from Iraq or Afghanistan to Germany, those missions are usually very busy and stressful because you can have 60 patients on the plane. You usually have only three nurses and four medics, so everyone stays very busy. You have to stay on top of giving meds and reinforcing dressings and constantly checking on everyone. You have to also make time for patients who are emotionally upset about all they've gone through. Many of these young people have seen their young friends die. Many have catastrophic injuries. It may be starting to sink in that their lives are now changed forever. You don't get to sit down since the work is constant."

Erin continued, "I had an alert mission into a FOB with 14 patients to be airlifted. Half of them had been involved in the same IED explosion. Everyone was asking about his buddies. It was a continual effort to try to get them to calm down. With combat injuries like this, the troops are needier. They need more reassurance that we will get them to the hospital. We not only gave a lot of physical care on that flight but lots of emotional care as well. Sometimes, we had to wait for patients on the tarmac to come from surgery. We'd get fresh postops on the plane because they want to get them to Germany as soon as possible. Many of these patients would have more surgery in Germany before they return to the States. It was high-intensity nursing on those flights. It was very draining both physically and psychologically."

Major Fran

Another stressful situation that a few nurses encountered was having an ill family member at home while they were deployed. Fran, an Air Force combat stress team leader, recalled, "I had to take emergency leave in the middle of my tour of duty in Iraq because I was notified by the American Red Cross that my father was dying. My father had Alzheimer's, so I'm not sure he really knew where I was. He died the day I came home from Iraq. I was waiting for a flight in Kuwait. I talked to the nurses at his hospital. He

[had] kidney failure and had some tumors in his belly. We didn't want to put him through any more. I got home just in the nick of time. He died later that day. I was glad that I made it home in time, but it was very stressful trying to get there."

Major Olga

Olga, an active-duty Army nurse assigned to a fast-forward surgical team in Iraq, recalled, "My older sister was diagnosed with breast cancer while I was in Iraq. She got good treatment, and our relatives were very supportive, but I just wish I could have been with her through the surgery and chemotherapy treatments. I am the only nurse in our family. I think I could have made the whole ordeal easier for my sister and our family. I was torn between feelings that I was needed in Iraq and that I was needed back in Texas. I kept having this inner conversation with myself about family obligations versus work obligations. I reconciled my dilemma by reminding myself my country was at war, and I was in the military. I also kept reminding myself my sister was very proud of me and supported my decision to be an Army nurse. Down deep inside, I always felt the need to justify my actions and decisions. I felt guilty about not being with my sister in her hour of need. Our late mother would have called this 'Catholic guilt.' To be honest, I think it's more than that. As a woman, I feel that I was brought up with an unwritten sense of 'trying to be all things to all people.' I also think that the nursing profession, the helping profession that it is, feeds into this."

First Lieutenant Leah

Leah was an Army Reserve nurse assigned to combat support hospitals in Mosul and Anbar province, Iraq, for 15 months. Leah was deployed to Iraq as soon as she completed Army Reserve combat training in Wisconsin. This training commenced immediately after her college graduation. She hailed from New England. Leah had been in this Army Reserve medical unit in an enlisted capacity before and during college. Her first combat assignment was working in the intensive care unit (ICU) at the hospital in Mosul, Iraq. Leah recalled how her environment contributed greatly to her stress. "There were mortars launched into our base every night. We would be awakened every night, and we'd have to go out into the bunkers. Not only was it frightening, but most of us were chronically sleep deprived as well."

Leah commented on her life since returning home. "Since I've been home, I suffer from PTSD. I feel guilty because I was not out there getting shot at. I'm amazed how many of us still can't get back into our lives because we are so affected by this experience. Fifteen months was too long to be away from everything you know and love. When I came home, I didn't know why I was depressed when I should be happy. I could not sleep. I was sleeping only about 3 hours a night. You can imagine how that affects you. You are trying to be happy when everyone is throwing you a party or taking you out to dinner. You are trying to smile when you haven't slept in 2 weeks. I kept thinking I should be sleeping and satisfied I made it home. I cried every day right from the start. I didn't know why any of these things were happening. I didn't know I had PTSD. Sometimes, I'm having flashbacks. I can close my eyes, and I'm right back in Iraq. Hot days take me right back there. Loud noises make me hit the deck. We got mortared almost every day in Mosul. I wonder if I'll ever be who I was before I went to Iraq. I actually mourn the loss of the person I was before. I guess after an experience like war, you are never quite the same, and I must accept that."

Many nurses reported difficulty sleeping after they came home from the war. Leah related, "I just felt very different when I got home. I had trouble falling asleep and staying asleep. I didn't know if I was overwhelmed by the change in environment, but I was crying every day, and I knew I was not happy. As a nurse, you try to manage everything on your own rather than seek help. You think, 'Okay, I'll try to get into a sleeping pattern and have a routine at bedtime.'"

Leah related, "PTSD can start at any time. It can start years after a war. Mine started right away, but I didn't know it, so I claimed insomnia on my VA paperwork. I just knew I was not sleeping. I thought, 'How ridiculous, I just came home from war.' I've not slept in months. However, because I didn't go to the doctor over there saying I was not sleeping, I don't have proof, and the VA won't accept my claim.' I thought, 'Wow, that's ironic. Why would I have to see a doctor? I mean, I have doctor friends. I could just talk to them.' Many of us had trouble sleeping. We are at war, so you almost expect it. I wasn't gonna run to the ER and say, 'I cannot sleep.' We had Benadryl accessible. You knew you'd be going home eventually, so you just thought you would get better. That was another frustrating thing. I didn't know if my experiences with dying patients or too many rocket attacks on our base were why I didn't sleep very much. Sometimes, I would fall asleep for a couple of hours. I would wake up drenched in sweat. I'd be sore when I'd wake up from being so tense. My muscles were so tense."

Leah reflected on how she believes the length of her deployment contributed to increased stress. "I think it was too long. Fifteen months of a rigorous and tortuous life was just too long. I can do it for 6 months at a time every other year, no problem. However, for 15 months to be away from everything you know and love. I didn't go around thinking, 'Oh, my God, this mortar could kill me.' I don't think I felt that way then, but now

I feel paranoid that I'm gonna die. I think the adrenaline is gone, and now I'm left with, 'I can't believe it, and I can't believe that I am suffering all this depression.' You expect to be so happy when you come home. You think, 'I'm having a little difficulty sleeping, and I'm a little irritable, but when I'm home in my own bed, I'm gonna feel so good. I'm gonna be so great, and life is gonna be so good.' Then you get home, and it's not that way. You're dealing with all these pent-up emotions you couldn't show over there. When somebody died, that's the way it was. You couldn't cry because you wanted to be strong for your soldiers, and you wanted to be strong for the soldier's friends who are looking at you. Well, this is something that I completely didn't expect. I still don't sleep, and I still have nightmares. I can't even explain it or say why. I think it is underrated how much war changes your life, and I didn't think it would. I've seen death before. I've seen crazy wounds before. An Army doctor died in Mosul from a mortar last month. The same type of mortars we were getting. Wow, that could have been me! I don't know if it's the realization I could have died or because it's horrible for all of those who did die, and now I'm back home safe."

Leah reported, "I'm also hearing from a lot of soldiers I know. Most of them are on medications for PTSD. Most of them can't sleep and have been diagnosed with PTSD. PTSD is definitely one thing I didn't expect. I've always been a well-adjusted, easygoing, 'go with the flow' person, but I didn't expect this. It's very disheartening."

Some nurses reported self-medicating themselves before they sought outside help. Leah recalled, "We always try to fix things ourselves. We take Benadryl or whatever we can find to help us sleep. It took months for me to realize I needed other outside help. I went to the VA system. My husband kept saying, 'You can't live like this. When are you gonna give up and go for more help, not just your own help and self-diagnosing?' I said, 'The VA is too overwhelmed to give the medical care which they need to.' Then I did get a call about a post-deployment health assessment we are supposed to do. This was several months after I came home. It was then I admitted I was depressed and having so much trouble sleeping. They ask you questions. Are you depressed? Are you having thoughts about committing suicide? You answer all these questions, and then they say, 'Here are the contact numbers. Please call these numbers.' In my professional opinion, this was way too late. At this point, I have gone 3 or 4 months without sleeping. I was extremely depressed even though I was trying to talk myself out of it. It was obvious I needed more help. I think even now that I am in the VA system, the system is too overwhelmed. I finally started seeing a therapist, and I've been home since October 2007, and now its January 2009. I hadn't seen a therapist through the VA till now. I had only seen doctors who kept trying to throw drugs down me. Now, I actually go for therapy. Before that, it was doctors saying, 'Try Celexa' or 'We can try Lexipro.' As a medical person, you want more than that. You want therapy. You want to work through it. You don't just want to cover it up with meds. By the time you get into the VA system, and they realize that you need therapy, it's always, 'In a month, you'll see this person, and then let's give you a therapy referral for the following month.' It is wait, wait, and wait some more! I'm thinking, 'Why am I going home to cry myself to sleep for 4 weeks before I finally get a damn appointment with a therapist?' To make a long story short, eventually, I got into therapy. I'm making progress. In my opinion, it took way too long to get into the system. Once I got paired with a therapist, things have improved. I have depression medication and anti-anxiety medication. The meds are helping, but it's only been 6 weeks. I'm definitely a lot better than I was a year ago."

Leah continued, "There are little things I notice. I have this fear that I am going to die. It's silly. In my head, I know I'm being overly alert or paranoid, but I still have the thought of dying. I think that someone is breaking into my house if I hear a noise at night. I get very anxious. Even though I know I am being silly, that's what I refer to it, as 'being silly,' it's still hard because I'm not big on taking meds. I'm also supposed to take Klonopin daily on an as-needed basis to help me sleep."

Some nurses diagnosed with PTSD found their family and friends to be supportive and helpful. Leah shared, "When I started researching PTSD, I thought, 'Oh my God, I have every single one of those symptoms!' The insomnia, the depression, and the anxiety, I had them all. It was weird because the depression was the biggest thing in my mind. Now that I've been working on controlling the depression, the other symptoms of being anxious and paranoid have come out more. I think they were hiding behind the depression because that was so overwhelming. So, I'm thinking I'm finally getting a handle on the depression, and now I'm feeling the anxiety and paranoia."

Leah reported, "I have to give credit to my husband. I can't imagine if I was married to anyone other than my husband how we would still be married. My husband is wonderful. He knows now I'm overly sensitive. If he does or says anything a little bit hurtful or annoying, he gently lets me know I'm overreacting. For example, if I'm getting angry over an eyeball roll or something, he knows just to talk me through it and just let me know I'm being overly sensitive by getting mad at something silly. He'll talk me through it because I can go from being in a good mood to a deep depression from some little thing that I get mad over. He is very patient and loving. I can't imagine not having a husband like him. I married the right one! However, it also makes me feel guilty because I feel he is not married to the same person who he married before my deployment. He thought he was marrying this wonderful woman, and then I come back from Iraq completely different, at least emotionally. I'm so emotionally labile. He is wonderful, and I feel bad for anyone who does not have such a supportive partner or one who doesn't understand. He's in the military, too, so he can understand my frustrations with the military. We have that bond. He can understand, and he's just very kind and loving. I'm so thankful my marriage is strong and good. It's because of him. He's put in the time and effort just talking me through things. I'm very happy."

Captain Penny

Penny was an active-duty Army nurse assigned to a fast-forward surgical team in Afghanistan. She recalled, "We were deployed out in the middle of nowhere. The rocket attacks would be sporadic. We'd be attacked with four rockets and then nothing for several days because they had to launch them from some remote place out in the countryside. After an attack, they would pack up their little truck and run. It wasn't like Kabul or another big city where the bad guys would be resupplied to launch every day. It was very stressful because we never knew when we'd be attacked. We felt constant tension over there."

Lieutenant Colonel Victoria

Victoria was a seasoned active-duty Army nurse who found herself doing a detainee care mission on her second tour of duty in Iraq. Victoria reported, "We had 13 rocket attacks that hit our FOB [forward operating base]. The first time it happened, I was getting out of a vehicle in front of the hospital with my supervisor. She was a Vietnam vet, so she hit the ground instantly. I said to her, 'What was that?' She said, 'A rocket just went over your head.' After you hear it for the first time, believe me, you will recognize it the next time. It was daylight, and I just lay there on the ground petrified."

Victoria recalled, "From one rocket attack, we had 77 casualties in 15 minutes because it landed in the middle of the detainee stockade. In my last 4 months, I felt like I was going to die over there in this dirty pit of a place. I'm sure a lot of people felt the same way, but we didn't talk about it. We kept these kinds of feelings 'close to the vest.' I was in a position as assistant chief nurse where I really didn't have any peers. We had Army, Air Force, and Navy folks on the forward operating base, but all of us were commanders of troops, so it could be very lonely at the top."

Victoria went on to described her frustration and added stress from higher headquarters' expectations. "We were not perceived well or treated well in my mind by our higher headquarters. The hospital was here, and all around us were detainee compounds. We had to walk in full 'battle-rattle' because we had to have all of our gear with us. There were riots within our compound. The first 6 months I was there, we had riots among the detainees regularly. At one point, we were in the hospital, and we heard a noise, so we went outside. The detainee compound across the street from the hospital was engulfed in flames. The detainees had lit it up. We had a lot of detainee-on-detainee violence. When they rioted, it was directed against us. This detainee stockade was air-conditioned and had running water and beds. When they burned it down, they all ended up in tents in the hot July sun without air-conditioning or running water. So they were only hurting themselves."

Victoria recalled, "When I first came back to Iraq for my second tour of duty, my anger returned. It is still there now 13 months after I came home, but it is getting better. I was mad enough at the Army that I wanted to get out. After I had been doing detainee care for about 3 months, I was talking to my husband on the phone. I told him I was going to get out when I came home. I was approaching 18 years in service, but I had had it, or so I felt at the time. Our higher headquarters had one quarter of the number of detainees we had, and they had a lot more staff. There was a huge discrepancy in what we were caring for versus what they were caring for. They didn't know our business at all, but they were going to tell us how to do our business. We had poor computer access. I would be told that I had to send something up to them. Well, the attachment files were too big, and they would not go through. I think sometimes they thought that I was willfully 'just blowing them off.' One day, the chief nurse from higher headquarters came down for a week. He was trying to show me on the computer how to get to the higher headquarters' website. He got very, very frustrated when he couldn't get through. He kept hitting keys, and nothing happened. He said to me, 'Is it always like this?' And I said, 'Yes, sir, every single day.' They didn't believe it until they came down and saw it for themselves. I'm still not sure they believed it. We had higher headquarters telling us we had to document every patient visit, which averaged 18,000 visits per month, on an SF 600 [Standard Form 600]. We didn't have paper to do this, let alone somewhere to store these forms once they were filled out. Headquarters did not live in our world, so they never understood our world."

Victoria reported that she felt her anxiety peak while still in the war zone. "I got really anxious a couple of weeks before I was to go home. I just felt that something bad was going to happen. Between Thanksgiving and Christmas, we had more than one occasion with incoming fire and mortar attacks. We had several rocket attacks during that period. Then we had a British artillery battery with us around the Christmas and New Year's season.

The British artillery troops decided it would be entertaining to shoot tracer rounds out, and they didn't tell us ahead of time. I'm lying in bed Christmas Eve. I went to bed early because I had a headache. All of a sudden, I hear these rocket sounds. I roll out of bed, and I'm on the floor under my cot. I'm trying to get my gear on, and I'm waiting to hear the sirens go off. I'm not hearing the sirens. I get up, finish putting my gear on, and I walk outside the tent. Someone walking by says everything is 'okay.' I walk back to my cot. I just feel that we're all going to be killed, and I'm never going home. All of sudden, being here, being vulnerable to rockets and mortars, just got to me. I was so close to going home. The danger just got to me in that instant. I was over there for 10 months before I came home on R & R. Things like dumpster lids slamming would make me hit the deck. The first 4th of July after I came home, the dog and I sat in the bathroom alone because the fireworks noise bothered both of us. It brought me back to the mortar and rocket attacks, so it wasn't such a good night for me. I kept telling myself I was at home, not in Iraq, and I didn't have to get on the floor. It has gotten better for me since then, but sometimes, loud, unexpected noises still bother me. I think I have some PTSD."

Victoria expressed anger and frustration at the weight of responsibility she and others had to shoulder while deployed as senior officers. She explained, "I've been home from my second deployment to Iraq for 13 months. There was a lot of anger that built up in me while I was over there and even after I came home. Anger over the way business was done. Anger because our unit had some issues. There was misbehaving. When you take a bunch of young kids where there is not really a thing to do when you are off duty, you invite misbehaving. We talked to our counterparts who were stationed in Baghdad. They talked about going bowling or going to the pool. If we wanted to sit outside and watch a movie on a big-screen TV at night, that was the only planned recreation we had other than going to the gym. Otherwise, there was nothing for these kids to do. As a result, some of them got into relationships and behaviors that were inappropriate and against regulations. I am a senior officer, so this was very stressful for me. I had to charge these folks with regulation infractions, yet I couldn't offer them a better environment to decompress and blow off some steam. It was a tough situation all around."

First Lieutenant Joy

Joy was an active-duty Air Force nurse deployed to Bagram Air Base, Afghanistan. She said she found herself getting used to the mortar attacks in the vicinity of their base. She reported, "When I left for Afghanistan, my biggest fear was for my personal safety. I thought the patient care stuff would be routine since I'm a critical care nurse. I was assigned at the Air Force's biggest medical center in Afghanistan. I received some training at the shock-trauma center in Baltimore before being deployed. I've seen blood and guts before. Well, let me tell you, it quickly changed. It flipped 180 degrees. It got to the point where we heard mortars coming in, and I'd sit on the floor and read the paper waiting for it to be over. It got routine. You just didn't think about it all the time, or it would drive you crazy. You'd get a little nervous when you heard small-arms fire. I remember coming home one night, and there was a bullet hole in my B-hut. You can't dwell on it."

Captain Abby

Abby was an active-duty Air Force medical-surgical and critical care nurse who deployed to Afghanistan with about 50 medical and nursing personnel from her hospital in the United States. Abby reported two stressful situations. She did not anticipate encountering soldiers committing suicide or being injured or killed by an accidental weapon discharge. Abby reported, "You expected to care for dying soldiers and severely wounded and burned soldiers from the battle. I was shocked when I had to care for soldiers with wounds from a suicide attempt. This happened to me three times during my year in Iraq, and all three of these soldiers died from their wounds. She added, "There are two situations I can recall that were accidental discharge of weapons. One was when a soldier was cleaning his weapon. It accidently discharged, hitting him in the leg. The other one was an accidental discharge of someone else's weapon that went through the tent and hit a guy in the chest. Of these two situations, one we were able to save, and the other, we were not. These situations were devastating for everyone in our compound."

Major Millie

Millie, an active-duty Army operating room nurse, told how the emotional toll of the war was paramount with the nurses. She stated, "We got back in June of 2006. Overall, with the whole war, I think that time is going to tell how significantly people were impacted with posttraumatic stress disorder [PTSD] and emotional issues. We saw a lot of it in the acute phase because we also treated civilian casualties. We had a number of instances where innocent civilians were shot by soldiers on patrol because they happened to be in the wrong place at the wrong time. The poor kid [soldier] makes a snap judgment to fire on a car because the driver doesn't respond to his command to stop or get out. The emotional toll on the troops in the field is tremendous. It is going to show up a lot later, but we saw the acute anxiety on the part of the soldiers. It is going to show on the medical folks, too, because we had to care for children and families caught in the crossfire of the fog of war. You just don't expect to have to deal with little kids all shot up, missing limbs, and severely burned from explosives."

Major Derek

Derek was an Army reservist from New York. He was assigned to Camp Bucca Detainee Center Hospital at the beginning of his tour of duty in Iraq. Later, he was transferred to the hospital at Abu Ghraib Prison. Derek opened up about the problems and issues he faced after returning from Iraq. He stated, "I had problems when I got home. I became a real serious person over there. Before deploying, I was much more lighthearted and easygoing. I came home with the feeling that everyone should have the same perspective as me. I felt if you didn't have the same perspective as me, 'Well then, I'm gonna tell you about it.' My attitude affected my relationship with my wife, my kids, and some of our relatives. Very often, things ended in a lot of conflict. Having an attitude as the one I did doesn't make you a good dad or husband or a good nurse. Fortunately, I got counseling that was helped by being on active duty for a few weeks after I returned home. It might have been more difficult if I had to go back and deal with a civilian job. Other sufferers were all around me, and things were more readily recognized. There is a huge benefit to having that military family around you."

Derek continued, "I recently started going to a VA hospital because I'm having anxiety and panic issues at work. I found my reserve for empathy and compassion was drained. Anything could set me off, make me mad and verbal. Before I went to Iraq, I was a laid-back person. I didn't let a lot bother me. Now, I'm increasingly bothered, and it seems to only happen at work. It would sometimes spill over toward my wife when I got home, but it was work that really set me off. I did have some issues. We are a level-one trauma center. Some patients came in with traumatic amputations. It was the kind of stuff we saw over there, and it really bothered me. I work in a PACU and surgical ICU. Now, I am actually thinking about moving away from the bedside. I never thought I'd want to do that, but there are a lot of possibilities in nursing."

Derek went on to report, "I sought treatment at the VA. I'm on some medications to help with the anxiety. It has been effective so far. Before that, I was almost obsessive about Iraq, and I would constantly think about it. It wasn't even that something would set me off. If I just had a moment,

I would just start thinking about it. I would replay certain situations in my head. They would come to me just out of nowhere. It wasn't like a smell set me off, or a sight set me off. It was that these thoughts just intruded whatever I was doing or thinking about 15 times a day. Every day, I would spend a significant amount of time just going over things about Iraq in my mind. I felt that this just wasn't right, so I went and talked to the doctor at the VA."

Captain Robert

Robert was an Army reservist from Maryland. He was assigned to hospitals in Tikrit, Mosul, and Anbar Province, Iraq. Robert commented on the milieu of his unit. "We would just sit around at the desk, play games, watch movies on the computer, and play cards when things were quiet. The lieutenant colonel would be upset if someone was sleeping during their shift even though there was nothing to do. He wanted you to sit there 6 days a week. This was an active-duty Lieutenant Colonel assigned to our unit, and he was a nurse. He was one of those guys who you can kind of tell right away that he was very politically minded. If he were a civilian, he would probably make a very good used-car salesman. He knew what to say. He had the contacts, and he sounded great. If you looked at him, you got the feeling right away that there was something shifty about him. The angles were always his angles. Whatever was done was done to better his career."

Robert reported that he and other nurses felt their anger come to a head when they returned from deployment. He recalled, "When I got back from Iraq, I was very angry and resentful because very few of us, the ones in uniform, were bearing the burden of this war. I spent a year in this God-forsaken shit hole called Iraq. I get back after a year, and I've had friends injured and killed. I come back after a year, and all the selfish people are worried about is the price of gasoline! I was very angry. This was because I think a very large part of the population does not really realize what is going on. People only care about the price of gasoline! I must admit that some people would come up to me and say, 'Thanks for your service.' I'd be like, 'Okay, but encourage your kid to join the service.' They don't want that. Service is not a valued thing. I'm better about some things now. It's just in our culture that service is not valued the way it once was. I'm very cognizant of that and am very resentful about that, but I try to not let it come out in public. Now, I just say things like, 'Thank you,' whereas I used to say things like 'When a recruiter comes to your kids' high school, don't picket it!' I came home with a lot of anger."

Captain Olivia

Olivia, an Army reservist, stated, "I have been diagnosed with posttraumatic stress disorder. I go to a psychologist, and I go to a psychiatrist, too. The psychologist is the one I actually sit down and talk to. The psychiatrist prescribes the meds. I'm on Zoloft, and he adjusts the dosage. I think the Zoloft is working. If my brother doesn't tell me I'm a miserable bitch, then I guess it is working. On Sundays, we try to have a big Sunday dinner at my aunt's house. If I'm really quiet, my cousins will ask me if I'm alright, if I'm taking my meds, and if I think they are working. I have not returned to my civilian ICU job. Right now, I'm in the Wounded Warrior Program because I got hurt over there. I hurt my shoulder, tore my rotator cuff in three places, and had surgery. I'm still rehabbing now. I'm still on active duty. I visit my friends at the civilian ICU where I used to work. My friends there say they can tell I'm doing a lot better now. Some of my ICU friends call and check on me."

Captain Marie

Marie, an Army reservist, recalled, "When I got home, I didn't think I had PTSD, but I think I had some type of adjustment reaction. A lot of people said I was a little different, a little withdrawn. I did not talk about my experiences right away. I had a lot of painful experiences. I worked in the ER a lot in Iraq, and we never knew what was coming through our door. I took care of many troops and civilians with just catastrophic injuries. I had people die right in front of me. Later, when I got home, I opened up a bit to my military friends. I found that every time I told my stories, it got easier and easier. I never did seek any counseling. Part of it was the stigma and potential repercussions on my career. In retrospect, I think I could have benefited. I could have worked through things a little bit easier. Just telling my stories, and doing things such as this interview, has made it easier and easier. Now, people tell me I am back to my old self."

Captain Richard

Some nurses reported stress and conflict with a few of the senior leaders at their hospitals. Richard, an Army reservist, reported, "Our chief nurse was big on rotating people through all the clinical areas, which was good. However, a lot of times, you got someone who you felt comfortable with what they were doing, and you felt they were competent. You didn't have to watch them all the time. Then they were moved to another area, and you had to start with someone else. Frankly, some of the people who came through didn't have the skill set to do what they were doing. Some didn't have the attitude to listen and learn, so we had a few instances of poor patient outcomes due to the care these novices provided. That was a little disheartening. No matter how many times we spoke to the chief nurse, she didn't want to hear anything about it. I had the opportunity to be the interim ICU head nurse, and that was when I tried to get her to change her approach. On the one side, it was a positive that we got to teach and mentor our young enlisted medics, but on the other side, it could be a negative because some people didn't want to learn."

Major Yvonne

Yvonne was an active-duty Army nurse assigned to an airborne infantry brigade in Afghanistan. She also filled in at a combat support hospital to keep her critical care skills sharp. Yvonne stated, "I found that a few married people developed inappropriate relationships while we were deployed. Some people took the attitude that 'what happens in Afghanistan stays in Afghanistan.' I am a married senior officer, and I found this behavior totally offensive. It made me sick to see people sharing photos of their children and spouses at the dinner table with their colleagues and then, later the same night, engaging in adulterous behavior with another married person. The physicians seemed to be the biggest offenders. To be honest, I don't know if this was a reaction to the stress of war or if these guys behaved this way during their whole careers."

In spite of all the stresses, the hardships, and the emotional toll of the wars, most nurses stated they would go back again, if needed. Several have completed two, three, or even four tours of duty in the war zone. Yvonne summarized the sentiments of many. "If they asked me to go back, I'd go back in a heartbeat. I know we are over there because we all raised our hand, and we are doing our part because it is our job. We believe in the cause because we did raise our hands and take an oath. However, the fact that we are over there and people are getting killed and shot at is the part that I don't like, but I know it is part of the job. So if all this is happening, I want to go over there and help them out."

13

Kinship and Bonding: My Military Family

Many nurses had positive things to say about the people they worked with and met while deployed in Iraq or Afghanistan. It was the first wartime deployment for some, whereas others had deployed two or more times since the wars began. There are not many occupations like the military, where you frequently end up living with the people you work with. This is a reality not just during deployments; military members also live together during field training exercises and temporary duty assignments away from home and while attending military courses. It is a unique way of life that most people outside the military have not experienced. Without one's military family, and the closeness, cohesion, and bonding inherent in that "band of brothers and sisters," deployment might be more stressful than it already is. Many of these relationships are often difficult to describe. Deployments, working in harm's way, and field training away from home in austere conditions are but a few of the differences between military service and a civilian job.

Captain Holly

Holly was an Army reservist assigned to the Abu Ghraib prison hospital in Iraq. Holly recalled, "There was friendship. I still have some good friends I met over there. I met another nurse before we deployed. She ended up being my roommate and best friend. You end up depending and relying on each other so much over there. We were roommates for 2 months before we really realized we could help each other and open up to each other. We developed a supportive relationship quickly after that. Before that, we were like two ships passing in the night."

Holly related, "I get emotional when I think about my friendships. With my roommate, it was a friendship that became deep, but we felt very differently about our jobs. She was, 'My country, right or wrong.' I felt differently. If I see something going on that is wrong, I'm going to jack them up about it and question it. Although we had different viewpoints about some things, we were and still are best of friends."

Lieutenant Colonel Judd

Judd was an Army Reserve nurse practitioner who served at the coalition hospitals in Tikrit, Mosul, and Anbar Province, Iraq. Judd remarked, "I remember telling my wife that performing this job was probably the most rewarding one in my career. If I could have the same job back in the States with my family there, I'd never leave it because of the camaraderie and the sense of teamwork. Working with the soldiers was the best. I've never seen doctors and nurses work so well together. You're all in the same situation. You are working together to get through the year. The bonding of our military people will always stand out in my mind. When we were getting hit with mass casualty traumas, everyone pulled together and worked so hard to save lives. The teamwork was just phenomenal."

Captain Trudi

Trudi was an older Army reservist assigned to the coalition hospitals in Mosul and Anbar Province, Iraq. "I met a wonderful bunch of people in Iraq. The media sometimes says bad things about the younger generation, but it is just not true. The young marines were wonderful, and the rest of them—the Army, Navy, Air Force, and coalition forces—were all wonderful. These young troops really rose to the occasion. I can tell you, young people in the military really have their act together."

Trudi went on to describe the kinship she felt toward the U.S. troops. Trudi stated, "Working with the American troops was a definite high point for me. Being a 40-something-year-old woman, I was much more prepared to be in a war zone than these 18- and 19-year-old kids. American soldiers I came across that were injured and in my ER [emergency room], I took a real piece of every one of them home with me. They were very grateful for everything they received. They were just great people."

Captain Suzanne

Suzanne, an active-duty Air Force nurse assigned to the aeromedical staging facility at Balad Air Base, Iraq, reported, "We helped a lot of people over there. We helped our soldiers, women and children, Iraqi soldiers, and some older people. We set up clinics to care for the nonsoldier population. We worked well together as a team. Some of the nurses were very young and inexperienced in both the military and in nursing, so it was challenging. Many of them got the hang of it. They would show up for duty ready to go when they knew there would be incoming casualties from the mortar attacks. We kept busy most of the time with construction projects, too, because a lot of things needed to be built. The people in my unit always pitched in to help."

Major Christina

Christina, an active-duty Air Force flight nurse, described how nurses relied on each other and other medical personnel to handle the uncertainties of war nursing. She recalled, "Nursing care for air evac can be very difficult. You don't know what you are getting a lot of the time. Air evac is not an easy job. You don't know what situation you are flying into. When you get there, you don't know what kind of injuries you are going to have to care for most of the time. They give you this report before you take off. You cover it in your briefing to the crew. Then you land, and it is frequently a different story. You think you are going to pick up 4 patients, and you get 10. You think you have a stable patient, and then all of a sudden, things are out of control. There's this element of the unknown with air evac. You try to focus on how you are going to plan your care. You get to your patients and come out with a whole different set of injuries. You have to be ready for anything. I can tell you the people on our air evac team really worked well together and always helped each other out. It was a team effort. We problem solved to handle many unexpected situations together. This was teamwork at its best!"

Captain Marie

Marie, an intensive care unit (ICU) nurse and Army reservist assigned in Iraq, exclaimed, "The camaraderie helped because after the 'mass cal' went through the ER, the flow of casualties would come to the ICU, and we'd have an influx of 8 or 10 patients. I'd just grab other nurses from the ER and bring them back with us because we didn't have enough staff. They'd come willingly. They wanted to help. They wanted to be involved. We'd even have nonmedical people from our hospital staff running through and taking out the trash and restocking our saline and supplies. As a nurse, we didn't want for anything. Everyone was very helpful. The nursing experience in Iraq was surreal. It was sad but great."

Captain Robert

Robert, an Army reservist assigned in Tikrit, Mosul, and Anbar Province, Iraq, remarked, "Meeting folks from all over was very positive for me. From the trauma surgeons who were with us to the lowest enlisted member, they were just great people. You get close to the people you work with. I will never forget them. They were terrific. I was in the Navy for 3 years, and now I'm in the Army Reserve. In both, the medics are just the best people alive."

Captain Erin

Erin, an active-duty Air Force flight nurse, told of how her coworkers and other people from her base helped fill the void left by leaving friends and family back in the United States. Erin reported, "Everyone knew they were going to be away from their family. Even if you might not have been a friend back in the U.S., you were their friend over there because everyone was separated from their loved ones. Everyone needed a friend and became friends. It was hard to be over there and away from everybody back home. I left on the best of terms with my supervisor and everyone I worked with who wasn't deploying. It was hard to be deployed over there without them. I had to make new friends and kind of get out of my comfort zone. However, I found the people in my air evac unit and at the hospital in Bagram, Afghanistan to be just great people. I quickly developed a bond with them even closer than with my colleagues back home. We lived, ate, played sports, and socialized together. They were just a great group."

First Lieutenant Leah

Leah, an Army reservist assigned to the coalition hospital in Mosul, Iraq stated, "The nurses and other people tended to help each other. You go into a facility where you don't know anyone. Once you are there, you work together side by side. Sometimes, you don't have a day off. Sometimes, you work day and night. Management is still the same as we have back in the U.S., but assignments are different. The Army nurses have to do guard duty as well as nursing care. Some of the Air Force nurses have to do LN duty, which means local national duty running humanitarian clinics outside the wire. We were soldiers and airmen first and nurses second. That is the basic difference between military nurses and civilian nurses. It is a 24/7 deal to be in the military. It was a good decision for me. I have loved my time in the military. I have loved the professionalism and the teamwork."

Captain Olivia

Olivia, an Army reservist, talked about her colleagues as if they were family. "I developed a lot of good friendships while I was in Iraq. In a war zone, your friends actually become your family. Therefore, I now have a huge extended family. I have my family and relatives here at home, but then I have my Army family. I trust my Army family just as much as I would my own brother and my cousins and my aunts. It is a big trust thing. If you don't have trust, then your deployment and the situations you find yourself in are going to be much worse. It is not going to be very good for you."

Major Millie

Millie, an active-duty Army operating room nurse, talked about the teamwork necessary to save lives. "Every patient that made it to us alive, and then made it to the operating room alive, is at home and alive today. We had a 100% track record if they lived to make it to the operating room. I'm pretty darn proud of our team. I had a lot of positives about my experience in Iraq. It was all about making sure our troops got the very best care possible in a war zone. It was about working as a team, and we did truly work as a team."

Millie went on to describe people giving of themselves. "If people heard there was something going on during their day off, they just showed up at the ER to help. I've never worked with a more giving group of people. Moreover, this was not just the nursing and medical staff; it was the administrative clerks, the lab technicians, the X-ray folks, and anyone else who thought they could help. If the infantry guys and the truck drivers heard we needed blood, they would come in and line up at the lab. If the guys and gals in the motor pool heard we had incoming casualties and we needed litter [stretcher] bearers, they just ran to the helipad or the triage area to help. The cooks in the mess hall would cart over meals for us if they heard we were working nonstop with the casualties. I truly saw teamwork at its best during this deployment."

Major Fran

Fran, an Air Force mental health nurse and combat stress team leader assigned at Tallil Air Base, Iraq, remarked, "We really enjoyed caring for the troops, and many of them we saw were from the front lines. We really had everything we needed. We had good equipment, adequate supplies, enough manpower, and solid support. We were sometimes surprised at all we had. Although we were a small hospital in Tallil, Iraq, we had the right mix of surgeons, nurses, and support personnel to carry out our mission. Everyone got along well and helped each other. The teamwork was truly inspiring. The rest of the military folks on the base supported us well, such as the civil engineers, the food service contractors, and the transportation troops. I worked a lot with various unit commanders and first sergeants on the base and at the nearby FOBs. They were all truly supportive to us medical folks and to their own troops as well."

Major Olga

Olga was an active-duty Army nurse assigned to a fast-forward surgical team in Iraq. She stated, "We did what we had to do. Our hospital was the best example of this. We had only nine people on our team. Everyone had to learn a lot of nonmedical as well as medical tasks because we were a small unit. We all learned how to drive a 5-ton truck and a Humvee. If someone didn't do their part, we would be in trouble. We all worked together and knew what each other could do. We were an awesome group."

Captain Alice

Many nurses spoke of the fondness and admiration they felt for their soldier-patients. Alice, an active-duty Air Force critical care air transport team nurse, stated, "I think the positive thing for me was being able to do my part as an American as I served my country. I guess the reward for me was to bring those guys and gals home. Wherever I may be taking them, it was a step on the path to bringing them home. They are my brothers and sisters. The air evac team I worked with was a super group of people, who cared so much for our patients and for each other."

Captain Meaghan

Meaghan was an active-duty Air Force critical care air transport team nurse assigned to medical evacuation duties in Afghanistan. She recalled, "Knowing that every one of those troops we can get onto that plane, we are taking an important step in saving their lives. That was hugely significant for me as a critical care nurse. Being able to bring them home to their families was the biggest positive for me. When I came home, some people said, 'You are a hero.' I said, 'The heroes are those folks who went outside the wire looking for the bad guys; they are my heroes."

Lieutenant Colonel Heidi

Heidi, an active-duty Army nurse researcher assigned in Baghdad, Iraq, recalled, "We were there to do a job, to keep them healthy and strong, to take care of them if they got hurt, but the troops were our heroes. They go in harm's way every single day. They are on a 300-mile convoy. They get hit with fire; they get hit with IEDs; they have to pick up their wounded, get back in the convoy, and scoot to the nearest military medical facility. That was their job. They just had to keep going. Try to keep safe, heed your training, and then just do it. I just love them and their spirit."

Captain Vanessa

Vanessa, an Army reservist assigned to the detainee ICU at Abu Ghraib Prison Hospital, related, "I joined the reserves in 2001 after the 9/11 terrorist attacks. I was green to the military. I didn't understand the military really is based on the 'grunts.' The enlisted side of the house is the backbone of the military. A lot of these kids come from poor, uneducated families from Middle America, and they are totally patriotic. They will put their life on the line. You don't have to ask them twice to go do something dangerous. I loved these kids and found them so sincere and so authentic, not like some of the people back home that are so self-centered and selfish."

Vanessa continued, "You may hear negative things about the local people in Iraq, but that was not my experience with the locals who worked at our hospital. We had interpreters, housekeepers, and Iraqi soldiers as guards. I got to know many of them over my year there and found them to be helpful and trustworthy. I know that may not have been everyone's experience, but it was mine. They made our jobs easier, especially the interpreters."

Major Michelle

Michelle was an active-duty Air Force nurse anesthetist assigned at an Afghan national army hospital in Kandahar, Afghanistan. Michelle recalled, "The folks at my hospital shared everything. If my roommate got brownies from home, she brought them in to work and shared them with everyone. If other nurses got a care package of female hygiene wipes, or Tampax, or sanitary pads, they put them in the supply box in the women's latrine so others who needed them could have them. We started a movie and music library at the hospital, so other folks could share the tapes or DVDs that were sent from home. If we needed extra clothing for our patients, we just emailed home for a box of tee shirts or toothbrushes or 20 pairs of socks, and within about 2 weeks, they would arrive."

Commander Josie

Some nurses described good working relationships with local people employed at their hospitals. Josie, a career Navy nurse assigned to a 16-person mentoring team at an Afghan national army hospital in Mazer-e-Sharif, Afghanistan, exclaimed, "For me, this deployment was one of the most rewarding experiences of my life. The people were wonderful. We had very loving people at the hospital. One housekeeper at the hospital, Zora, would come running down the hall every day to hug me. We had this wonderful man at the hospital who was the optometrist when I got there. Then he became the pharmacist, and finally, he became the dentist. He did all the jobs well. He was just amazing and so helpful. He spoke very good English and taught me my first Afghan phrase. The Afghan food at the hospital was wonderful. We all enjoyed the food. I was just so happy while I was in Afghanistan. My mother even said, 'I've never seen you look so happy in pictures than your pictures from Afghanistan. Your eyes have never been brighter or sparkled so much.' I was just in my element there, and I would certainly go back. I am even considering, when I retire from the Navy, going back to do some humanitarian work there. The people at that hospital were awesome. They were so loving and so kind."

Captain Liz

Some nurses reported how important it is to stay in touch with the people they were deployed with and what these relationships mean to them. Liz was an active-duty Air Force flight nurse assigned first to Iraq and later in her career to Afghanistan. Liz stated, "I keep in touch with the people I worked with over there. The bond between us is very strong. When you are deployed, you get very tight with your team. The camaraderie was just awesome. We supported each other and helped each other so much. From our commander on down, these people were just the best. I just couldn't imagine being there with any other group of people. Tomorrow, I'm headed to Washington, DC to have a mini reunion with this group of people because one of the men is getting promoted. We are all going to his promotion ceremony and have a reunion. I haven't seen them since last August, when I left Iraq."

Captain Tina

Tina, an active-duty Air Force nurse assigned to Balad Air Base, Iraq, and later at FOB Salerno, Afghanistan, exclaimed, "The people I worked with were so special. We felt a kinship and brotherhood I can't even explain, except that is was deep, respectful, and committed. We worked so hard together, hung out with each other, and looked out for each other, making sure everyone was doing all right with the deployment. We relied on our overseas military family for the time we were deployed much more than our current stateside military family. When you are deployed, you don't have the same layers of support from your immediate family, relatives, and neighborhood friends. Those support systems are far away. All you have by your side when you are deployed is your military family. Luckily, I was in Iraq with a great group of people from three different stateside Air Force hospitals and a group of Army nurses who came to work with us for 4 months of their 12-month deployment. These people were very high quality, and I saw their commitment to our country and to serving others every day. They were such a fun-loving yet very professional and caring group. I made a connection with those people that I wouldn't have met anywhere else because we were from four different stateside groups. We now stay in touch by email, phone calls, and I've taken two mini vacations with five of the nurses I was with in Balad. We are all scattered around the U.S. now, but we go the extra mile to stay in touch."

Major Derek

Lastly, many of the nurses reported that they would go back to their deployment location if they were needed. An Army Reserve major, Derek, shared, "I'd go back if I was needed. I don't think I'll have to go back, although I am always ready. At my rank, there has to be a need for someone like me. I set up clinics and managed an intermediate care ward at a detainee hospital. This is my second time in the Army. Years ago, I was on active duty in the field artillery branch. I got off active duty to go to nursing school. I came back in the reserves as a nurse. In Iraq, I feel we are making a difference as we assist the Iraqi people to build their nation. I like the teamwork in the military. I like to be part of something bigger than myself. In my civilian job back home, we don't have the same sense of belonging, commitment, and teamwork."

Commander Rita

Rita, a career Navy officer and nurse anesthetist assigned to a fast-forward surgical team in Iraq, remarked, "If I was needed again, I'd go in a heartbeat. That's what I'm trained to do. The military paid a lot of money to train me to do anesthesia care. How could I say no to 20-year-old kids coming in with all kinds of combat wounds, legs blown off, and shrapnel in their belly? It is my privilege to serve."

First Lieutenant Lisa

Lisa was a critical care nurse assigned at the coalition forces combat support hospital in Mosul, Iraq. Lisa reported, "What I remember most is the wonderful gang of people I worked with. Everybody pitched in to help, whether we were taking care of casualties or cleaning the ER and ICU after a mass cal. Even some of the doctors mopped the floor if it needed to be done. They were just a great group."

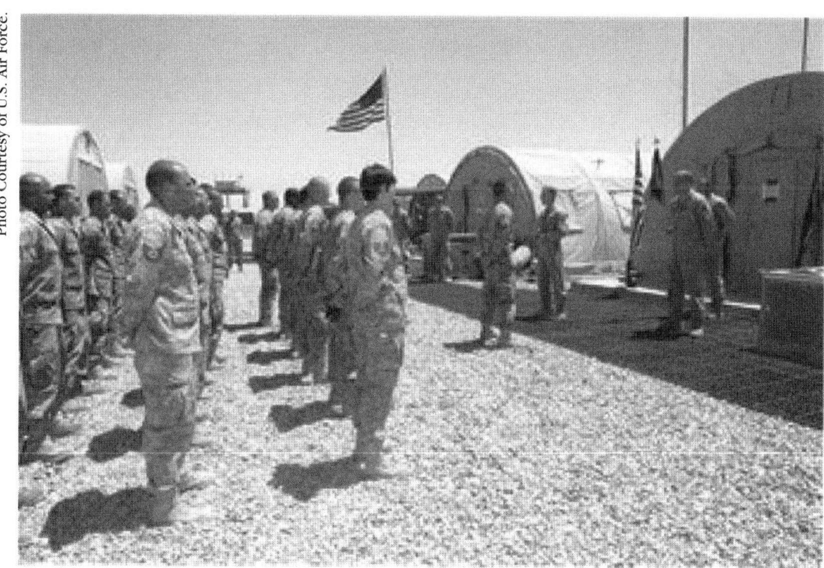

Photo Courtesy of U.S. Air Force.

Air Force hospital staff, Iraq.

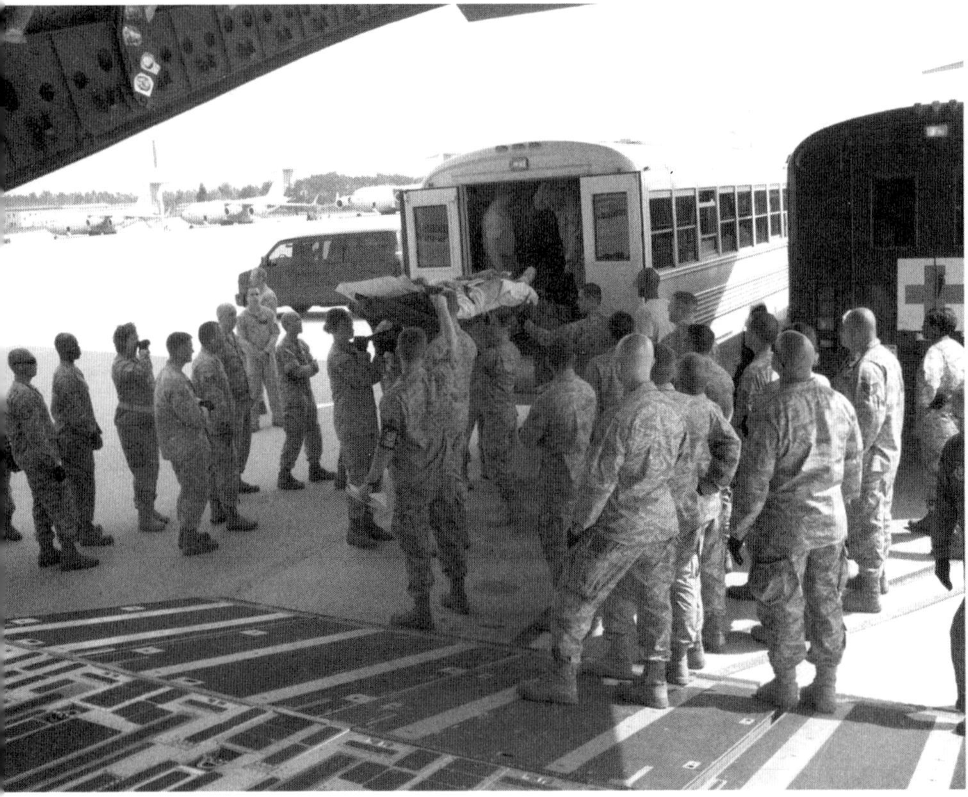

Photo Courtesy of U.S. Air Force.

Volunteers offloading patients from air evacuation ambulance bus (Ambus), Ramstein Air Base, Germany.

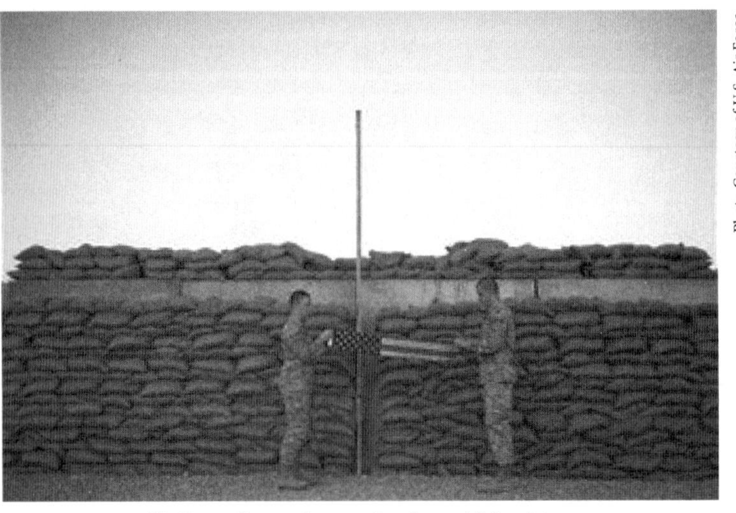

Photo Courtesy of U.S. Air Force.

Air Force forward operating base, Afghanistan.

14

Professional Growth: Expanding My Knowledge, Skills, and Abilities

Nurses admitted that war zone nursing duties afforded a significant opportunity to hone trauma, critical care, and surgical nursing proficiencies. They learned to live in a foreign culture and to work with their coalition brothers and sisters in providing nursing care to anyone who needed it. Although war results in terrible injuries and deaths, from a medical perspective, it also provides a great opportunity for learning. Nurses learned from each other and from the clinically challenging circumstance of having to care for people with catastrophic injuries.

Nurses further developed their leadership skills while deployed as they learned more about the military services, the combat environment, and themselves. They learned up-close-and-personal how to survive in a war zone environment such as convoy risks, ambush tactics employed by insurgents, and survival strategies. They made do with fewer creature comforts while improvising to get by. They learned more about themselves in terms of pacing their rest, relaxation, and private time away from work.

Captain Abby

Abby, an active-duty Air Force nurse, recalled, "I was deployed as a medical–surgical nurse. I was there for 6 months at the hospital at Bagram Air Base, Afghanistan. At first, I worked on an intermediate care ward. Then they had a need for ER [emergency room] nurses, so I ended up working in the ER for the remaining duration of my tour of duty. It was a great experience professionally because I learned so much. We saw some amazing wounds, orthopedic injuries, and burns, and I gained so many skills. It is an unfortunate thing we have to have so many people get hurt, but as a nurse in terms of skills, you learn the most in a combat zone. War nursing is a great opportunity for learning. I learned an awful lot about trauma care and emergency medicine. I had never been involved in trauma care before. I had never worked in the ER and never worked in the ICU [intensive care unit] before. This was the most eye-opening experience I have ever had in my life. I saw things in terms of trauma that I will never ever see again in my life. I saw injuries that no one should ever have to see or care for. It was just an awesome clinical experience."

First Lieutenant Joy

Joy was an active-duty Air Force nurse assigned in Afghanistan. She remarked, "It was a real growth experience because I had not been a nurse for very long. I didn't quite know what to expect and didn't have any preconceived notions. We really did learn a lot. We really grew as nurses and as leaders. We had to rely on each other as team members. We relied more on our own nursing judgment because the doctors weren't around that much. We learned a lot from each other, and we developed new skills. It really helped me to develop more clinical skills and the confidence that goes with that. I also learned more about the military being over there. In the medical field, you don't always get to learn military things as much as the nonmedical military personnel do. Over there, we learned a lot from the troops and learned about what it was like for them outside the wire. Clinically, I got to care for trauma patients and fresh critical postop patients, who helped me gain new skills as well as confidence."

Lieutenant Commander Clare

Even nurses who were experienced in stateside trauma care stated that they gained valuable experience and expanded their specialty learning. Clare, an active-duty Navy nurse assigned to a surgical hospital in Anbar Province, Iraq, recalled, "We were always learning. Even as shock-trauma critical care nurses and physicians, we learned a lot over there. We all had enough training and experience, but what we saw and had to deal with in the war zone was just the worst trauma you could imagine. We saw injuries we had never seen before. We had to deal with the added element that we were also under fire. We cared for U.S. military personnel, coalition forces, and local women and children caught in [the] crossfire of war. We had to deal with seeing an age-diverse and culturally diverse group of patients as well as the psychological sequelae of traumatic war injuries. We saw people physically ripped apart from gunshot wounds, blast injuries, chemical injuries, and the like. So we had a lot more to contend with than the average inner-city level 1 trauma unit."

Captain Christina

Flight nurses described the autonomy with which they practiced in Iraq and Afghanistan. Christina, an active-duty Air Force flight nurse, reported, "I did tours as a flight nurse in both Iraq and Afghanistan. We don't normally fly with a physician onboard. We fly with standing orders for our patients. Essentially, it is two or three flight nurses and three air evac technicians. The senior flight nurse calls the shots. We may have 70 patients on the plane. If there is a very critical patient, we may have a physician on board, but usually, we don't. Flight nursing is a very autonomous specialty. Being able to be autonomous as a nurse was a big plus for me. I had the resources to radio a hospital on the ground, if I need to confer with a flight surgeon or if I need special orders for meds or whatnot. Most physicians are willing to give us whatever orders we need to take care of those patients. Flight nursing is a gutsy specialty for the best nurses in the Air Force. It is not for the novice or those who don't like adventure or those who don't feel at home at 35,000 feet. Even though we all served as flight nurses in the States, nothing will ever compare to the skill level we developed taking care of combat-injured troops in Iraq and Afghanistan. It was a challenge. Every mission posed new types of injuries and new clinical situations."

Lieutenant Colonel Judd

Many nurses described their expanded role of nursing practice in the war zone. An Army Reserve nurse practitioner recalled, "The Army was building a new hospital in Anbar province, and this was during the surge, so they needed me there. I was a nurse practitioner, but they needed me in surgery as first assistant. I said, 'I don't do ORs [operating rooms]; I don't even know what an OR looks like!' They said, 'Don't worry. We'll teach you!' Therefore, they taught me. The whole experience was a positive challenge for me because I was doing something I never thought I would do in a lifetime. I never thought of myself working in an operating room, cutting off someone's leg to save his life. I was needed to do a job, and I contributed everything that I could. I stayed very busy because there were many amputations."

Major Yvonne

Some nurses had the opportunity to perform humanitarian missions outside the walls of their hospital and base compounds. Yvonne, an active-duty Army nurse, recalled, "Although I served as a brigade trainer for our airborne brigade, I got to do some missions outside the wire. Doing the humanitarian aid missions was a very rewarding and new experience for me. We'd distribute a lot of clothes and shoes that were donated by people in the States. Working with the South Koreans and Egyptians was rewarding and getting to see how they provided medical care. We also got to work with some of the coalition forces and had dinner with the commander of the forces from the UAE [United Arab Emirates]. We got to see what their culture was like and to eat their food. We spent time on other coalition compounds in the Bagram, Afghanistan, area. We got to meet our coalition medical and nursing counterparts from Poland, United Arab Emirates, South Korea, and Egypt. Most of these folks spoke English and readily welcomed us and toured us through their facilities. It was a wonderful learning and sharing experience."

Captain Penny

Nurses described aspects of their expanded practice. Penny, an active-duty Army nurse assigned to a forward surgical team, recalled, "Some of the procedures I did in the war zone, I can't do here. I've put in chest tubes. I've done lots of endotracheal intubations. Nurses don't do those procedures here in the U.S. When you have only two surgeons and you have 15 critical patients, you end up doing more than nurses do in a stateside ICU or trauma unit. I've seen more and done more than my ICU nurse manager, and she has been a nurse for 28 years. In the emergency area, we were debriding wounds, exploring wounds and removing the shrapnel, inserting chest tubes, suturing wounds, and other procedures primarily reserved for the surgeons. It was a big adjustment period for me coming back home to Fort Bragg, North Carolina. Your scope of practice is definitely expanded when you are deployed."

Major Alene

Alene was an Army reservist assigned to the hospital at Bagram Air Base, Afghanistan. Alene related, "It was a great learning environment. When it came to medical skills, I got to intubate people, and even my LPN [licensed practical nurse] medics got to intubate people. I got to explore wounds and remove shrapnel. I got to insert arterial lines and do two tracheotomies in the triage area. We took advantage of any training opportunity that arose. This was really rewarding because civilianwise, that's not in your job description, but in the military, it's different. If you have had the training, and were signed off on a skill, you can perform the procedure. The physicians were eager to teach. It was really a necessity to learn so you could help when the physicians were inundated and overwhelmed with fresh casualties. You were another pair of skilled hands."

Alene went on to explain, "I have been in two wars, Operation Desert Storm in Iraq and now the war in Afghanistan. I must say that I am very proud to be an American. In addition, I would do it again. I feel very strongly about taking care of our soldiers. This is important for me. We made a difference over there. We saved a lot of soldiers and a lot of Afghanis, as well. We truly made a difference in so many lives. It was very rewarding to see that we made a difference. I got to know some of my patients pretty well. I knew that without the care we provided, they would have surely died. I also believe we certainly did our part to ensure our soldiers got back home to their families. It was definitely a good feeling for me to know I played a small part in caring for our soldiers and giving them the care they needed to make it home."

Major Michelle

A few of the nurses were assigned to special programs in Afghanistan to mentor the local Afghan national army medical and nursing staffs at the Afghan military hospitals. Michelle, an active-duty Air Force nurse anesthetist, explained, "They didn't know how to effectively manage a big trauma. They didn't know what adequate fluid resuscitation was. They didn't know how to keep a patient warm in the operating room and to monitor vital signs. They never wrote anything down. I actually got them to chart. I developed an anesthesia record to help them document the fluids, what medications they used, and vital signs. I kept telling them that if you didn't write it down, you didn't do it. I learned so much about reinforcing the basics and in setting milestones for people learning a new skill. There were many frustrations for me, but there was also progress."

Michelle went on to discuss the mentoring role. "Our mentoring role was huge. They had no background in anatomy and physiology training. When you are doing anesthetics and the patient is intubated, one of the gold standards we use is to verify the tube is in place, oxygenation is good, and the patient is being ventilated in a satisfactory manner. I don't know how I pulled this off, but I managed to find two gas analyzers from a warehouse up in Kabul. We heard from our medical logistics folks that there was some medical equipment in this warehouse. They had no inventory documents;

everything was just piled into this warehouse. We went up there and found them. They were old analyzers from Bagram. They weren't using them anymore because the Air Force hospital at Bagram had all new anesthesia machines. The U.S. forces had given them to the Afghan national army, but they had just sent them to this warehouse because they didn't know how to use them. When I found them a couple of years later, I took them back with us to Kandahar and hooked them up to our anesthesia machines, and they worked. It was one of the best days of my deployment when these gas analyzers actually worked. They made a huge difference because everything I was teaching them, they could now see. They could read the measurements, and it made sense to them. The 'light bulb' went on for these folks. I got them to the point that they were almost meeting the anesthesia standards we have in the U.S. This was a huge accomplishment for the Afghan medical folks and for us as their mentors."

Michelle reported she pondered the question, 'Did we make a difference over there?' She shared her answer. "I think we did. It was much better when we left than when we got there. If the U.S. continues to 'babysit' them with mentoring teams in Afghanistan, things will continue to improve as far as medical care. However, if we leave them on their own, the hospital will crumble and go back to the deplorable conditions we found when we arrived. They also have to dramatically fix their logistics, or things will not progress. You can't run a hospital without medicines and supplies. We [the mentoring team] pushed them. We pushed the Afghans to strive for something better. In addition, they had to respect you, and like you, or you got nothing from them in terms of work and cooperation. We had to constantly push them to do things, like to change dressings and chart things, and monitor their patients more closely. They didn't like to change dressings; the wounds were mostly dirty wounds from IED blasts, and the dressings needed to be changed. The pieces of shrapnel were dirty. There was dirt in the blast injuries, and the dressings needed to be changed on these infected wounds. I know we saved a lot of people who wouldn't have been saved. I can only hope, 10 years from now, that I hear about this hospital, and it is thriving. I hope in 10 years, they are still doing what we taught them. Then I will truly feel gratified and know we truly made a long-term difference."

Commander Josie

Not only did nurses assigned to mentoring duty believe they made a positive difference in the lives of the people they trained in local hospitals and clinics; many other nurses assigned to all levels of care facilities believed they made a difference in the lives of their patients. Josie, a senior Navy nurse assigned to an Afghan national army hospital near Mazer-e-Sharif,

Afghanistan, reflected, "We gave medical care not just to military members but also to a lot of local Afghans. If we were not there to give medical care, those people would have died. We saw so many children injured by the fighting or because they stepped on land mines. The positive thing for me was saving the lives of local people, including many children, as well as caring for our soldiers. If we were not there, so many people would have died. We made a huge difference."

Major Lee

Many nurses reported enhanced professional confidence and self-esteem because of developing improved clinical proficiency and acquiring new clinical skills. Many of these skills were reserved for physician practice in stateside trauma centers and intensive care units. Lee, an Army reservist, remarked, "It was a good experience. I've worked in an inner-city ER in Philadelphia for 20 years, and my experience in Iraq was a change and a challenge. For example, in the beginning, I was in charge of the ER. I had to get with all the surgeons and make sure we had the equipment we needed. We inventoried the equipment, and then I ordered more supplies we thought we might need. I got to set up trauma stations and felt good when things worked smoothly. I gained confidence that I could be more than just an ER staff nurse. I never aspired to be in charge of an ER, but I found I really had an aptitude for it."

Captain Trudi

Trudi was an Army reservist from New England. She stated, "My deployment gave me confidence as a nurse. Before this assignment, I had worked in primary care, on general medical-surgical units, and very rarely in the ER. Being able to jump into the ICU at Mosul and learn about ventilators and the camaraderie of the other nurses there with ICU experience was special. In addition, the fact that they accepted my lack of ICU experience and taught me was such a big positive for me. They took me under their wing and were there for me. If an American soldier came in and it was close to change of shift, the outgoing shift would stay to make sure everything was good, especially when our census was full. The day shift would stay to help the night shift to make sure everything was set up for those patients. The American soldiers were our priority. Sometimes, you had to step away from your Iraqi patient to be with the American soldier and make sure he or she had everything they needed right away. I came home after 1 year as an experienced and confident trauma ICU nurse, when I had no critical care skills other than basic CPR before I went to Iraq. This was such a positive change for me. My nursing experiences in Mosul enhanced my self-esteem as a nurse and person."

Major Olga

Olga was an active-duty Army ICU nurse assigned to a fast-forward surgical team. She reported, "The skills I learned with all the traumas were very beneficial. I got to do things as a nurse I will probably never get to do again. At the FOB, working on a forward surgical team, I got a lot of experience. I had never seen trauma like that before. The trauma was fresh from the field. I didn't know how I'd handle it, but I learned quickly. Now I know that no matter what is thrown at me, I can handle it. By the time I left, I was able to handle any war trauma that was thrust into my care. That was a confidence builder. I definitely came back a more confident nurse."

First Lieutenant Leah

Leah, an Army reservist, recalled that studying coupled with hands-on clinical experience was necessary to master new skills. "I hit the books over there. I learned a lot about vent settings. Some of the stuff I didn't really understand at first, but I studied, and it became clear. I definitely came out of there a more confident nurse. I learned quickly and had the right skills."

Captain Erin

Erin, an active-duty Air Force flight nurse, summarized how the underlying philosophy of the military to "leave no soldier behind" added to her confidence and self-esteem as a member of the military medical services. "Something I am very proud of, and don't completely understand, is our country's philosophy and practical application of the sanctity of human life. Perhaps the best way to describe it is that we'll have soldiers in a vehicle that goes out on a patrol, flips over, and burns because of rolling over an IED [improvised explosive device] in some obscure location in either Iraq or Afghanistan. Three soldiers were onboard. Two are dead. The one remaining soldier is gonna require a lot of help to live. We'll send out help into harm's way with bullets flying and bad guys everywhere just to save that 18-year-old soldier. We spent a few thousands of dollars training him and another few thousands of dollars getting him his gear. We pay him less than $2,000 a month. We'll send out three other vehicles with 12 soldiers in them to bring him back, even if we think there is little hope of survival. We will put all of those soldiers into this fight to go pull that injured soldier out of there. They will drive anywhere and do anything to get that injured soldier out of there. They will render any kind of aid needed since we train everyone in the military to be first-aid providers. They'll literally do everything humanly possible to keep this kid alive. We'll launch three helicopters, two of which will guard the third one, which has an actual medic on it. They'll go and land under fire to save this one soldier. These helicopters cost millions and millions of dollars with the pilots, who are officers and other crewmembers. It has cost millions of dollars to train all these people who are going out to save this one kid."

Erin went on to describe the medical care. "They'll do lifesaving procedures on the helicopter, get him to a field hospital, and perform surgeries that don't even exist outside of a U.S. military hospital in Iraq or Afghanistan. They'll perform procedures that will be written about several years from now in medical journals. Then, they'll fly a plane in harm's way, with the soldier being cared for by flight nurses in back, to a large theater hospital like Balad, Iraq, or Bagram, Afghanistan, and perform numerous other surgeries. Then, he may be transported to Germany and then back to the U.S., where he will go through rehabilitation. The story keeps going on. In addition, let's face it, this amount of effort and attention is foreign to almost every other civilization. This preservation of life principle is completely and utterly mind-boggling. Here we are in a culture where we kill people with handguns in the major cities of the U.S. We have this incredible juxtaposition of ideals where life is so cheap on one hand, and then we have this preservation-of-life principle in the military. The whole thing is literally mind-boggling. It's a positive thing to me. It is very difficult to understand. It's also very powerful. I'll tell you why it is so powerful. It is so powerful because every troop we have understands. They know our health care system in the military will do quite literally anything to get them through it. These guys and gals know that we will do everything possible for them. Their belief in me motivates me to do the best job possible. They are motivated by what I do, and I am motivated by their faith in me. Therefore, it's a very reciprocal relationship, and that's very positive. This is why our military can be successful when it's allowed to be successful."

Major Samantha

Another aspect of providing care that enhanced the nurse's repertoire of professional skills was the emotional support and encouragement they provided their patients. This was an especially difficult task because the vast majority of the combat casualties they cared for were young soldiers and local children. Samantha, an active-duty Army nurse assigned in Afghanistan, exclaimed, "I felt like I did a lot of good being there for the soldiers and providing their nursing and emotional care. I held their hands and let them know we cared about them and that we were going to get them home safely. Being there for them and dressing their injuries was so important. I will never ever experience this again. It was the worst thing I'd ever done, and it was the best thing I'd ever done."

Samantha went on to describe caring for injured children, "Seeing little kids when they first came into the hospital was so troubling. Some were so critically injured. However, rehabilitating them was very rewarding and challenging. They are there for months on end. These were mainly the burned kids. They were so grateful. You could see it in their eyes. They came back from the recovery room, and you recognize them. You give them a nickname because their last name is so long. The names would stick. We'd keep track of the kids as they came out of the OR. We'd monitor their progress. To see the child discharged after 4 or 5 months was very gratifying. They'd get so emotional leaving us. We had become part of their family. It caused all of the nurses there to cry. We were so grateful. We'd just hope for the best outcome when they would leave our base and go back to the little village where they came from. I remember one child we called 'Fez'. Fez would come back for outpatient visits. He would make sure to come and greet us each time. That was certainly one of the positives. I was not a big fan of pediatrics before I deployed."

Major Millie

Not only did nurses report professional and clinical growth experiences, but several reported how the experience of their deployment to a war zone helped them grow personally as well. Millie, an active-duty Army operating room nurse, remarked, "I learned a lot about myself personally. I grew as a leader over there. I had been an OR nurse for a long time, but the trauma was never to the extent of what I saw in Iraq. It was good for me to see myself doing the clinical side again. I had been doing the administrative and education side of OR nursing for some time. I went right back to the clinical side in Iraq, and it was a positive experience to jump right back in. It was a good thing for me. I learned that I had the skills and abilities to do the clinical, administrative, and educational sides of operating room nursing. I truly liked having these abilities. My leadership was valued by my colleagues. I felt intrinsically valued, confident, and important to our mission. I felt fulfilled over there as a nurse and as a person."

Millie described some personal learning experiences. "I learned a lot about how I handle stress. How I am when I have no sleep. I think on my next deployment, I will have a better handle on things. I learned more about how stress and lack of sleep affects me. I learned it is important to remember to take care of yourself. If you can't take care of yourself, you can't take care of anybody else."

Captain Suzanne

Suzanne, an active-duty Air Force nurse assigned to an Aeromedical Staging Facility in Iraq, explained what she learned about herself. "The wealth of knowledge I gained, not only the clinical nursing stuff but the knowledge I gained about myself, was so important. I learned when 'the shit hits the fan,' I know what I'm doing. I don't freak out. People have said they can look at me, and they can see that I'm 'in the zone,' and I just go with it. Afterwards, I have to write things down. I was so methodical about what I did with our patients. The best thing I learned about myself was to develop a system that worked and to stick with it."

Captain Alice

Alice served as an active-duty Air Force critical care air transport team nurse. She exclaimed, "Because of my deployments to Iraq and Afghanistan as a CCATT nurse in aeromedical evacuation aircraft, I am by far a better nurse, a better leader, and a better human being. In both war zones, I can say I have changed people's lives. I am not just talking about taking care of Americans; I am talking about taking care of Afghanis and Iraqis as well. I also learned a lot about myself as a person, a leader, and a nurse. I grew in so many positive ways because of my deployment experiences. For me, the positives of deployment far outweighed the negatives."

Lieutenant Donna

Donna, an active-duty Navy nurse assigned to the coalition forces hospital in Kandahar, Afghanistan, reported, "You know, I miss the action of deployment. I just want to get back somewhere now. It gets in your blood. I don't care where I go as long as once I get there, my job is taking care of soldiers, sailors, airmen, and marines. It's what I want to do. Now, I can see why some people spent eight or nine years on and off in Vietnam. It's just something you want to do. There's something special about it. We all have our roles to play."

Donna went on to further explain her feelings, "I felt like I was doing something very important over there. What can be more important for a military nurse than taking care of wounded troops? That is our mission in the military nurse corps. Everything else we do is secondary to that mission. I would go again in a heartbeat. As a nurse, I have gained skills I would have never gotten a chance to attain and master if I had stayed in my regular job back in the States. Yes, there was danger. Yes, I was scared. However, I have to admit that I learned so much as a nurse and as a person. In retrospect, I wouldn't trade my time in Afghanistan for anything. I really matured over there. I learned what it means to be in the military, to be in harm's way serving my country. I feel a sense of professional and personal pride. I have a renewed confidence in my skills and in my judgment."

15

Women's Health and Hygiene Experiences

With most military nurses being female, women's health and hygiene experiences were paramount in the lives of the deployed nurses. A myriad of topics under this heading echoed in the voices of the nurses. For example, many women found the bathroom and shower facilities to be dirty, primitive, lacking in privacy, and sometimes far from their living quarters. Sometimes, they had to clean the bathrooms themselves. Other times, bathrooms were closed right after breakfast and lunch for cleaning by contractors, which were the most inconvenient times. Nurses noted definite differences in the quality and quantity of facilities depending on the year they were deployed, 2003 to 2010, and whether the location was on a large U.S. compound, a smaller forward operating base, or elsewhere.

BATHROOM FACILITIES

Lieutenant Colonel Victoria

Victoria, an active-duty Army nurse, provided a descriptive account of her two deployments to Iraq. As a women's health care provider herself, she was acutely tuned in to female deployment experiences. She referred to night trips to the bathroom as "a walk on the wild side," focusing on the imminent danger of a mortar attack or the possibility of being jumped on the way to or from the bathroom in the dark.

Victoria compared and contrasted her 2003 and 2008 deployments to Iraq, stating, "When I was in Iraq in 2003, the bathroom facilities were limited, poor, and primitive. The toilets were a board of plywood with holes in it. It had one of those big basins underneath, which was cleaned out on a daily basis. They poured the urine off and burned the feces right behind the latrines. Of course, things were a lot better in 2008." *She added*, "During my second deployment to Iraq, the toilets and showers were better than before, and they were permanent facilities, but you still had to walk quite a distance to get to them. Otherwise, near the hospital and our sleeping tent, you had to use port-a-potties. They were supposed to be cleaned twice a day, but sometimes, they were horrendous. At nighttime, if you had to go to the toilet you had to use a port-a-potty. You had to make sure you had a flashlight with you to check out the port-a-potty before you used it because people missed the hole a lot, so there was urine sprayed all over in there, not to the mention bugs and, sometimes, exposed feces. It was gross, absolutely disgusting." *She added*, "If you wanted to use the permanent toilets in the middle of the night, you had to walk across the whole compound at 2 a.m. It could be dangerous. Women could be taken advantage of if they went out at night in the dark."

Captain Abby

Shortly after being promoted to the rank of captain, Abby found herself working in the emergency room and on an intermediate care unit at the Joint Theater Hospital in Bagram, Afghanistan. Her remarks about life in Afghanistan were laced with frustration as she recalled, "Everything was just inconvenient in Afghanistan, whether it was taking a long walk to the permanent latrines at night or having to clean our own showers and toilets. It was just so primitive. The trailer latrines were cold in the winter and hot and smelly in the summer. I used to wonder if they could have made it better for the women, or maybe the decision makers just lacked that kind of awareness. I just don't know."

Major Christina

Christina stated that she was "living her dream as an Air Force Flight nurse." She joined the Air Force Nurse Corps several years after completing college with the hopes of being sent to the Flight Nurse Program. After completing two assignments at Air Force medical centers in the United States, she was selected for flight nurse training. Later, she was deployed to Germany, Iraq, and Afghanistan as a flight nurse. She reported, "I flew all in-country missions in Afghanistan as well as to Germany and to

Iraq and Pakistan. I covered the whole Middle East. When you are on an aircraft, you can have a mission that goes for 15 hours. On the back of a C-130 aircraft, the only bathroom you have is a honey pot, a bucket with a shower curtain in front of it for privacy. I could not believe this setup in 2008; it really made me mad." *She added*, "It is well known in the Air Force that all personnel, especially females, avoid using makeshift bathrooms on the aircraft. You only go to the bathroom in-flight if absolutely necessary. You try to hold it until you land, and then you run to the nearest bathroom."

First Lieutenant Lisa

Lisa was an Army reservist assigned to the coalition forces hospital in Mosul, Iraq. Lisa recalled, "What bothered me most was having to wear your combat gear all the time in the heat and then having to go into a smelly bathroom. I doubt the bathrooms were cleaned as often as they needed to be with the high volume of female soldiers using them. I felt like it took 5 minutes just to get my body armor off and sit down on the toilet. By that time, I felt sweaty and dirty. It was such a negative experience. It made me feel gross."

First Lieutenant Joy

Joy was an active-duty Air Force nurse assigned to the Joint Theater Hospital at Bagram Air Base, Afghanistan. Joy reported, "The local Afghans seemed to be cleaning the bathrooms whenever we needed to go in there, like after breakfast and after lunch. You know, you need to get in there right away after your coffee kicks in. The timing of the cleaning was frustrating. You felt like you had to plan your whole day around the bathrooms being cleaned."

Major Alene

Alene was an Army reservist assigned to the coalition forces combat support hospital in Mosul, Iraq. Later in her career, she was deployed to Afghanistan. Alene related, "The port-a-potties were disgusting. I hope I never have to use a port-a-potty again as long as I live. What bothered me the most about them was the smell. They smelled to high heaven of urine, and urine was on the floors and toilet seats all the time. I was afraid to touch anything in there, and I always brought my own roll of toilet paper because, often, there was none. I always carried a packet of antiseptic wipes in my pocket so I could clean my hands afterwards."

SHOWER CHALLENGES

Shower facilities and the supply and temperature of the water depended on location. The condition of the facilities, the issue of privacy, the water supply, and water temperature were of significant importance to the nurses.

Major Vivian

Vivian, an Air Force reservist, attributed her "survivalist attitude" in dealing with living conditions in Iraq to her love of camping and the outdoors. She recalled that a major complaint of her nurse colleagues was the shower facilities. She stated, "We were allowed a 3-minute shower every day. However, we didn't have hot water every day. You had to get in, get wet, lather up, rinse off, and get out. That's what most of us did. Some people took longer than 3 minutes, but most of us respected the fact that there would not be enough water if we weren't quick about showering." *She added,* "I could live with the 3-minute shower partly because I have short hair. It wasn't a big deal for me. However, it was a big deal for many of the girls, especially those who had long hair. They couldn't get all the shampoo and conditioner out of their hair. It could be a definite challenge. Sometimes, little things like this could get to them. It was bad enough that we were in a war zone, seeing injuries and fatalities every day, but having to work in a hot, dirty environment without a chance to really feel clean was a morale buster."

Lieutenant Colonel Victoria

A seasoned Army nurse, Victoria, told about her first deployment to Iraq. "In 2003, when we arrived, we did not have the infrastructure there ahead of us to take care of anything, like shower facilities. I literally went weeks on end without anything that remotely resembled a real shower. I learned how to bathe and wash my hair in about a liter of water. We were given 6 liters of water a day. Therefore, you could drink it, bathe with it, or do your laundry with it. It was a real toss-up! I became the queen of what was referred to as the 'poncho shower.' Therefore, what we would do is strip down as much as we could under our rain ponchos and give ourselves 'bird baths.' *She added,* "From April 2003 into May, we just didn't have any water for bathing. Therefore, I called myself clean if I didn't smell as bad as my patients did. It was a real downer; it really sucked."

Captain Erin

This active-duty Air Force flight nurse in Afghanistan related, "Sometimes, when I wasn't flying, I'd help out at the hospital. We didn't have enough water, and your choice was to either flush the toilet or take a quick shower. If you had a particularly difficult day at work with an action-packed flying mission or mass cal event at the hospital or a bunch of injured children, having to forego a shower because of a water shortage simply added to your stress. When you were feeling down in the dumps because of your workload or the sad situations you had to deal with in your job, creature comforts became more important as an escape or a little respite at the end of the day."

Captain Meaghan

Meaghan, an Air Force nurse who flew on aeromedical evacuation flights as a critical care air transport team nurse, stated, "One of the biggest things that stands out for me was that we were not able to take showers for a week. It was horrible! There was a broken pipe or something. It was a hardship for me." *She furtherer commented*, "The showers in the Bagram hospital area were pretty disgusting. What was supposed to be a new shower trailer had been up and running for maybe 7 years or longer. It had electricity, heat, and running water. There was a nasty little shower curtain, and the walls were covered in a greasy green slimy nastiness, and the floors were, too. You had to wear shower slippers, and everything was always wet or at least damp. There was no room to bend over in the shower stall, and you were only a few feet from the main door looking onto the street." *She added*, "In the winter, we had to deal with ice and snow right outside the showers. It was freezing outside. I remember a colleague describing our whole experience as 'living in your garage,' and I agreed with her. It was pretty horrible; I expected better."

First Lieutenant Leah

Leah was an Army reservist deployed to Mosul, Iraq. She recalled, "You had to walk down the streets to get to the showers. So, you had to be fully dressed from head to toe all the time." *She added*, "The water was from the Tigris and Euphrates River, and it was very dirty water. You couldn't open your eyes or mouth when you were in the shower. You could not even brush your teeth with the water. It was for bathing only. You had to use bottled water to brush your teeth."

First Lieutenant Lisa

Lisa, an Army reservist in Iraq, reported, "In Mosul, we had a long walk to the showers. We had to carry all our own shower supplies and a change of clothes. Taking a shower was not a relaxing experience over there. When I get home, I think I'm going to start taking long, relaxing baths."

First Lieutenant Joy

Joy was an active-duty Air Force nurse deployed to Afghanistan. Joy reported, "I must admit that I thought the shower facilities for women would be better. The shower stalls were small, and the floors were always wet and slippery. I felt that the shower stalls were a breeding ground for mold and mildew. It made you appreciate what you had back home; you know, the creature comforts."

TRYING TO STAY CLEAN

Women in both war zones expressed concern and frustration with trying to stay clean while working and living in these countries. Many were creative in their attempts to stay clean. Some felt that their efforts were a monumental task.

Lieutenant Colonel Heidi

Heidi, an Army nurse deployed to Iraq, described her cleanliness challenge, "I never really felt clean. You never felt fresh like you do at home. The biggest hygiene issue for me was sweating. The sand of the desert caked in my armpits and chafed the folds of skin in my crotch like dirty, wet sandpaper." *She added,* "I sweat so badly. It would run down my back, through my butt crack, and pool. At times, I would wear a sanitary pad just to catch the sweat. It was between 120 and 130 degrees at times." *She went further to say,* "I've lived in lots of places but have never encountered such heat, humidity, dirt, and sand like this before. It was unreal."

Lieutenant Commander Clare

Clare, a Navy nurse serving in a tent hospital in Iraq, described her experience. "It was very hot, and we worked in a tent. Outside, it would be 140 degrees, and inside the tent, it would be 150 degrees, so we would be constantly sweating, dripping wet. We felt dirty and disgusting. We knew we smelled awful. I just wanted to crawl in a hole and not show my face." *She added,* "I must admit that as nurses and as women, we were concerned about our own health and hygiene. You don't feel that great about yourself when you are a sweaty mess. It was an unhealthy environment for both patients and nurses. The heat and humidity compounded everything. I felt like I was doing nursing in a sauna. Most of us asked our families to send feminine hygiene wipes in our care packages from home because we were constantly sweating."

Major Christina

Christina, an Air Force flight nurse, commented, "I think my flight nurse training prepared me well to be aware of women's health and hygiene issues that I would be faced with while deployed. We always pack extra underwear, socks, T-shirts, and an extra flight suit to change into if necessary. Sometimes, we'd be landing at 2:30 a.m., it would be over 100 degrees, and the tarmac would be hot. You had a set of dry clothes to change into. You are out in the desert, you are loading patients, and it's hot. You get totally drenched. Luckily, our flights suits dry quickly."

Lieutenant Colonel Victoria

Victoria, a seasoned Army nurse, reported, "I showered every day during my second deployment to Iraq for a whopping 4 minutes. I'd run in the morning, so I'd shower in the morning. At the end of the day, I would go to bed feeling pretty disgusting and dirty because it was 120 to 130 degrees outside. I was pretty hot and sweaty at the end of the day. Well, that's what they made baby wipes for, right? Therefore, in the evening, it would be a 'baby wipe wipe-down' before I got between the sheets. In addition, I was probably the only person on my FOB [forward operating base] who laundered my sheets once a week. There were probably guys who didn't wash their sheets the whole time they were there. But that was not the case with me."

Major Lee

Lee was an Air Force reservist who deployed to Iraq and Afghanistan. Lee commented, "We not only battled the enemy; we battled the dirt, dust, sand, and sweat on a daily basis. Then, feeling clean was always very short-lived. In Iraq, we also had to deal with the sand flies and their bites."

Captain Liz

Liz was an active-duty Air Force flight nurse. She served tours of duty in Iraq and Afghanistan. Liz recalled, "With all the flying I did, I felt grubby and sweaty a lot. Some missions were so long. It seemed like we were always busy. I feel like we worked nonstop."

Captain Holly

Holly was an Army Reserve nurse from New York. She was assigned with a large cadre of reservists to the Abu Ghraib prison hospital in Iraq. "Working in a prison hospital was a challenge in itself. The prison was overcrowded with filthy detainees with horrible body odor. So, when they became patients, we tried to clean them up. Needless to say, I felt pretty dirty and sweaty myself."

Captain Alice

Alice was an active-duty Air Force nurse deployed to Afghanistan. She commented, "Being a CCATT nurse, I was extremely focused on the life-sustaining care I was providing to my patients. To that end, I kind of forgot about myself. I probably looked pretty awful at times, like I needed a shower."

MENSTRUATION ISSUES

Deployed females were faced with the decision to continue their menstrual periods or to suppress them by using continuous oral contraceptives or Depo-Provera injections. Women were provided with this information in pre-deployment health briefings and in printed health promotion literature. This decision brought about numerous thoughts and feelings regarding future reproduction and overall health in the deployed nurses.

Commander Josie

A Navy nurse and mother of three, Josie deployed to Afghanistan in the later years of her career. She reported, "I didn't use menstrual suppression because I didn't think that would be a healthy thing for me to do. I actually used sanitary pads rather than tampons because I felt that tampons could get dusty and dirty from the primitive environment even before I used them. I didn't want to risk toxic shock syndrome or an infection using tampons." *She added,* "When I first arrived, there were about 45 women in a big open tent where I lived. I would say that about 30 of these women were suppressing their periods with either birth control pills or Depo-Provera injections. Most of these women were younger than me. I don't know if that might have had something to do with their decision to suppress their periods. I'm kind of an old-fashioned gal."

Major Diana

Diana was an Air Force reservist assigned to the aeromedical staging facility at Balad Air Base, Iraq. Diana consistently reflected how proud she was to serve in Iraq. She also had strong feelings about menstrual suppression. She stated, "Managing menstrual periods was definitely a problem for many women. I purposely chose not to have my period while deployed. I went and got Depo-Provera and brought a few shots with me. I had other nurses give me the shots when I needed them. It was very important to me not to be distracted by my period when I was engaged in such important work. The heat and dirt were enough of a bother; I didn't need my period to make me more miserable. I felt that it was my duty to make myself as comfortable as possible so I could take care of my patients to the best of my ability and with a smile on my face."

Lieutenant Colonel Heidi

Besides being an Army nurse, Heidi was a nurse-researcher who worked on several research studies during her time in Iraq. She gave her perspective on having one's menstrual period during deployment to a war zone with her comments. "I went into the combat zone thinking that it would not be necessary to suppress, but when I got there, it was a different situation. The heat, humidity, and sand definitely contributed to a woman's comfort level, and when she had her period, everything became magnified. I'm glad women have options. Granted, menstrual suppression is not for everyone, but people need the education piece to make informed decisions about their health. The climate and weather in Iraq, not to mention the combat conditions, can cause women to keep their options open on this important issue."

Major Christina

An Air Force flight nurse, Christina recalled, "I went on continuous birth control pills when I deployed so I wouldn't have to deal with my period while flying and because of the heat, dirt, and dust." *She added,* "There was no real bathroom on the plane, no private place to deal with your period."

First Lieutenant Joy

Joy was an active-duty Air Force nurse assigned to an intensive care unit in Afghanistan. Joy remembered, "Most people dealt with their periods the same way that they would at home. There were plenty of supplies available. The base provided everything you would need. There were also plenty of CARE packages from charitable organizations and women's groups, too."

INFECTIONS

Deployed women were at risk for a variety of infections such as urinary tract infections, vaginal infections, and skin infections. They also reported exacerbations of acne, outbreaks of rashes, and athlete's foot. The heat and the dusty, dirty environment as well as spartan shower and bathroom facilities added to the unhealthy conditions.

Major Olga

As an active-duty Army nurse, Olga recalled forgetting about her own personal needs when providing nonstop nursing care on a regular basis. She stated, "During the day, many of us learned to hold off emptying our bladders because of being busy at work, having to take off all of our combat gear in order to go, the long distance to the toilets, and the lack of security around us." *She added*, "In theory, we all knew that we should not neglect our own health or put our health at risk. However, in reality, the hours flew by as we attended to critically injured patients. This was simply how it was."

Lieutenant Donna

Donna, a Navy nurse, mentioned, "Several of the women I deployed with had GYN [gynecological] problems while we were deployed. There were cases of bacterial vaginosis, lots of rashes from the heat, and many women had yeast infections because of sweating so much. I also remember people with athlete's foot, probably from the wet floors in the showers and bathrooms. There were many people with bug bites as well."

Captain Vanessa

Vanessa was an Army reservist assigned in Tikrit and Abu Ghraib, Iraq. She commented on being shocked at some of the infections she encountered while deployed. She stated, "There were actually more STDs [sexually transmitted diseases] than I expected. There was gonorrhea, and I even heard of a case of syphilis. Given the general order, 'There will be no sex in theater,' I was surprised at the number of cases of STDs." *She added*, "Of course, the number of infected males outnumbered females, and the number of infected enlisted personnel outnumbered officers. However, the whole scene was a bit shocking to me. I didn't expect so much of this in a war zone."

Major Michelle

Michelle was an active-duty Air Force nurse anesthetist assigned to mentoring duty at the Afghan national army hospital near Kandahar, Afghanistan. Michelle talked about her routine in the operating room (OR). "When I was doing a case in the OR, I just held it. I put off going to the bathroom for hours. I stopped drinking coffee before my shift, too. I really didn't think about using the latrine until my work was done. I guess I put myself at risk for a UTI [urinary tract infection]. This was not a good practice, and I guess that most of the OR crew was guilty of doing this. It's not that we set out to do this. We just all get very caught up in our work, especially when there is emergency case after emergency case. During a mass cal, sometimes it is like assembly-line surgery. We save so many lives that would not have made it during Vietnam. We've come that far. Yet as medical people, we should know better than putting ourselves at risk for UTIs."

Major Christina

Christina, an active-duty Air Force flight nurse, lamented about elimination issues while flying. She stated, "When I was flying, I'd try to hold off going to the bathroom because we had to use the honey bucket. I'd try to wait until we landed. Then, when we landed, all the females would run across the flight line to the nearest bathroom to pee. It was amazing to see how dark and concentrated our urine could be when you withheld fluids while flying and became dehydrated. Sometimes, I'd end up with a dehydration headache as a result. As nurses, we knew that we should not allow ourselves to become dehydrated, but we refused to use that horrible honey bucket on the plane. I don't know why the military planes can't have tiny bathrooms like commercial planes."

Numerous nurses from both war zones complained of a host of ailments, many of which they attributed to the heat, humidity, dirt, and sand as well as the lack of water for proper bathing. Some mentioned acne flare-ups, ringworm, insect bites, and a plethora of skin rashes. Many developed athlete's foot for the first time in their lives, owing to the constantly wet shower and bathroom floor. A nurse reported, "My athlete's foot was so bad that the deepest cracks in my feet actually bled, and some pieces of skin peeled off like a bad sunburn."

Captain Holly

Holly was an Army reservist deployed to Abu Ghraib prison hospital in Iraq. Holly related, "With all the dirt, dust, and sand around us, infections were commonplace. Iraq was the perfect breeding ground for them. Bacteria grows most easily in a warm, dark, moist environment. Welcome to Iraq! I remember lots of rashes, ringworm, and fungal infections."

First Lieutenant Joy

Joy was an active-duty Air Force nurse assigned to the hospital at Bagram Air Base, Afghanistan. Joy related, "Sometimes, there was a problem with GYN care. For example, there was a physician's assistant [PA] designated to provide GYN sick call. The PA was male. So, most of the women did not want to go to him. Then, we got a Navy nurse-midwife who provided GYN care, and all the women flocked to her." *Joy added,* "I remember working with an older nurse, who told me that they made her take a pregnancy test with everyone else even though she told them she had a hysterectomy a few years ago. Both she and I thought that was crazy—no uterus, no more periods, but you still have to take a pregnancy test."

UNINTENDED PREGNANCIES

Unintended pregnancies occurred in both war zones, and once a pregnancy was identified, the woman was sent back to the United States. Some of these pregnancies may have been an attempt to be shipped home from the war zone. Others were simply wartime surprises or the result of a R & R (rest and relaxation) vacation leave.

Captain Marie

An Army Reserve nurse, Marie, commented on the unintended pregnancy situation as she saw it in Iraq. She had spent her tour of duty in Iraq in three locations as a medical-surgical and intensive care unit nurse. She stated, "I think as the war progressed, there was an increase in sexual activity. Male-female social encounters increased as we moved from the desert to a more urban setting. There was more socialization, the environment changed, and there were more opportunities. People were lonely, horny, and some had a devil-may-care attitude. Don't get me wrong; this was certainly not everyone, by any means. However, some people definitely took advantage of the situation. It was hurtful when you knew that the person had a family back in the U.S. waiting for them as they were carrying on with someone else. Some MDs were notorious for this behavior. It made me sick. The unintended pregnancies made me sad."

Commander Josie

Josie was a seasoned Navy nurse and mother of three grown children. Josie stated, "When it comes to sexual activity in a war zone, it is basically, 'Don't ask, don't tell.' *She added,* "However, when a pregnancy occurs, many other factors come into play, and the military does not want pregnant females to remain in a war zone." *She recalled two situations in particular involving female soldiers. She related,* "One young woman got pregnant by a German soldier, and another young Air Force gal got pregnant by a U.S. contractor. Both women were sent back home as soon as the pregnancies were documented. Situations of this nature are problematic for everyone involved. Not only is it breaking rules, but also, each unit loses a valuable worker, and a new human life waves in the balance. This definitely puts those involved in a crisis mode."

First Lieutenant Leah

Leah, an Army Reserve nurse stationed at the coalition forces hospital in Mosul, Iraq, recalled, "I remember a soldier who had an ectopic pregnancy and required immediate surgery. This could have been a very dangerous situation if it had not been diagnosed early. I also remember a pregnant medic who was sent home. The medic was a very important asset to her unit, and people were upset at her abrupt departure. In addition, a few women discovered their pregnancies soon after taking an R & R leave. They spent their midtour break vacationing somewhere like Hawaii with their husbands or boyfriends and returned to the war zone pregnant." *She added,* "A friend of mine became pregnant toward the end of her deployment. Her husband was with her in Iraq, and they planned to start their family soon. They found out when they had about 2 weeks left. So, my friend ended up going home with the rest of us."

Major Vivian

Vivian was an Air Force reservist who served in Iraq and several years later deployed to Afghanistan. Vivian stated, "We had three expectant moms who were soldiers, not nurses. As far as I know, their pregnancies were not intended. However, someone could have gotten pregnant to leave the country. I guess if someone hated being in Iraq that much, they could view pregnancy as a plane ticket home. Yet, there would be repercussions with their job, their military rank, and future promotions. However, in my opinion, this pales in comparison with having to decide about carrying the pregnancy or aborting it."

Major Millie

Millie was an active-duty Army operating room nurse assigned in Iraq. Millie related a story that she deemed "unforgettable," stating that it was her "ultimate wartime shocker." She stated, "We delivered a baby in the OR. It was an Army soldier, who claimed that she did not know that she was pregnant. She came to the ER with abdominal pain, and she was assessed to be in active labor. Apparently, no one else in her unit knew she was pregnant because if the pregnancy was determined earlier, she would have been sent back to the U.S. She gave birth to a healthy, full-term baby. She evidently got pregnant during the deployment, not before going to Iraq. She had been in country for 11 months and now would return to the U.S. with her baby as soon as they both were stable enough to fly."

SAFETY ISSUES

Besides the dangers of mortar attacks, IEDs (improvised explosive devices), RPGs (rocket propelled grenades), enemy ambushes, car bombs, and the like, many of the nurses mentioned fearing the risk of a sexual assault by male military personnel, workers, or enemy troops. Women were warned about not taking any unnecessary risks while deployed and the importance of traveling with a 'battle buddy' at all times.

Lieutenant Colonel Heidi

Heidi, an active-duty Army nurse researcher assigned near Baghdad, Iraq, reported, "In my job, I was privy to some sexual assault cases from 2005 and 2006. I got my team together and told them, I know how sexual assault happens. It happens because there is access. If we prevent access, we will cut down the number of sexual assaults." *She added,* "Our female OB-GYN physician would tell me some horrific stories about sexual assault. She was seeing a lot of stuff that broke her heart."

Major Vivian

Vivian, an Air Force reservist, had deployed to Iraq and Afghanistan. She reported, "In both places, women were encouraged to take a buddy with them to the bathroom at night. They'd tell us, 'Don't go anywhere by yourself at night.' I've heard of people being attacked in the showers or bathrooms in both Iraq and Afghanistan. *She added,* "I don't know which fear was worse—being hit by a mortar attack or being jumped on your way to or from the bathroom in the middle of the night. The nurses that I was with were good about not taking chances with safety. We really subscribed to the buddy system."

Lieutenant Colonel Victoria

An active-duty Army nurse with two deployments to Iraq under her belt, Victoria recalled, "During my first deployment to Iraq, we convoyed from Kuwait to Mosul, which ended up being a 2-day convoy. When we were allowed to get out of the vehicle to go to the bathroom, we could only walk about 6 feet off the road because that was all the space that had been cleared for bombs and IEDs. It was awkward, but it was also very scary. With that experience, the danger of being in a war zone began to sink in, even though I had yet to see the enemy. I came to learn that it wasn't as if the enemy was even recognizable. A bomb could be planted on an old farmer or even on a child. As nurses, we always want to help everyone, but we learned to be careful."

First Lieutenant Leah

An Army Reserve nurse, Leah recalled being mortared for 17 days straight when she was assigned to the hospital in Mosul. She told of how her sleep was often interrupted and how she would have to leave her trailer and take cover until the attack was over. She told of a colleague who resorted to urinating in a bottle in her trailer at night so that she did not have to make trips to the bathroom in the middle of the night. Leah mentioned being at a post-deployment conference where the guest speaker was a female soldier who told her story of being gang raped by three male soldiers while she was deployed. Thus, Leah saw the safety issues up close and personal, with mortar attacks and with physical and sexual violence. She related that she is her reserve unit's post-deployment representative for violence against women.

The aforementioned recollections and stories of the nurses illustrate the various challenges, concerns, frustrations, and fears that were linked to their deployment experiences. Not only were these women at risk for enemy encounters; they were also faced with safety and security issues on their own military compounds. The stress of the war zone and all that goes with it readily consumed their thoughts, affected their feelings, interrupted their sleep, and interfered with their lives.

16

Parental Separation

Nurses reported that leaving their children to deploy to war was the hardest part of this military mission. Some left toddlers, whereas other left teenagers or young adults. The challenges depending on the age of the children were different, but the stress and worry was the same. All of these parents found ways to cope, but the pain of being away from their children was real.

Child care arrangements during deployment were like putting the pieces of a puzzle together. Some nurses had stay-at-home spouses or grandparents care for their children. Others had to hire caretakers or find after-school programs for their children because their spouses worked later than normal school hours. Each nurse–parent found a way to put the supports in place to provide adequate child care.

Nurses found creative ways to stay in touch with their children. The mail, Internet, videos, and telephones were used, when available. In the earlier years of these wars, connectivity with family was more difficult than in later years, as technology improved even at the smallest of outposts.

One aspect of the wars that hit hard for several nurse–parents was caring for other people's wounded and dying children. The nurses found these circumstances especially heartbreaking and difficult, as the memories of their own precious children remained vivid in their minds. Lastly, amid the pain, worry, and heartache of being separated from their children, these nurses answered the call and stepped up to the challenge.

LEAVING MY CHILDREN BEHIND

Captain Marie

Nurses experienced a plethora of emotions when they deployed and in the weeks leading up to deploying. Marie, an Army reservist, recalled, "I thought I was strong and that this was going to be an adventure. I was going to handle this fine mentally. Well, that last week before I deployed, I had indigestion every day, and I had psychosomatic symptoms. I couldn't lie down without dreaming about what Iraq was going to be like without my children. I was sick that whole week. I would cry. I didn't think I would respond that way at all. I was very shocked. I didn't think I would miss them that much, but I did."

Lieutenant Commander Clare

Clare, an active-duty Navy nurse, recalled, "Telling my kids that I was getting on a plane and going away to war was just so tough. I had trouble sleeping for over a month before we left for Iraq. I wasn't worried about my safety, or at least, it wasn't foremost in my mind. What was foremost was leaving my kids behind and not really knowing when I would see them again. The week before I deployed, my mind was racing. Was the child care plan going to work? Were my relatives really going to help my husband and fill the void? Did we really have all the support systems in place? When would I hold my kids again?"

Major Michelle

Michelle was an active-duty Air Force nurse anesthetist deployed on mentoring duty at the Afghan national army hospital in Kandahar, Afghanistan. Michelle recalled, "I don't think there is a word that can describe the feeling of leaving my kids behind. Gut wrenching maybe comes close. Of all the things I went through on this deployment, leaving my kids was the hardest. It was the hardest thing I've ever gone through in my life. The stress and worry I experienced during this separation got to me more than seeing the injured and the dead. It was so hard to leave my kids. I can't describe the tension in the pit of my stomach. Looking back now, with all the trauma and horrible injuries I saw in Kandahar, what I thought about and worried the most about was my kids. It was always my kids. Separation from my kids was the biggest price I paid in this war."

Major Vivian

Vivian, an Air Force reservist deployed to Iraq and Afghanistan, recalled, "In 2006, when I deployed to Iraq, I had three children. The oldest was 19, the middle one was 16, and the youngest was 12. My husband was on active duty, so it was a real eye-opener for me to think that we both could be deployed, and the kids left with relatives. I was really in denial since the wars started. I had never deployed anywhere before, and I was a major with 6 years to go till I was retirement eligible. I was in shock when my reserve unit got selected for deployment. It was really upsetting for all of us to have me deployed. My son was commuting to his first year of college, and the others needed me even more. I am proud to have served, but it was the hardest thing in my life to leave my kids and go off to war."

Major Yvonne

Yvonne, an active-duty Army nurse assigned in Afghanistan, stated, "I was a single parent with two teenagers. The thought of deploying at such a significant time in my kids' lives really upset me. All I could think of was missing a high school graduation, my son learning to drive without my help, and all the pressures on kids today. I'd conjure up all types of terrible things in my mind that could happen while I was gone, like my daughter getting pregnant or raped, or car accidents. How would my family manage without me? Luckily, my sister and her husband took in my kids as if they were their own. My ex-husband also took the kids almost every weekend. He is a good father to them, but he works in a different city, so he couldn't take them full-time. Teenagers can be difficult, but my kids are pretty mature and responsible. We lived on a military post, and the military doesn't really put up with unruly kids. If kids are chronically in trouble, a family can get kicked out of military post housing. The military takes breaking the rules seriously."

Lieutenant Colonel Victoria

Victoria was an active-duty Army nurse who deployed twice to Iraq. She reported, "I spent 7 months near Baghdad, Iraq, on my first deployment at the beginning of the war in 2003. At that time, I had two children. My son and daughter were both enrolled in middle school. It was just so tough to leave the kids. My husband was on active duty with the Army, too. Two years after I came home from my first deployment, I got sent back to Iraq for another 15 months. At that time, my husband was still on active duty, but he had a medical condition that prevented him from deploying. At least I knew he would be there to take care of the kids. It was hard on my husband because he still had to work every day, but at least he could be home in the evening to fix their dinner and attend their sports games. He didn't get a break for those 15 months except for meeting me on my R & R [rest and relaxation] leave. He and the kids met me in Orlando, Florida, for 10 days over Christmas. Then we had to say good-bye again, and I returned to Iraq. It was very tough being over there for 15 months with my husband and kids back in the States. I sure missed a lot of holidays and birthdays."

Lieutenant Donna

Donna was an active-duty Navy nurse deployed to the coalition forces hospital at Kandahar,Afghanistan. She recounted, "My baby girl was only 2 years old when I deployed to Kandahar in 2004. Leaving her back home was the most difficult thing I have ever had to do. She was our only child, and I worried about her the entire time I was gone. I worried about her more than I ever worried about my own safety in a combat zone. It was just so tough getting on a plane and leaving her behind."

Lieutenant Colonel Heidi

Heidi was a career active-duty Army officer assigned to Baghdad, Iraq, as a nurse researcher. She recounted, "Leaving my kids was the hardest part. We knew I'd eventually have to deploy. The Army let me push it off as long as I could. I have three sons. My little one was in preschool, the middle one was in second grade, and the oldest was a high school freshman when I deployed. It was just so tough to have to leave them behind. I wondered at the time if I would ever see them again. I was only gone for 7 months, but it was during a very unsafe time in Iraq, and my sons knew that."

Heidi continued, "We lived in Washington state. We were having so many funerals for the Stryker battalion guys. So many were being killed, they started to batch the funerals. My oldest son's best friend's dad died the day I flew from Kuwait to Baghdad. I didn't know he was killed because I didn't have any contact with anyone back in the U.S. for my first 2 weeks. When I found out, I felt really bad. I knew the son pretty well. It was a typical military family where the dad was a sergeant who was always gone. I knew the son because he would travel with us to ball games and fishing at the lake. The son stayed at our house several times. I knew this death would cause more worry for my sons because now Mommy was in Iraq. I worried how this death would affect my sons."

Captain Olivia

Olivia, an Army reservist assigned to Mosul and Anbar Province, Iraq, recounted, "It was very difficult to leave my kids back home. I worried about both of them, but my daughter was really too young to know what was going on. I understood my son knew the realness of what was happening and that I was in a war zone. That was hard. There was no innocence to it; he just worried and worried. My daughter was younger, totally innocent, and just worried about who would tuck her in at night. Since my husband was a stay-at-home full-time parent and I travel a lot even when I'm not deployed, my husband is the one to tuck her in anyway. She didn't experience much of a disruption. She actually had a similar life while I was gone. It was more my son who concerned me. He knew every day what could happen, and he had to live with that [crying]. I didn't tell my husband about all of the mortar attacks and stuff like that until I got home because I thought it would make him worry too much. He actually got angry because he felt I had fooled him into thinking I was safer than I actually was. He worked through it quickly. He's never been in the service. My husband is very supportive, and he's so proud of what I do."

Major Alene

Alene, an Army reservist deployed to the coalition forces hospital in Mosul, Iraq, reported, "The more I talked with my kids on the phone, the more difficult it was, and I started having a hard time. I missed them, and you think of those milestones that are gonna come up and you are gonna miss, but there's nothing you can do about it. I think it's just as hard on boys as it is on girls. My little one slept with my husband the whole time I was gone and to this day. It's been 3 years, and we still can't break that habit with him. We're still having a hard time with it. He still comes into our room every night, and he's 9 now. He still does this every night, and it started with my deployment. We are now going to probably have to go for counseling because this behavior has just not resolved."

Captain Richard

Richard was an active-duty Army nurse assigned to the detainee center hospital at Camp Bucca, Iraq. Richard recalled, "It was tough leaving my son. We were very close, and he was only 10 years old when I deployed. I worried that he might give up Little League because I was the coach, and now someone else would have to take over. He's a quiet kid but a good athlete. Sports were always something we did together. I knew my wife would attend his ballgames. I knew my son needed my encouragement to hang in there when he struck out or committed an error. He was sensitive about the mistakes he made, and I always boosted his morale and let him know I was proud of him."

CHILD CARE ARRANGEMENTS: PUTTING THE PUZZLE TOGETHER

Putting the pieces of child care arrangements together was a challenge for many deployed nurses. Several nurses reported they were married to other members of the active-duty military or reserve forces. Some nurses were able to work with their spouses to alter work hours to provide for child care, whereas others had to elicit the help of extended family, babysitters, day care centers, and after-school programs. Each nurse–parent found a way to make child care arrangements adequate, but many worried about the stresses their deployment placed on their children.

Major Michelle

Michelle, an active-duty Air Force nurse anesthetist deployed to an Afghan national army hospital near Kandahar, Afghanistan, recalled how her family arranged their child care. "My husband took care of our two preschoolers while I was gone. My husband and I were both active-duty Air Force. He had just returned from Iraq 2 months before I was deployed to Afghanistan. He had it harder because I was gone more than twice as long as he was in Iraq. We both understand what it takes to deploy and what it takes to be the sole working parent at home. The kids were very attached to me. When I was gone, it was very hard on my husband. He had to have the kids in day care. The child development center was down the street from our house. When I was gone, he still had to work. He had a long commute to work, and it was hard. One of the hard things about being on active duty is that you usually don't have relatives close by to help you when your spouse deploys. The spouse at home rarely gets a break. The hard part was that he had only been home from Iraq for 2 months when I left for Afghanistan. He never had time to decompress from his own deployment before he had to ramp up to take care of the kids."

Major Derek

Derek was an Army reservist assigned to Camp Bucca Detainee Hospital and Abu Ghraib Prison Hospital in Iraq. Derek stated, "My kids were older, but it was still a challenge to leave. All along, I felt like we had a good handle on things as a family. I didn't really worry too much. My wife worked part-time, so she could keep close tabs on our 15-year-old son and 13-year-old daughter. We have good kids, so I was only minimally worried about leaving for a year. I think my family was more worried about me going to Iraq than I was about them being home without me. My wife was always good with minor household repairs. My son knew how to mow the lawn and change the oil in the car. I figured that if anything major came up with the house, my wife would ask her brothers for help. She also always took care of paying the bills, so I didn't have to worry about finances. I figured we would all miss each other, but things on the home front would be okay."

Derek went on to report, "Things ended up working out well. My wife managed very well, and the kids helped around the house. Now, I'm home and teaching my son how to drive a car. I think being deployed has brought us closer together as a family. Although I've been a reservist for quite some time, this was the first time I deployed. We all learned a lot, and don't take anything for granted. Overall, I'm glad we could do our part for our country. People don't realize how great things are in the U.S.A. until they go to a war-torn poor country like Iraq."

Captain Abby

Abby, an active-duty Air Force nurse deployed to Bagram Air Base, Afghanistan, stated, "Luckily, my parents only lived about 2 hours away from our house. I knew Mom and Dad would help my husband out with child care and chauffeuring the girls to Girl Scouts and soccer practice. Their elementary school also had an after-school program for parents who had to work late. Believe it or not, the thing I worried about the most was my husband learning to fix dinner. Other than grilling steaks or chicken on the barbecue, he didn't really know how to cook. I sure didn't want them to be out eating fast-food every night."

Abby recounted, "Looking back on how things went, I believe that my husband and parents did a very good job of keeping things together while I was deployed. Mom ended up teaching my husband how to cook some of the kids' favorite meals. That was nice because now that I'm home, we share more kitchen chores than we did before I left. He gives me a break from having to cook every night. My kids have also developed a closer relationship with their grandparents."

Captain Holly

Holly, an Army reserve nurse assigned to Abu Ghraib Prison Hospital in Iraq, recalled, "I left for Iraq in the middle of a very nasty divorce. I had gotten married very young. I lived either with my parents or with this man for almost 20 years. I joined the military reserves. I was told, 'You will probably never get deployed.' I got deployed within 2 years of signing up. As much as I missed my daughter, and it was hard being away from home, it was a time I learned that I could do it. I can do just about anything on my own. I learned there was nothing I needed to be afraid of. My daughter was 9 when I left and 11 when I came back. My ex [ex-husband] took care of our daughter when I was gone. Even though the marriage was over, he helped as a parent. He is actually a great dad."

Captain Robert

Robert was an Army reservist assigned to Takrit, Mosul, and Anbar Province, Iraq. Robert recalled, "I worried about my wife managing our teenage son without me since he was 14 and could be difficult. Maybe we were too permissive with him over the years. I had several talks with both of them before I left. In retrospect, they became much closer, and he really stepped up in helping her around the house. He matured a lot while I was gone. I think he took 'being the man of the house' seriously. When I left for Iraq, I was nervous the first few months each time I talked with my wife on the phone. I was afraid she was going to tell me how difficult our son was being; you know, like not calling when he was going to be home late, or refusing to get a haircut, or acting like a rebellious teenager. Now that I'm home, I'm very proud of how well he did while I was gone. He now wants to apply to West Point or Army ROTC [Reserve Officer Training Corps] to embark on an Army career. This was a real turnaround for him in the last few years."

Captain Marie

Marie was an Army reservist from the Boston area. She described the difficulties she first encountered when trying to arrange care for her two preschool-aged children. "When I was first notified of the deployment, I asked my husband how he was going to manage the kids while working at the same time. All I got were vague answers. Finally, I said, 'You need to speak to your supervisor, get a concrete plan in place, and see what they can do for you in terms of your schedule.' Well, the people he worked with were positively wonderful. They said he could come in late to work. He works as a law enforcement officer. They let him sell off some of his shifts so other people could work. He only had to work three shifts a week. Since I had only worked part-time in my civilian job, my Army pay was going to increase my salary substantially. He formulated a plan with three shifts a week and going in late on those 3 days so the kids could get off to school. I have to say it turned out to be a good plan."

Captain Tina

Tina, an active-duty Air Force nurse who deployed to Iraq and Afghanistan, remarked, "My Mom lives with us, so that gave me some extra comfort knowing she was there. I don't mean that my husband couldn't handle the kids, because he could, and he is very good with the kids. I had planted the seed early, probably a year ahead of time, that I'd probably be deploying in the future. I talked to them a lot about it. Even with being apart from them, the transition was smooth. It could have been a lot worse than it was."

Captain Suzanne

Suzanne, an active-duty Air Force nurse assigned to the aeromedical staging facility at Balad Air Base, Iraq, recounted, "I have one child, a daughter. She was 2 years old when I deployed to Iraq, and now she is 8 years old. The hardest part was the day I left. It is hard when they are not with you. They're just not there. Our family support made it so much easier. My daughter stayed with her dad, and we had a wonderful babysitter. Our babysitter was like a grandmother. I always felt my daughter was well taken care of. I think we were very blessed that we had good help while I was gone. My husband is also a very competent spouse. I was fortunate not to have to worry so much about the day-to-day stuff being done and if our daughter was being well cared for. I didn't have those worries, but I still missed my daughter immensely."

Lieutenant Colonel Victoria

Victoria, a career Army nurse who deployed twice to Iraq, reported, "On my first deployment to Iraq, my daughter was 11. I had no idea how long I would be gone, so we had a conversation about starting her menstrual cycle. We talked about that this might happen while Mom was gone. I gave her some written information, a drawer of supplies, and a list of people she could talk to if she had some questions or concerns. I told her that if she is comfortable talking to Daddy, who also happens to be a nurse, that is also okay. Therefore, we had this conversation just in case. I got to Kuwait about a week later. I managed to get a phone to call home to say 'Hey, I'm here.' When I talked to my husband, he told me our daughter had started her menstrual cycle. I burst into tears because this was a significant life event. I had only been gone for about 10 days. Even though we had the conversation before I left, I wasn't thinking this would happen at 11. It may have been stress related, too. I don't know."

Victoria further mentioned family events during her second deployment in Iraq. "During my second deployment, both of my children got licensed to drive. It was supposed to be a 12-month deployment and at a time when my son was a junior in high school. I knew I'd be deploying in early spring. I calculated that I'd be home for his last 2 months of his senior year. I'd be home in time for his graduation. Two weeks after I arrived in Iraq, they extended everybody to a 15-month deployment. I actually arrived in the U.S. 2 days after my son graduated. It was very distressing. I thought I had all this plotted out, and I thought I had control of things. Very early in the deployment, I lost control of things, and it was very difficult. Missing this milestone for our family was just very difficult."

Victoria added, "My son does not carry the disappointment of me not making his graduation with him. He's okay with it. We've had a lot of conversations about it. Finally, I can stop beating myself over the head about it."

Major Lee

Lee, an Air Force reservist deployed to Balad Air Base, Iraq, recalled, "Although I only deployed to Iraq for 5 months, I left behind four children ages 17, 11, 7, and 5. I can't imagine what it was like for some of the Army nurses who were gone for 15 months. My husband, with help from his parents, took care of our kids while I was gone. It was hard to leave, but I was more fortunate than a lot of people who were deploying. My husband's parents lived in another state. They were retired. They came and stayed at our house for 4 of the 5 months I was gone. They are wonderful grandparents and helped our family so much. I will always be grateful for the help we got. My husband didn't have to take any time off from work because of his parents' help."

Lieutenant Donna

Donna was an active-duty Navy nurse deployed to the coalition forces hospital at Kandahar, Afghanistan. She recounted, "My daughter was only 2 years old when I deployed to Kandahar in 2004. Luckily, I did have a good support system back home. Before I left, my husband and I were able to find a mature, older, and very experienced live-in nanny, who was truly the best. My husband was able to continue working and was not interrupted once he went to bed at night. This woman was a godsend for our family. Now that I'm back home, we continue to have her babysit when she is available."

WILL THEY REMEMBER ME: STAYING IN TOUCH

Nurses used a variety of methods to stay in touch with their children back home. On some of the more developed bases, Internet access was possible. However, in the early years of the war and on small forward operating bases, communication was a formidable challenge.

Commander Josie

Josie, a career active-duty Navy nurse assigned to mentoring duty at the Afghan national army hospital in Mazer-e-Sharif, Afghanistan, remarked, "My oldest daughter and I had a specific time we would use Skype to contact each other. It was harder for me to Skype because we had poor connectivity in Afghanistan. We had to use the civilian contractor's computers from the base Internet café instead of our own. My family could email me at my government email address during the day, and that was frequently easier for them. I also had a phone number where I could call Bethesda Naval Medical Center in Maryland, and the administrative specialist at the front desk would connect me to a DSN line, so I could call home. I called regularly that way, and so did everybody else. This worked out well. I have three daughters back in the States, and we were able to talk at least once or twice a week."

Major Lee

Lee, an Air Force reservist deployed to Balad Air Base, Iraq, recalled, "They really do try to keep you as connected as much as possible with your family while you're deployed. We had phones and the Internet available. They would videotape you reading a book to your kids, and they'd send it for you. Therefore, there were a lot of ways to stay connected. I can't imagine before all this technology how it would have been trying to keep in contact with my family and waiting to hear from them. I was very thankful for all of this technology. What really helped me was that I worked myself to death. I'd work, work, work, and then when I was done, I'd fall asleep. That's what I heard from a lot of my colleagues, too. Time passes much faster if you keep yourself busy. On the other hand, if you are not doing anything, you tend to focus on home and on the things that you are missing."

Captain Marie

Marie, an Army reservist deployed to Iraq in the beginning of the war, recalled, "In the beginning of my deployment, it was very hard to stay in contact with my kids because my base was pretty primitive, and the infrastructure was horrible. We always had problems getting the Internet. The one phone we had to call home was always busy or down. Therefore, the connectivity with home was always a problem. Even when I did get through, after a minute or so, I would get disconnected. Later in my deployment, I tried to do a video chat with my kids, but the bandwidth was terrible. I could only do video or audio but not both. I tried a couple of times to do a videocam with the kids on Saturdays, but it would cut out, and the kids would get upset, especially my daughter. I ended up getting a cell phone. However, often times, the cell towers were blown up, so then the cell phone wouldn't work. I quit trying to do videocams because it just got to be too dramatic, too hard, and too upsetting. Some of the bases had more capability, but where I was at the time I deployed was limited. About halfway through my deployment, the available technology vastly improved."

Captain Tina

Tina, an active-duty Air Force nurse, described how her family kept her abreast of her children's activities. "My husband sent me some of the kids' school work and their art work. I had it pinned up all around my room. The walls were just plywood, so I just used nails or thumbtacks to put up my kids' work. Before I left, my room looked like a day care center. My plywood shack at FOB Salerno was maybe 10 by 10, and it was covered with stuff from my kids. I got a lot of care packages from home, too. My husband was always good about that. When he and the kids made cookies or brownies, they also mailed me a tin of them. We also talked on the free phone about once a week."

Lieutenant Colonel Victoria

Victoria was a career Army nurse who deployed twice to Iraq. She recalled, "With my first deployment, we had almost no communication with home. It was difficult because it was 2003 at the beginning of the war. About once every 3 or 4 days, I could get on the Internet for a few minutes to send emails. On my second deployment to Iraq, I had a lot more communication. I had daily access to a computer. My two children handled it very differently. My daughter probably emailed me almost every day. When I would call home, she was always upbeat and talking. My son, who is a little more introverted, only sent me about half a dozen emails in 15 months. If I would call and he would answer the phone, some days, he would hand the phone directly over to his Dad or his sister. Some days, he was very chatty, but those days were less common than the others. I did recognize this was how he coped with my deployment, and I tried not to let it bother me. I tried not to feel bad, although it could be painful thinking my son did not want to talk to me. It was how he coped, and it worked best for him. Fortunately, I was able to understand. I had to respect that this was working for him. I had to leave it alone."

CARING FOR WAR-INJURED CHILDREN

Nurses described their experience in caring for other people's children injured in war. Several nurse-parents reported how it was especially difficult for them when they had to care for injured children, especially if the children in some way reminded them of their children back home. Some nurses stated they lacked pediatric experience before they deployed. Others admitted that pediatrics was one of their least favorite clinical areas of nursing.

Captain Marie

Marie was an Army reservist deployed to Iraq. She remarked, "I tried to cope with this deployment as best I could. I tend to think my coping mechanisms were good, but I would constantly think of my kids because of the pediatric patients we had. Actually, most of them were about their age. I had a fair amount of pediatric patients. Some of them were abused, but others were injured by explosions or gunfire. It was just so tragic. These hurt little kids really got to me. They reminded me so much of my own kids. Some nights, I would go back to my trailer and cry. Injuring children is such a heartless act."

Marie continued, "One of the boys that I took care of was shot with an AK-47 by his 4-year old brother. That's the kind of things we had to deal with, and this little boy was pretty sick. You'd have some that were dipped in hot water with burns [her voice got shaky], and it just makes you sick, and it makes you so angry. There is so much of that over there, injured and abused children. People don't realize how well we have it here in the U.S. until they see what goes on with people in other places."

Major Olga

Olga, an active-duty Army nurse assigned to a fast-forward surgical team in Iraq, remarked, "Sometimes, the situations with wounded children wouldn't hit me right away but bothered me when I went to bed. I would have a dream that something would happen to my daughter. It was frightening and was probably triggered by some of the pediatric cases I saw. Unfortunately, we took care of lots of kids with war wounds and burns. Kids would pick up unexploded shells, and then they would explode. We saw lots of devastating injuries to little kids over there. I can't imagine how the mothers of these injured kids feel. If my little girl was burned or blown up in an explosion, it would just kill me."

Lieutenant Commander Clare

Clare, a Navy critical care and shock-trauma nurse, recalled, "I absolutely dreaded taking care of wounded or burned children. Some of the nurses preferred taking care of the little ones. I dreaded it. It was just too close to home, too close to my daughter and son back in the States. It brought up too much baggage and memories for me. Every little kid I cared for in Iraq brought me right back to my own. I could see my own kids in every little injured kid. I could visualize my kids in every hospital bed in the peds [pediatric] area. I did what I could to avoid caring for kids. I swapped assignments with other nurses so I wouldn't have to do pediatrics."

Major Michelle

Michelle was an active-duty Air Force nurse anesthetist assigned to mentoring duty in Afghanistan. Michelle recalled, "I have two kids at home. Every time I saw injured children, it just tore me up inside. Injured children are one of the most terrible things that happen in war. Unfortunately, some of the most traumatic injuries happen to the children. I really felt for the mothers of these injured kids. They cried, and I cried with them. It was so senseless and so tragic. We did surgery on kids who lost hands from picking up unexploded ordinance. I used to think, 'What will happen to these kids in this society? What kind of life are they going to have?"

17

Homecoming: A Difficult Adjustment

Many nurses found homecoming to be more difficult than expected. Difficulties included insomnia and sleep disturbances, family role conflict, employment reintegration issues, parenting discord, fatigue and motivation issues, medical problems, and other individualized stresses. Some nurses described the experience of reunion with their children. Seeing their children again was an event many nurses dreamed about, and they counted the days until it was a reality.

Homecoming difficulties were generally unanticipated by the deployed nurses. Many stated that they figured they would just pick up their activities and relationships where they left off. It took some time after returning home to decompress and to realize that they had changed and their families had changed. Some reported that they thought with the happiness of the occasion and with family and community celebrations, the stressful memories of the war zone would quickly fade. However, most found that reunion and reintegration were just not that simple.

Major Vivian

Vivian, an Air Force reservist, recalled, "I thought I would just get home and be able to enjoy all the things I missed and fall right back in. Well, it was harder. The children grew, and they were older. They had different issues than before I deployed. My husband was the parent for 7 months. He had to step back, and he didn't know how much. We were really walking on eggshells for a longer time than I thought. It didn't even become obvious to me until I had been home for about 8 weeks. My husband had a keener insight into it than I did. He would say on the phone, 'You're coming home. I'm nervous.' And I'd say, 'What are you nervous about?' 'It will be great.' And he was thinking, 'She's coming home. She's going to expect this and expect that.' My friends and my family would tell me how nervous he was. There were financial issues that needed to be out on the table. In families, there are always issues. But, you know, we were very, very blessed."

Major Diana

Diana was a seasoned Air Force reservist assigned to the aeromedical staging facility at Balad Air Base, Iraq. Diana remarked, "My younger children came with my husband to the airport to meet me. My oldest son wasn't there because he wasn't able to get military leave at that time. Everybody was there at the airport to meet me. We came home and had a nice family time and dinner. Later, we all sat around the computer and looked at my pictures. We talked about what had happened while I was gone, and they asked me questions about my deployment. It was pretty awesome to be with them and to be home."

Some reservists reported problems reintegrating into their civilian nursing jobs. Diana explained, "I feel a 'nursing letdown' since I came back. Professionally, the stateside civilian nursing environment is a letdown. It is kind of boring. Patients at my civilian hospital are sort of self-centered, wrapped up in themselves and their own problems. I just can't get excited about caring for these patients on the medical-surgical unit I work on in a community hospital. On the other hand, the soldiers cared and worried about their buddies more than themselves. The soldiers would get up out of their beds and do something because they didn't want to bother you to do it. They were respectful. They didn't want to bother the nurses because they could see how busy we were. Returning to civilian nursing, this was not the case. I am very dissatisfied with civilian nursing after serving on active duty. Military patients just didn't complain about anything, and they cared so much for each other. You come back home and realize that some civilian patients have such a sense of entitlement."

Commander Josie

Josie, an active-duty Navy nurse assigned to an Afghan national army hospital, recalled, "I was wounded by an AK-47 [Russian semiautomatic rifle] round in my elbow, so I came home on an Air Force aeromedical evacuation flight from Germany. My girls were there when I landed. My middle daughter had picked up her sisters at the airport before I arrived on the medevac flight into Andrews Air Force Base. They were all there within the hour of when I arrived at Bethesda Naval Medical Center. They knew I had been shot and wanted to be with me. Two of my girls were with me the entire week I was in the hospital. My youngest had to return to her job, so she was only with us for the first weekend. It was great to have my babies there with me in the hospital."

Major Michelle

Michelle was an active-duty Air Force nurse anesthetist assigned to mentoring duty at the Afghan national army hospital in Kandahar, Afghanistan. Michelle related, "I was really nervous coming home because I wasn't sure how the kids were going to react. They met me at the airport. When they saw me, they just took off running and almost knocked me over. Everything I had hoped with the kids came true. My husband and I, however, took a much longer time to readjust. The first year and a half after I came home was very difficult. Things are much better now. I think a lot of it was that my husband turned out to have PTSD (posttraumatic stress disorder) that was untreated from his time in Iraq. We couldn't talk. He had angry outbursts. It was just frustrating for me. His moods would change. He ended up getting some therapy, and he's better now. Of course, my personality changed, too. I lived in fear every single minute I was in Kandahar. I became much more outspoken and assertive during my deployment. That carried over when I came home. My husband was always assertive. I was never shy or easily intimidated, but I definitely became more assertive in Afghanistan. I guess he was used to me being a bit quieter. I would just put it out there, whatever I thought, and that was not what he expected. He's very assertive anyway. Now, having me come right back at him was something he wasn't used to. Therefore, it caused tension. Now, he will always be way more assertive than I'll ever be, but we understand each other better now. But it was continuous tension for a while as we both adjusted."

Michelle continued, "I think there are different issues depending on the ages of the children when a parent gets deployed. My preschoolers were innocent about the dangers and problems of living in Afghanistan. I'm facing another deployment in the next couple of months, and I haven't told them yet. I'm a little worried about how hard it is going to be on the kids now that they are 7 years old and much more aware of war and dangers. I think it will be harder this time. They are wise and battle hardened since they've had both parents deploy. Besides my upcoming second deployment, my husband will probably also deploy again in the future. The kids are much more aware of war and the issues we must face since they are older now."

Michelle commented on her transition to life back in the United States after being deployed to Afghanistan. "Little things don't bother me as much anymore. I don't sweat the small stuff anymore. My friends or somebody will complain, and I'll just remind them that it's good to be home, not being shot at or living in a plywood B-hut. There are no IEDs or incoming mortars here. There's money in the bank; I have a job and a very loving family. Things that would have been a big deal before I deployed, I can now put in perspective."

Lieutenant Colonel Heidi

Heidi, an active-duty Army nurse researcher, recounted, "My husband and I looked at my return from deployment very analytically. Before I deployed, I went to the mental health clinic and picked up a copy of the family brochure for deployment/redeployment. I checked out all of their materials, and I read everything. My husband read everything, too. We tried to follow the evidence-based stuff that was recommended. My husband said to me on the phone, 'What do you think it is going to be like when you come back?' I was given a 'little battle book' about coming home that is put out by the Army. My husband and I read it over the phone. It brought up things, such as that I might want to go to my room and watch movies because that's what I did over there. In addition, my husband would say, 'Please work on that because we don't want you to do that, we want you to be back in the family. We love you and want you to do things with us.' I could also tell that my husband was worried that I'd come back as this PTSD person. He was just like on the edge of his seat wondering how messed up I was going to be now. I said to him, 'Look my big PTSD is gonna be if I'm standing in the middle of the kitchen with a plate and I'm going to have to get my own food.' My son was most worried about his video games where he shoots people because they make noise. I didn't like listening to that before I left."

Heidi mentioned some family stresses that she did not expect. Heidi stated, "I was gone for 7 months. I never considered that my husband and kids would go on to develop new routines while I was gone. My husband had assumed many roles like 'homework checker,' 'school lunch maker,' and 'bath monitor' that I used to do. When I got home and watched him do all these things with the kids, I felt kind of useless. The transition turned out to be harder than I thought. We worked through it, but it was not easy."

Heidi related how gratified she was by the performance of her research team in Iraq. "I do have a tremendous amount of personal pride over my performance and my team's performance. When it comes to how I reintegrated the experience with my life, I think part of it was that I did a job I liked, one that I volunteered for, one that I was good at, and one that I had adequate support in doing. I had family support. My husband and children were extremely supportive. Other family and friends were supportive, too. Total strangers were supportive. I cannot underestimate the effect and impact of total strangers. I received 93 packages and 350 cards and letters while I was deployed. A large part of this was from total strangers."

Heidi reported that her tour of duty in Iraq was less stressful in many respects than her life in the United States as an Army officer, a wife, and a mother. Heidi explained, "Homecoming was great because I really missed my family. However, there were some aspects of coming home that I did not look forward to. For me as a working mom, it was actually an easier job to be deployed to war than what I normally have to do because in Iraq, I only had one job. When I'm home, I have two! It was so much easier in Iraq. I didn't have to do any cooking, any cleaning, and any laundry! I did clean my own room, though. I didn't look out for anybody or anybody's schedule other than my own. I didn't have to drive anybody anywhere. In addition, somebody fed me, and it was all healthy, fresh food. They did my laundry for me, and I just watched movies at night in my room. I just did my job and worked out at the gym. I thought it was a really great life!"

Heidi added, "Another positive was having a job where everyone thinks what you are doing is important and that you are on the top of everyone's priority list. I mean, I really loved it! The extra money in my bank account was a great homecoming surprise. My husband didn't touch my direct-deposit pay while I was gone for a year. I made a lot of extra money because I was in a war zone. It was nice. I spent next to nothing while deployed. I won't give you the raw figures, but it was cheaper not to have me in the house for a year. We saved money on my car, the gas, the insurance, and all the other stuff. With me deployed, you don't pay for food, transportation, or anything. We were able to take a nice homecoming vacation about a month after I came home."

Captain Tina

Tina, an Air Force nurse, related, "Parental separation is a really painful thing as you know. I was out to lunch with a group of women, and one woman said something like, 'I don't know what kind of mother would or could leave her kids and deploy.' Some people are really quite oblivious. I decided to let it go, but probably a very small part of me still holds onto that comment. Some people are just clueless about the military and the sacrifices military people are asked to make for the greater good of our country and the freedoms we enjoy."

First Lieutenant Leah

Leah, an Army reservist stationed in Mosul, Iraq, told of her sleep problems after she came home. "I now need to take something to get to sleep but frequently wake up 4 hours later. When this happens, I think, 'Good Lord, I have to get up in 3 hours to go to work.' If I don't go back to sleep, I'll feel like crap the next day at work. I recently talked to a friend of mine, who was a medical technician in the ICU [intensive care unit] with me in Iraq. He said he couldn't sleep unless he leaves a fan on because he needs the noise to go to sleep. Our trailers where we lived were right off the helipad, and all the helicopters came in right over where we slept. Therefore, there was constant noise all day and all night long. There was no way to block out the noise unless you put yourself in a coma from Tylenol PM or something stronger. Before going to Iraq, I was the type of person who could fall asleep at the drop of a hat."

Captain Marie

Marie, an Army reservist, reported how sleep had become an obsession for her once she returned home. "Over in Iraq, the work was so stressful. You had to be alert all the time for subtle changes in a patient's condition and situationally aware because of the impending danger of rocket or mortar attacks. In Iraq, I followed a routine of trying to get to sleep early after my shift ended so I would be rested and refreshed. It was very important to me to exercise my 'sleep discipline.' Once I got home, I couldn't break that pattern of having to go to sleep. If I didn't get at least 7 hours of sleep, I felt like I couldn't function. I have now struggled with this for almost a year since I got home. Since I've gotten back, it is not that much different from when I was in Iraq in terms of this feeling of needing sleep. It is like an obsession for me."

Captain Penny

Penny, an active-duty Army nurse assigned to a fast-forward surgical team, remarked, "Since I got home, it is very difficult to sleep through the night. I keep rehashing things that happened over there, like the mass casualty situations or when we lost a patient. My mind is going a thousand miles a minute, and my heart is racing, too. I think I'm going to have to go for counseling because I'm constantly tired in the morning, even when I take an OTC [over-the-counter] sleep aid. I simply can't turn my mind off. I try to do relaxation exercises, but it doesn't work. I feel like I get my body relaxed, but my mind is a constant movie screen of images. Last week, my mother told me to have a glass of brandy or sherry before going to bed. Maybe I'll try that. I'm not a big drinker, but if it will help me get to sleep, I'll try it."

Major Millie

Some nurses reported adjustment and motivational problems after they returned from the war. Millie, an Army operating room nurse, recounted, "Since I came home, I don't have much tolerance for little things people complain about. When I came home, I really had to learn patience again. When I came home, I was so very exhausted. I just wanted to lie on the couch and do nothing. To get my motivation back was very difficult. Getting back to old routines has been a struggle. I was naive to think it was going to be easy and expecting everything would be the same as before. When I got back, everything sort of sunk in. I didn't process everything until I got home. After I was back a month or two, things started to fall into a more normal rhythm. I think the transition back was probably the biggest hurdle for me. It was unexpected. I thought that it was not going to be a big deal. I thought I'd just resume things. Well, the transition turned out to be harder than I thought."

Millie went on to report that her deployment experience also changed her in positive ways. "My experience over there has changed me for the better. My experience has changed my perception about a lot of things. I know it made me appreciate this country so much more than I already did. The little things that people complain about, I don't have a lot of tolerance for anymore. When I came back, I had to learn patience again. I can't expect people to understand what we are all going through while deployed and when we return. However, I know I am a better person and a more confident leader because of my deployment experiences. I learned a lot about myself and being a leader over there. Some other benefits that occurred because of my deployment experience were the fact that I am a less picky eater and less materialistic now. I shop less for clothes, jewelry, and things for my house. I guess I finally realized I have enough stuff for right now. I'd rather spend my money on a nice vacation on the beach or in the mountains. I'd like to see more of the U.S.A."

Captain Holly

Holly, an Army reservist assigned to Abu Ghraib prison hospital, stated, "I was divorced, so I had to leave my 7-year-old with her dad. It was hard transitioning back after I returned. Even though her dad did a very good job overall, he was much more permissive about letting our daughter stay up late, eat junk food, and spend time watching TV. Once I got home, I had to struggle with these changes with my daughter. I guess some of my expectations about maintaining my routine with my daughter were unrealistic."

First Lieutenant Joy

Other nurses, who did not have children left behind when they deployed, expressed their readjustment difficulties. Joy, an active-duty Air Force nurse assigned in Afghanistan, shared, "I thought it would be very good to come home. I thought everything would be normal again. Well, nothing is normal again. I'm having relationship problems. I'm having sleep problems, and I'm having work-related problems. I'm disappointed in a lot of people back here. I would be interested in learning how other nurses felt coming home. I felt a kind of letdown once I got home after the initial homecoming party. You can understand there is a certain amount of excitement being in the situation we were in. Then coming back to a normal stateside hometown can be a real letdown. I felt kind of down after the parties were over, a little low or 'in a fog' for a while. It is hard to explain, but I guess I got used to the adrenaline rush of our work over there. Nothing back here seemed as important or urgent when compared to what I had been doing for the last year."

Captain Abby

Abby, an active-duty Air Force nurse assigned to the Joint Theater Hospital at Bagram Air Base, Afghanistan, commented on her homecoming difficulties. "Homecoming was sensory overload for me. Brown and gray were the colors I saw in Afghanistan. Coming home and seeing so much color and beauty around you, and having so much freedom and choices, was very stressful for me. I had real difficulty adjusting once I got home. When I was in Bagram, my life consisted of 200 hundred yards, my room, the hospital, the dining facility, and the gym. There really wasn't a whole lot more than that because we were restricted where we could go. Now, I'm home, and I have choices of what I will wear, where I can go, what I can eat, and I can call people on the telephone, and I can drive my car. It was such a drastic change. For some people, it might be easy to slip back into an old routine, but I am very impacted by my deployment experience and very aware of what is going on in the world."

Lieutenant Donna

An active-duty Navy nurse, Donna was deployed to the coalition forces hospital in Kandahar, Afghanistan. She told about her difficult reentry into life back home. "Coming home was very hard for me. I missed being a normal person. It was very hard to come back. This may sound silly, but it was hard to make choices when I came back. I had difficulty choosing what to spend time doing, other than work. Over there, it was so intense, and you were either sleeping or working. It was almost as if I was on automatic pilot at work. I was a well-oiled machine doing nursing care. I was very focused on the tasks at hand. Yet, when I got home, I would just stare at the furniture and wonder what to do with myself. I'd try to pretend my household tasks were like my nursing tasks at work. You know, do laundry, buy groceries, and dust and vacuum. To a certain extent, that worked for me. However, when all the household chores were done, I would channel surf the TV, not knowing what to watch. It was a pretty bland and boring existence for a while. Maybe that was the way many of us gradually reintegrate ourselves into society after experiencing war. I don't know."

Donna further reported that she caught the wrath of her younger sister upon returning from deployment. She stated, "My sister treated me very poorly when I returned from Iraq. She said I overburdened her with having to grocery shop and drive our 75-year-old mother to appointments during the year while I was gone. She said she had to be at our mother's beck and call at all hours of the day and night and that she resented it. I guess this is what happens in a small family or if there are not a lot of relatives in the immediate geographic vicinity to help out. In addition, our mother prefers to have her daughters do everything and would never ask a cousin or neighbor for something. However, when I was deployed, I went away thinking relatives, friends, and neighbors would pitch in more with me gone."

Captain Trudi

A few nurses reported medical issues after their return home. Trudi, an Army reservist from the Cape Cod area, deployed to Mosul, Iraq in September 2006 and returned home a year later. Her unit was moved to Anbar Province 6 months into their tour of duty. When Trudi deployed, she was in her early 40s. Trudi related, "I came home with a few medical issues. I had vague abdominal cramps, fatigue, and some bouts of diarrhea. I had a colonoscopy done, which showed inflammation of some sort, which seems to be resolving now that I've been home for 3 months. I also had an issue with joint pains, which again seems to be resolving. So whether there has been an exposure to something, I don't know. I'm going to go way out on a limb and say this may be due to some sort of chemical exposure or the burn pits in Iraq."

Some nurses found that a few family members were upset with them for being deployed. Trudi explained, "I have five older brothers, and one of them was very angry I was overseas. He was very angry with me for going to Iraq. I never told my family we were being mortared. The Boston Globe came out with an article that said we had weathered many mortar attacks.

We all heard the article was going to be printed, and we were all scrambling to let our families know before they read it in the paper. This brother emailed me and told me I was selfish to cause our elderly relatives to worry and that I was selfish to stay in the reserves after the war began because I knew the potential for deployment to Iraq was high."

Major Fran

Fran was an active-duty Air Force mental health nurse assigned to a combat stress team in Tallil, Iraq. Fran shared that she never felt physically at her best while in Iraq. "Most of my symptoms started after I received the anthrax vaccine before deploying. I had fatigue, joint stiffness, and joint soreness. I became very tired with only moderate exertion. My blood work after I got back from Iraq showed borderline anemia. All of this was a big surprise to me because I am young and athletic, but I did lose more than 15 pounds while deployed. I guess the whole deployment experience was a bigger jolt to my body than I figured it would be. I certainly had to switch gears when living in Iraq."

Captain Vanessa

Vanessa, an Army reservist, discussed returning to her previous nursing position. "The transition to home has not been as easy as I thought. Going back to my job at the hospital here has been difficult since someone else has been doing my job for the last 7 months. It has really taken a while to readjust to my civilian work environment. Although the people at work were glad to have me back safe and sound, and there was certainly enough work for all of us, things seemed different. I think it was me, not them. I think I look at things differently now. I think I was a more serious person when I returned. I was less fun loving, less engaging, and less conversational. I didn't think I was clinically depressed, or suicidal, but I definitely had a changed outlook on life. War does that to you."

Major Yvonne

Yvonne, an active-duty Army nurse, reflected on homecoming after her first war zone experience and her disappointment with relatives. She stated, "Some members of my family acted like I had been on a vacation. They did not lift a finger to help me readjust and never asked how I was doing after a year in a war zone. I was simply incredulous at their behavior. Were they afraid to bring it up? Were they fearful that I would cry or pull out a gun? Were they angry I missed a wedding, a baptism, and a retirement party? Well, I guess they were too busy with their own lives. I was out of sight, out of mind. It made me disappointed and sad because I realized many people in the U.S. were out of touch with the two wars that were raging. I think because Iraq and Afghanistan were so far away, these wars were not on their 'radar screens.' Unless they had someone very close to them in these wars, like their son or daughter, or their husband or wife, they simply didn't relate to it. Yet, it was in the newspaper and on TV every day. So, I must admit, my cousins, aunts, and uncles were pretty oblivious to the fact that I had been deployed for a year."

Lieutenant Colonel Victoria

An experienced active-duty Army nurse, Victoria remarked, "My homecoming was wonderful. My husband and I are both active-duty officers. I have been in the Army for 21 years. We are a military family, and our children are used to one or the other of us being gone for periods of time. We lived in a big military community on the Army post, so a lot of the families had moms or dads deployed. I couldn't wait to get home. We had a very nice family dinner celebration. It was tough on my kids because some of their school friends lost parents in Iraq. They didn't tell me about the specific losses until I got home."

Victoria further related that she believed most active-duty nurses returned to a supportive home and military community environment. Deployments were commonplace, and troops were coming and going all the time. She stated, "When I came home, it was wonderful to see my family. I took 30 days' leave to spend quality time with them. I got back into midwifery. I took stock and realized I have a very diverse background and much to continue to offer the Army. I have had two deployment experiences in Iraq, but not many senior people have had these experiences. I'm a better leader for those experiences. I have greater currency and credibility with the young officers than many other senior officers because of my deployment history."

Major Samantha

A seasoned active-duty Army nurse assigned to the Joint Theater Hospital at Bagram Air Base, Afghanistan, Samantha discussed her homecoming. "Coming home was a positive experience for me. The deployment also brought me much closer to my husband. He was one of the first Rangers that went into Afghanistan after 9/11. He made it back fine with honors and all that, but in 2003, he had a bad training accident. I met him after he retired. Therefore, I never really understood what he had gone through in

Afghanistan. We've been together since 2004 and have been married for 3 years. I have this special bond with him. We've both been deployed. I think that's one of the reasons I've survived so well mentally. It was because of him. He'd talk to me on the phone saying, 'Honey, just put on one boot at a time, just keep moving, it will all fall together, just keep your head down.' I had my soldier husband supporting me 100% of the time. I was privileged to go to Afghanistan since that's where he had been."

Major Olga

Some active-duty nurses found homecoming especially stressful because they were given minimal time to move from their old stateside base to a new assignment location. Several nurses expressed how an impending move added to their stress and readjustment problems. Olga, an active-duty Army nurse, explained, "I think it is very important when people come back from a war zone they be given enough time to reintegrate. I got time off with my family when I returned home, but I also had to prepare to move to my next assignment within 30 days. It was simply not enough time to readjust to family routines, pack up our household goods, move across the country, start the kids in new schools, move into housing on a new base, and start a new job. I don't think senior people really understand what this added stress does to a family. It is just too many changes in too short a period of time. In hindsight, I would have rather stayed at my old base for another year and then moved to another base next summer."

Olga continued, "In my new assignment, I was in an office full of civilians, except for my boss. It was very frustrating for me. The civilians didn't understand what it means to deploy and what you have to give up. I worked for a colonel who was a hospital administrator. He had never deployed to a war zone and didn't understand what I was feeling or what my family had gone through. When people come back from war, they should not have to move for at least 6 months to a year. It's just too much change. My superiors put pressure on me to move right away to a new assignment. They made it sound like I had this important job waiting for me. This move was just too disruptive for me and my family. Now, I'm the token military person who has deployed in my new office, so I have to speak on behalf of everyone who has deployed. I suppose there's value in that, but it is very stressful to be 'the lone ranger.' You come back here to the States, and you have to move immediately. You are thrown into a new environment with people who have not experienced a war zone deployment. I felt very disconnected and isolated. I left a cohesive unit overseas, and I really miss the camaraderie and teamwork of living together and working together to save lives."

Major Christina

Christina, an Air Force flight nurse, talked about her spiritual growth while deployed. She stated, "I grew a lot spiritually. I think because it was a hard time, and I had to cling to God more than I would have had I stayed back in the comfort of North America. I am also more tolerant of human diversity after living and working in close quarters for over a year in a foreign country."

Christina remarked, "People have been absolutely wonderful since I got home. When I am in uniform, people are very respectful. I've never had so many people thank me for my service." Christina summarized the sentiments expressed by many. "Now that I'm home, I'm gaining a new perspective on the world. I'm realizing how much we have here and how fortunate we are. I am very proud of our country and our military. I saw so much oppression of women and generalized poverty during my deployments to Iraq and Afghanistan. We are so lucky to be Americans and to be free."

Photo Courtesy of U.S. Air Force.

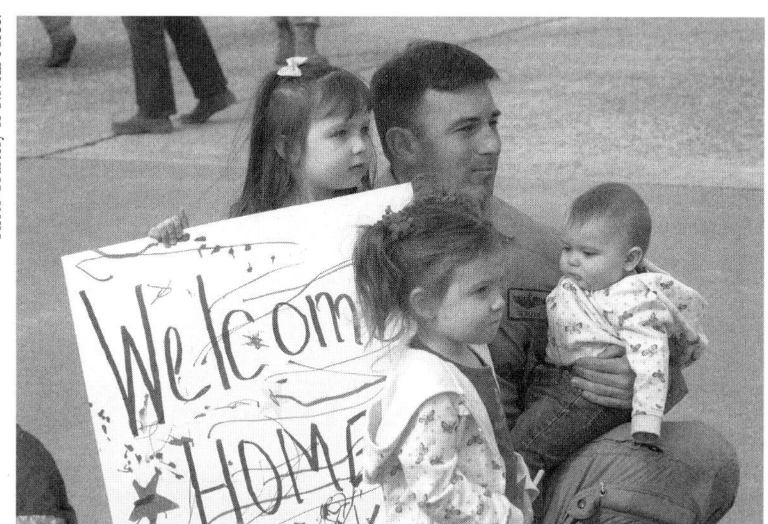

Air Force pilot and children.

Photo Courtesy of U.S. Navy.

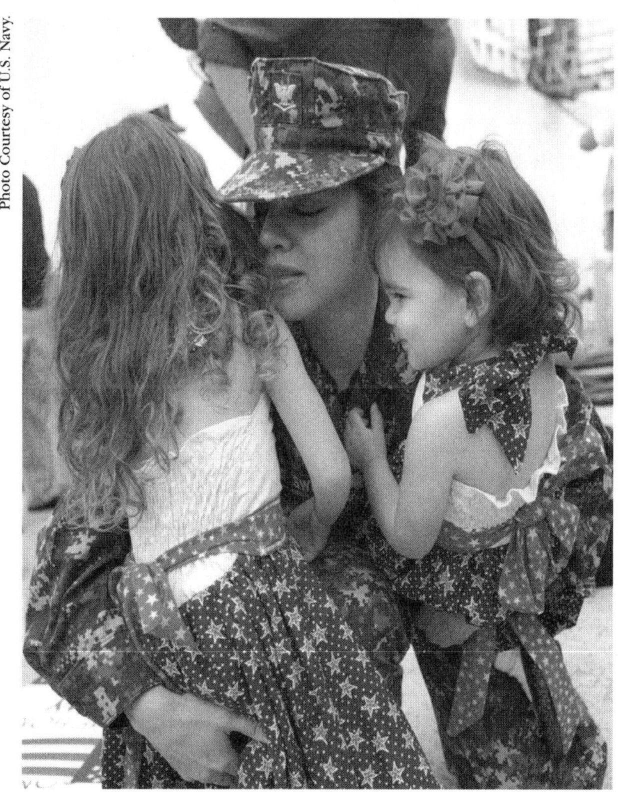

Navy Hospital Corpsman returns home.

18

Listen to Me: Advice to Deploying Nurses

Nurses imparted advice to help future deploying nurses. The nurses focused their advice on deployment expectations, the mission of military nursing, pride of service, and having outlets away from work. They cautioned deploying nurses to expect hardships and to reach out for support from loved ones back home as well as their colleagues overseas. They also stressed that training and preparation for deployment needs to be realistic and that deployment training should include dialogue with nurses who have returned from war. They further advised to keep nursing skills sharp, to start a journal while deployed, and to talk about their experiences while overseas and after they return home. Nurses advised that one's location of deployment would dictate living and working conditions.

Major Diana

Some nurses looked back on their deployment as a great and rewarding experience. Diana, an Air Force reservist assigned to an aeromedical staging facility in Iraq, stated, "I've talked to nurses, and I encourage them to volunteer for Iraq. I tell them, 'Honey, if you want an experience that you will never have as long as you live, go to Iraq."

Diana went on to relate, "It was a good experience for me. It is a sad thing to talk about a war, with all these soldiers coming home with their lives changed. However, putting that aside, it was a good experience for me as a nurse. I certainly learned a lot. We had enough staff to do what we had to do and accomplish the mission. We worked hard, but we were able to do what we had to do. It was very rewarding."

Diana further reflected, "I have a 22-year-old son. When each of those helicopters came in, I treated every one of those troops as if they were my son, or my brother, or my husband, or my father. You can't help but get wrapped up in what you are doing. You can't help but get close to those 'young-ins.' It just pulls at your heart. It makes you a stronger person, and it makes you a better nurse."

Captain Tina

Other nurses reflected on what it means to be a military nurse. Tina, an active-duty Air Force nurse who was assigned in Iraq and Afghanistan, related, "For me, being part of the Air Force is very important. I love the Air Force. I grew up in the Air Force, and I always wanted to do something in the Air Force. I'm actually doing something far more than I expected to do, taking care of our troops in a combat zone. I never expected to be in a war. I love the people I work with and our patients, too. I feel like I'm making a real contribution."

Major Millie

Millie, an active-duty Army operating room nurse, stated, "I think every military nurse needs to go through an experience like this in a war zone. They need to see what war is about, to see the injuries, to see what these young troops are going through. They need to see the women and children and what they are going through."

Millie related, "War injuries are truly the most horrific injuries, the worst trauma a nurse will ever see. I'm a very experienced surgical nurse, but war injuries were a new experience for me. I had never seen people blown apart from fragmentation grenades. I had never seen limbs blown off with the person's joint ligaments hanging like strands of rubber bands or limp spaghetti noodles from where a joint and limb used to be. I had never seen a face completely wiped away with empty eye sockets still smoldering from an IED blast that cremated four soldiers in a Humvee. These are the horrors of war, and military nurses need to know what can happen."

Commander Rita

Rita described her career as a military nurse. "I came into the Navy 25 years before I left for Iraq in 2003. I spent my whole career training to go to war. That's our primary mission in the military, to go to war. Your whole career in the military is geared toward taking care of troops on the front lines. Being in the medical field, that's exactly what I did. I spent many deployments on ships. I've been overseas doing humanitarian missions. I've been on the USNS Comfort, one of our hospital ships, during the first Persian Gulf War. I had put in my retirement papers in July 2002 before the war in Iraq started. However, I got called to deploy. I told my surgical team I would go to Iraq and stay till our mission was over, and it was time to go home and retire from active duty. We went as a team, and we came home as a team. The last patient I took care of on active duty was in Iraq. He was a staff sergeant, and I took care of him in a tent. He was my very last patient. I got on the plane and came home and retired. I feel like I had a helluva great career. Everything I wanted to do in my career, I did do."

Major Christina

Some nurses described what it takes to be a military nurse and the price they perceive to be paid as a result. Christina, an active-duty Air Force flight nurse, remarked, "I would recommend military nursing to anyone, but deployment is not easy. Its 100% deployment for nurses, especially if you are intensive care qualified. It depends on what base you are from. You come back different after being in a high-stimulus situation every day for 6 months or more, and many people come home with behavioral issues because of what they dealt with in providing nursing care and living in a war zone. Many people do not understand this until they go there themselves. You need to seek support when you get home. Don't expect to have your life be exactly the way it was before you left. War changes you. Deployment can change your family, too."

Lieutenant Colonel Victoria

Victoria was a seasoned career Army officer who served two tours of duty in Iraq. She related, "When it comes to nursing in the military, you have to have a strong personality, and you can't be real[ly] emotional. You have to know yourself. You have to be a leader, clinically proficient, willing to take orders and be a cohesive member of a team. What you see in the news may not be true. What you see out there is the truth."

Victoria recounted, "I think my two deployments to Iraq made me appreciate the things I have, like being an American and being a nurse. I have a greater appreciation of the military since I came home. I have a great appreciation for the nurses who deploy. I am in the Army, but I learned a greater appreciation for the Air Force, Navy, and Marines because I have seen what those folks have to endure. We are all in these wars together, brothers and sisters together across all the military services."

Victoria went on to describe how at first she underestimated her abilities to endure and adapt to her deployment environment. "I think during my first deployment, I found out I was a lot heartier than I thought I was. Before going to Iraq, my idea of camping was really staying at the Holiday Inn. The first time I deployed to Iraq at the beginning of the war, we didn't have much water. I can't tell you how many weeks I went without showering. After we set up the hospital, I convinced myself that I was clean because I used a couple of baby wipes. The one day we finally got water to shower in, and I'm washing and watching my tan go away! However, I found out I was a lot heartier than I thought I was. I quickly found out that although I didn't like it, I could do a lot of things that I had to do."

Many nurses emphasized how important support and communication from home were in facing the challenges of life and work in a war zone. Victoria commented, "I had great family support. We had some folks that struggled at my combat support hospital. Fifteen months was a long time to be gone, and the mission was hard. On my first deployment to Iraq, one of the most rewarding things about it was taking care of soldiers. So my second deployment taking care of detainees was not very rewarding. About a third of the staff had deployed before, so in previous deployments, they had taken care of the soldiers, too. We had a really hard time now taking care of the 'bad guys,' the detainees."

Victoria continued, "I had family support, so I had it pretty good. I knew my children were being well taken care of. I didn't have to have mail forwarded because my husband was paying the bills. I just picked up my stuff, and I went to Iraq. I knew my husband was going to take care of everything at home. My daughter emailed me every day, my son emailed not quite so often, but we did pretty well because I knew everything was taken care of at home. I had two children who took driving lessons while I was gone, which I didn't have to deal with. While I was deployed, my two children also had fender benders, which I didn't have to deal with. My mother wrote me a letter every day. I asked my mom to send some toilet paper, so she sends a case. I said that I needed baby wipes, so she sends a case. I realized quickly that some of the people I deployed with didn't have nearly the support that I did. If I even hinted I wanted something, my husband had it in the mail to me immediately. Yes, I had tremendous support. My husband is also a military officer, so he knew what I needed. He knew what our kids needed, too."

Lieutenant Colonel Heidi

Nurses talked about the realities of future deployments for military nurses. Heidi was an active-duty Army nurse researcher assigned in Iraq. She stated, "You joined the military, so be prepared to deploy. I think that you need to be prepared. Don't listen when the rumors say you're not going to go. Be ready; have your personal affairs in order. It is not if; it is when. As these wars continue, just about everyone will eventually deploy. Enjoy the time you have with your family. Remember it is your job to prepare your family as best you can. Have a family plan, and line up supports for them long before you leave."

Commander Josie

Josie, a career naval officer, stated, "The military operations deployment tempo has been high since early in 2003, and this pace is going to continue indefinitely. That is the reality our military faces today. Where our troops go, our military medical assets go, too. Therefore, if you are a military nurse, you will mostly likely find yourself in harm's way sooner rather than later. The military is an all-volunteer force, so if you step up and volunteer as a nurse, you need to understand deployment is very probable. If you can't live with or stomach that fact, then you are working for the wrong organization."

Josie emphasized for future deploying nurses to cultivate friendships while overseas. "My roommate and other friends I made there kept me going. We certainly learned a lot, and we were able to keep our sense of humor. You get very close with the people you are deployed with. You depend on these people for everything. There is a huge bonding with the people you serve with. I flew out to Ohio a couple of weeks ago to get together with some of my buddies from Afghanistan. You might not see each other for a year or two, but as soon as we got there, not a second went by, and we were right back where we were together. I think military people in general have a very special bond with each other that kind of withstands time. The people I met over there are just very special. They may not have been the person you thought who would become your best friend. They may be people with different outlooks or reactions or ways of behaving, but all of a sudden, they become your lifeline. I tend to be friends with quiet people because I'm kind of loud and try to be funny, but who knows until you reach out to people. We all became close and supported each other over there. Now, we are still strong supports for each other back in the States."

Lieutenant Donna

Several nurses gave advice about having outlets in the deployment environment. Donna, an active-duty Navy nurse who deployed to Kandahar, Afghanistan, indicated, "I would tell them to make sure they have some outlets so they get a break. When you get in country, plan some activities for yourself, whether it is journaling, reading, watching movies, or playing sports. You need to find something to keep you occupied and some way to keep in touch with your family. For me, the computers with the webcams were a way to keep in touch with my family online. I even helped the kids with schoolwork and reports online. Get comfortable with computer technology; you will use it as a lifeline over there. Some people I deployed with joined chapel activities, book review clubs, and enrolled in online courses. I took online courses while I was in Afghanistan. But I don't think until you are deployed you can truly be prepared for that environment."

Major Samantha

Samantha, an active-duty Army nurse assigned in Afghanistan, recalled, "We were off 1 day a week, but we'd usually spend it back there at the hospital because we'd want to be with the people we knew. We could come in and call our families, watch TV, talk to the patients, and help our coworkers. Sometimes, we'd come in and watch movies together or play cards. Nurses need to know ahead of time that there really isn't anywhere to go, even if you get a day off. It is not like time off back in the U.S. Your base compound is pretty much it. If you are lucky, there may be other coalition compounds nearby where you can visit and socialize. You need to find things to do to occupy your time off."

Captain Abby

Nurses frequently described physical activity as an outlet. Abby, an active-duty Air Force nurse assigned in Afghanistan, recalled, "A bicycle was a luxury over there. I made friends with somebody who had a bike. When I didn't want to run anymore, I'd bike around the perimeter of the air base. I got to see what else was out there. A lot of people were on their computers all the time. The rest of the people were always at the gym and lifting weights and trying to stay in shape. There weren't a lot of things to do. I would tell anyone who was deploying to make sure you have some type of outlet so you get a break, and your work is not all-consuming."

Major Yvonne

A few nurses described keeping a journal as an outlet for their thoughts, feelings, and experiences. Yvonne, an active-duty Army nurse, recounted, "I kept a journal, and my thoughts and feelings are there. It now helps me to process my experience. Journaling was a good outlet for me while I was in Afghanistan. It helped me unwind when I finished up my 12-hour shift. It took me a full year till I was able to read my journal once I got home. It was quite shocking, and it chokes me up a bit when I read about my experiences, but it is definitely getting easier to comprehend and ponder what that year was like. I want nurses to be able to talk about it, and keeping a journal facilitates talking."

Captain Meaghan

Meaghan, an active-duty Air Force nurse assigned to a critical care air transport team, recalled, "I journaled through a Word document on a thumb drive. My journal ultimately turned out to be 44 pages long, and everything is there; all my thoughts and experiences are there. I highly encourage folks to keep a journal during deployment. It will really help you make sense of things when you get home."

Another piece of advice imparted by these deployed nurses centered on the location of where they were deployed. Some nurses were assigned to large base compounds such as Balad Air Base in Iraq and Bagram Air Base in Afghanistan. Others were assigned to small fast-forward mobile surgical teams or small forward operating bases with a small surgical hospital.

Major Michelle

Michelle, an active-duty Air Force nurse anesthetist assigned to mentoring duty at an Afghan national army hospital, reported, "Working at a big hospital versus a mobile one is going to be different. Big bases are more developed. You will find more facilities and infrastructure on a big base. Those who deployed in the earlier years experienced more primitive conditions than those who went in 2006 or later. Living conditions and meal options have become better as time progressed."

Michelle went on to explain some differences based on location. "Being in a mobile unit or on a small FOB will most likely be much more bare bones in terms of creature comforts. You have to be able to live in an austere environment. You have to be secure with roughing it. You just don't have everything there in a war zone, and you have to improvise. You have to be able to live in that kind of environment and go without sleep sometimes. You have to make do with what you have. You need to know how to take a shower out of your canteen. You have to be a flexible person. Things are going to be quite different on a small FOB compared to a big fixed base with an airstrip."

First Lieutenant Leah

Nurses who deployed cautioned future nurses who will deploy to expect all kinds of hardships. Leah, an Army Reserve nurse assigned to the intensive care unit (ICU) in Mosul, Iraq, stated, "Expect hardships ahead of time, so you won't be surprised. Expect to live in primitive conditions with very little privacy. Expect the bathrooms and showers to be down the road from where you sleep. Hot water will most likely be a luxury. I lived in an 8-by-10-foot room in a plywood building, so I was really living in a type of poverty. I was there for 15 months. All you have is your uniform. You can't wear anything else. You have to wear wraparound tennis shoes and your combat boots. So, you actually downsize on everything. Then you come back to what we call 'luxury' here in the U.S. You have proven to yourself you can really live without these things. You can have a very simple life if you have to."

First Lieutenant Joy

Some nurses advised to always maintain a professional demeanor with your patients and to try to avoid getting personally involved. Joy, an active-duty Air Force nurse assigned in Afghanistan, commented, "You have to disconnect. You can't get overly attached to patients because they get transferred out quickly. I kept it professional, not personal. I did not want to get attached to anyone over there. On any given day, someone you knew could be killed, so I was very distant while I was over there. I just wanted to do my job the best I could and then to get the hell out of there. I was close with other hospital staff but not with patients."

Joy went on to reflect, "Sometimes, it was frustrating seeing all these young people injured and then not knowing what eventually happened to them when they were shipped out. You just have to learn to keep busy, stay professional, and take care of yourself."

Captain Marie

Marie, an Army reservist assigned to hospitals in Balad, Mosul, and Anbar Province, Iraq, commented on the importance of staying in touch with family back home. When she deployed to Iraq, she left a husband and two small children behind. "Being away from family was hard, but communicating by mail, email, and occasionally video conference really helped. It was so great to have communication such as telephone lines and the Internet, when we could get connected. Our kids were both preschoolers when I left for training at Fort McCoy, Wisconsin. My husband was able to mail me their artwork since getting mail was not a problem most of the time. The post office at Balad Air Base was open 7 days a week. They really tried to make everything convenient for us. Mail was free. My family sent me many packages and letters. It really gave me something to look forward to and added the nice element of surprise."

Major Derek

Another important piece of advice from nurses who deployed was that training needs to be as realistic as possible and should always involve input from nurses who have deployed. Derek, an experienced Army reservist, reflected, "If training is going to be realistic, nurses who have returned from wartime deployments need to do some of the training and tell folks what it's really like and answer questions. People who are deploying need to have this dialogue with those who have gone before. Classes on specifics are fine, such as clinical procedures, PTSD [posttraumatic stress disorder], endemic diseases and infections, [or] weapons training, but there needs to be a dialogue besides these skills classes. A PowerPoint presentation just doesn't cut it by itself; there needs to be dialogue."

Derek went on to report, "What you are seeing with your eyes over there, the blood, the death, and the emotions you are feeling, I mean, who teaches you that? You can click through a PowerPoint slide presentation on Iraqi culture. Well, give me a break; that just didn't do it for the emotional side of your experiences over there. I truly think people going over there need to hear this kind of stuff, the stuff I am telling you. They need to know this is what you are going to feel or you may feel. It's a normal response to an abnormal situation! You're not going crazy. I wish I was more prepared. I think I would ask for better training in this regard from the military. I think this needs to be discussed and described by nurses who have been there."

Derek went on to discuss some realities of homecoming. "I think that one of the things we need to do in our training before deployment is to let people know that homecoming can be almost as hard as going. Another thing is that most people tended to pull together when the going got tough over there, but not everyone did. There will sometimes be people who are angry at being there and take it out on everyone around them. Nurses who are going to deploy need to know this stuff. They need to be made aware of the range of behaviors they may see. I think we owe this to them."

Lieutenant Colonel Judd

Nurses could not emphasize enough that it is crucial for all military nurses to keep their clinical skills current. Judd, a Vietnam War veteran and Army Reserve nurse practitioner, remarked, "I don't care if you do a desk job in the U.S., like quality assurance, risk management, infection control monitor, or nursing research coordinator; you have to find a way to keep your clinical skills current. We don't need a lot of nursing administrators on a deployment; we need people with sharp clinical skills who can hit the ground running."

He further commented, "Every military nurse is a clinician first, so nursing skills are very important. Nurses need to have some good solid clinical experience before they deploy. I was thankful I had a lot of ER experience. As a nurse practitioner, my assessment skills were very sharp. Working in the ER is a great background because I am familiar with most heart medications, with caring for trauma patients and patients in respiratory distress. You have to handle all kinds of illnesses and injuries in the ER. An ER background is good to have in your pocket going into a war zone. It is just good to have these critical care and assessment skills."

Captain Liz

Liz, an active-duty Air Force flight nurse, remarked, "I think the thing that I was least ready for was burns. As flight nurses, we had to be ready for anything. I didn't have very much experience taking care of burns. Some of those skill things were nobody's fault. We didn't know what we didn't know. It all worked out, though; we all learned, and we got it together. It just goes to show how important it is to have the clinical skills because you never know what type of injuries you will be tasked to care for."

Major Fran

Fran was an active-duty Air Force combat stress team leader and mental health nurse assigned at Tallil Air Base, Iraq. Fran remarked, "My primary specialty is mental health nursing, but I had not worked in mental health for 6 years prior to going on this deployment. Therefore, it was a little bit of a struggle for me. I had been in various administrative roles. We went for a week of mental health training with the Army folks prior to going. Then we went for a month of training on how to fight a war. They had us out there on the firing range shooting the 9-mm, the M-16, the 50-caliber machine gun, and throwing hand grenades. Therefore, nurses need to expect to refresh their combat arms training before they deploy. Luckily, I had many years of mental health nursing experience, even though it wasn't very current experience. However, I had kept up with my continuing education studies in combat stress and general mental health areas."

Captain Olivia

An unpleasant occurrence for several of the nurses when they deployed was witnessing infidelity. Olivia, an Army reservist, recalled, "This was my very first deployment. Some of the married people over there behaved badly. There is a huge problem with fidelity over there. What goes on over there, well, there's a saying that 'what happens TDY [on temporary duty] stays TDY in the military.' It's like 'what happens in Vegas stays in Vegas.' I could not believe how rampant it was even though there were rules in place. For example, you weren't supposed to be in your quarters with a member of the opposite sex. It still happened, and there was no way to control it with so many troops. I mean, there were thousands of us over there. In addition, if you got busted for it, it becomes everybody's business, and everybody knows. Yet, people were willing to take risks over there, and I was just stunned by it. When the sun goes down over there, there is this whole other world. You would have situations where both people fooling around were married to others back in the U.S. I couldn't believe my eyes, just lots of infidelity. It was shocking! It wouldn't happen so much in big-tent or open-bay dorm situations because you do have four people to a room or cubicle. It would happen in plywood huts and smaller trailers where you have your own 10-foot-by-4-foot room. For the most part, people kind of kept it to themselves. However, I can tell you, there were married officers as well as enlisted troops involved in adulterous relationships over there. I guess I was naive, but I was just so shocked by this kind of behavior."

Major Alene

The nurses advised future nurses who deploy to talk about their experiences while deployed and when they returned home. Alene, an Army reservist assigned in the emergency room (ER) and ICU in Mosul, Iraq, recalled, "Every time I tell my stories, it gets easier. In my little group of friends, we talked about it. We talked about what we were seeing and doing. We shared our experiences and feelings with each other. It helped because you then knew you were not alone, and others were experiencing the same things and had the same feelings. It really gave me a reality check that I wasn't going crazy, that others were feeling some of the same things."

Alene went on to describe other things that were discussed. "We also talked about why we volunteered to go to Iraq instead of a safer place like Germany. I think it made us better nurses and stronger people. It made us attuned to what was going on in the world and to understand better what the soldiers have to go through before they get home again. People need to find folks to talk to while they are over there. Venting what is bothersome and troubling is a type of mental hygiene that people need. You are seeing some terrible injuries, and you are witnessing threats to your safety, like mortar attacks. You need to have folks you can talk to because most of us did not share the most stressful stuff with our families while we were deployed, and a year or 15 months is a long time to hold it in. Holding it in is not healthy."

Major Olga

The nurses proclaimed that nurses who deploy should feel a sense of pride in their military service. Olga, a career-minded active-duty Army nurse, remarked, "I was very proud to go. My husband is so proud of me, and my family is so proud of me. My husband is a retired Army Ranger, who also did a tour in Iraq. I am proud that I was able to accomplish my mission, to deploy for a year and work on a fast-forward surgical team. I'm proud of my family, too. I always knew we were strong, but now I know we are really strong. This is what I joined the military for, to take care of American troops and anyone else caught in the crossfire of war."

Olga went on to state, "I would like to go back again if I was needed, but because of my family situation, I will probably be retiring in a few years. I would not mind going back again. My mom is old and needs my help now. For my family, going once was enough. If I was by myself and didn't have family responsibilities, I would volunteer to deploy again."

Captain Alice

Alice, an Air Force nurse assigned to a critical care air transport team, served tours of duty in Iraq and Afghanistan. Alice exclaimed, "I'd go back in a heartbeat, and I've already spent 6 months in Iraq and 7 months in Afghanistan. Both were such rewarding experiences. I learned so much in terms of trauma nursing over there. The patients were so appreciative of everything we did for them. I would really like to go back. I have actually volunteered to go again. It is a great place to practice nursing, and the best job in nursing is taking care of soldiers and working in a flying ICU. It is very rewarding. I'm looking forward to going back, and I've been told I'll get to work in an ICU in a hospital or be a CCATT nurse again."

19

Conclusion

In writing this book, we embarked on a fascinating journey that took us to numerous towns, hamlets, cities, and villages across the eastern United States as we interviewed many active-duty and reserve nurses who served in Iraq or Afghanistan during the war years 2003 through 2010. Talking to nurses about their wartime service brought back memories of our generation's war, the Vietnam War. During the Vietnam War, we both graduated from college and began practicing as registered nurses. As we pondered nurses' experiences in the current wars, we could not help but look back at U.S. involvement in our generation's war. In listening to the deployment and homecoming experiences of today's military nurses, we were reminded of the glaring differences in deploying to and returning from the current wars as opposed to the Vietnam War. What were these differences?

Well, for most of the Vietnam War, troops were not usually deployed as a specified unit. They were sent as individuals to replace someone scheduled to leave Vietnam or to expand the size of a unit already in country. With this type of deployment, it was not possible for unit bonding to occur until an individual arrived in Vietnam and was eventually assimilated into a unit. On the other hand, in the current wars, most military members deployed to the war zone as a unit, such as an infantry battalion, a combat support hospital, or a fighter aircraft squadron. The greater majority of active-duty folks and reservists usually trained as a unit and deployed as a unit. For example, some Army Reserve units trained at Fort McCoy, Wisconsin, and Air Force hospitals from Florida, Texas, Ohio, and California deployed a large number of personnel to air base hospitals in Iraq or Afghanistan. Training and then deploying together facilitates unit cohesion and collective identity.

Another difference between military troops, including nurses, in the current wars and those in the Vietnam War was the way they were treated by the American people once they returned to U.S. soil. For military personnel returning from Vietnam, there were few parades or public homecoming celebrations. Some people called Vietnam veterans "baby killers" and spit on them. Other times, people avoided Vietnam veterans because they were afraid of explosive and bizarre behavior due to posttraumatic stress disorder. Troops returning from Vietnam were advised by higher headquarters to change into civilian clothing in the airport once they returned to U.S. soil. Otherwise, if they remained in uniform, they might be attacked by angry people or antiwar protesters. Needless to say, despite this turmoil, individual families were generally happy to greet and welcome their family member home from the Vietnam War. On the other hand, our military members returning from Iraq and Afghanistan are welcomed by a grateful and proud American public. Parades and ceremonies are taking place on military bases and in hometowns across the United States. Troops in uniform are applauded in airports and openly thanked for their service. On some commercial airliners, military personnel are allowed to enplane and deplane ahead of all other passengers as a sign of respect. Handshakes, hugs, and pats on the back are extended by total strangers as troops pass through bus terminals, train stations, and airports on their journey home.

Another difference between these two groups is the way the military services acquired them. During the Vietnam War, although some men and women volunteered, most men were drafted to serve. When the United States withdrew from Vietnam, the draft ended. Shortly after the end of the Vietnam War, the United States instituted policies for an all-volunteer military. The United States still relies on an all-volunteer military today.

Why do we point out the differences in the way military personnel from the Vietnam War and the current wars were treated? One reason is that the voices of the Vietnam War nurses were slow to be heard. It was not until 1983, ten years after the United States withdrew combat troops, that *Home Before Morning* by Lynda Van Devanter and Chris Morgan was published. In this book, Van Devanter described her own Vietnam War experience as an Army nurse. This book helped awaken nurse veterans and other women who served in the Vietnam War to their own feelings and struggles. As you know, most Americans were against the war in Vietnam and viewed it as an embarrassment for the United States. For the troops who served in Vietnam, there was tremendous psychological pressure to suppress one's own painful feelings and try to move on. Shame, guilt, and regret were part of the collective American conscience. As a result, many who served in Vietnam did not talk about their experiences when they returned home. If they did share their experiences, it was usually only with other Vietnam veterans.

Some veterans thought that maybe if they did not talk about it, the unpleasant war memories would go away. There was a palpable stigma associated with Vietnam service. Therefore, for 10 years, the nurses of the Vietnam War were silent and invisible veterans.

In contrasting how U.S. military troops were treated in the Vietnam War versus the current wars in Iraq and Afghanistan, we can only hope that the American public has learned a valuable lesson since the end of the Vietnam War. Our military personnel carry out U.S. policy and are instruments of that policy; the civilian leadership of our country makes U.S. policy. We should not punish the military troops for any mistakes and missteps of our leadership in Washington.

The wars in Iraq and Afghanistan have been expensive not only in monetary terms but in human losses as well. The human toll of the last decade has been high. The number of U.S. troops who have died in the war in Iraq is close to 4,500, surpassing the number of military deaths in the Revolutionary War. The U.S. military death total for the war in Afghanistan has surpassed 1,700. This brings the total for the current conflicts to 6,200 deaths. The number of U.S. military personnel wounded in Afghanistan has reached 13,500, whereas over 32,200 have been wounded in the Iraq war (Tilghman, 2011). For the military nurses who have served in Iraq or Afghanistan, these aforementioned numbers are not just statistics. These numbers have faces and names. Many of these faces and names have crossed paths with the nurses on air evacuation flights, in triage areas, on fast-forward surgical teams, in aeromedical staging facilities, and in combat support hospitals.

Since the beginning of the wars in Iraq and Afghanistan, several books have been published detailing the experiences of combat soldiers, air combat controllers, and helicopter pilots. In comparison to what has been provided in the literature about soldiers' experiences in Iraq and Afghanistan, much of the nurses' experiences have gone untold. We think it is time to identify, describe, explore, and document military nurses' experiences in the current wars. We have undertaken three research studies to tell the nurses' stories, which has culminated in this book.

We feel a closeness to the nurses in this study. We sat in their kitchens, living rooms, and dens. We shared a pizza with one nurse in Brooklyn, bowls of clam chowder in Rhode Island, barbecue in North Carolina, and ice cream in Virginia as they told us their stories. We handed them a box of tissues in New Jersey and cried with them in Delaware and Cape Cod. We visited the grave of one of their friends at Arlington National Cemetery and then listened to the story of how he was killed while they were jogging together. One theme we heard repeatedly was how these nurses gained a deeper appreciation for their freedoms and way of life in the United States. The carnage and devastation of war left an indelible imprint on these nurses.

They truly learned how precious, yet fragile, human life is and how life can be snuffed out in an instant.

Serving in a war zone, with personal triumphs and tragedies, will always equate to a special and unique experience. In the nurses' perceptions, no human experience before or after will parallel this experience. Unlike the combat soldier or helicopter pilot who intermittently dealt with injured or killed buddies, these nurses lived with the constant trauma of war every day. They cared for young soldiers with bloody stumps for legs, Humvee passengers covered with hunks of charred flesh, children with disfigured faces and missing parents, and masses of people in pain crying out for help.

The voices of nurses who served in the Iraq and Afghanistan wars are heard loud and clear in this book. They told their stories, poured out their hearts, and tried diligently to make sense of their experiences. Some shared the circumstances surrounding notification of their future deployment and their personal and family's response to the news. Some deployed with active-duty units from Army, Navy, or Air Force hospitals, whereas others in reserve units were activated. Others volunteered as individual augmentees and joined units already in Iraq or Afghanistan or those scheduled for deployment. Some nurses wanted to go and felt a strong military obligation to serve in a war zone. Others wanted to serve but struggled with family issues and responsibilities.

The nurses experienced the Iraq and Afghanistan wars as frightening, austere, and clinically challenging. The element of danger was always present, and it followed them to the gym, to the chapel, to the mess hall, and to work. Rocket and mortar attacks were always a threat, especially after dark. A stream of wounded warriors with severe mutilating injuries ebbed and flowed and sometimes gushed into their triage areas. Yet, the nurses actively worked to recreate "home" and add some semblance of normalcy to their lives. They sought creative outlets such as forming a choir or a country line dance group, writing in a journal, or taking an online academic course.

The customs and language in both countries were foreign, living conditions were primitive, and the lack of privacy was stressful. Yet, nurses volunteered for humanitarian missions to bring health care to women, children, and the elderly in nearby villages and towns. Nurses were quite vocal, airing their discontent about bathroom and shower facilities in the more remote locations. Privacy issues also depended on location: one nurse having a trailer of her own versus another nurse sharing a large tent with more than 50 others.

The nurses experienced time as moving too fast and in short supply during mass casualty situations. Conversely, time almost stood still as the end of one's combat tour drew near. Time was measured by the calendar and the clock, by letters and emails from home, by formed or lost relationships, by events in the war theaters and back in the "world," and by the dawn and darkness of each day. Time was something busy nurses and dying patients had too little of and severely burned and maimed soldiers had too much of.

Many nurses could not escape the tangled web of thoughts, dreams, emotions, and physical sensations. Living in a war zone gave way to a heightened awareness, a hypervigilance. The nurses' visions centered on the casualties: many limbless, mindless, paralyzed, burned, and disfigured soldiers, nationals, and children, who were mere shadows of their former selves. The nurses will carry these memories with them forever. Memories of being ankle-deep in blood, seeing people with their faces blown off, holding human brain tissue in your hands, and being with a marine as he breathed his last breath and then accompanying his body to the morgue. It is difficult to let go of these memories.

In their stories and recollections, the nurses vividly recalled the smells and sounds of war. Odors from the burn pit, the latrine, and the operating room comprised one's reality. The pounding of the helicopter blades, the thud of incoming mortar rounds, and the human cries of pain signaled an onslaught of casualties and another night without sleep. The cascade of emotions ranged from an adrenaline rush, which enabled the nurses to perform life-saving procedures and work long hours without a break, to feelings of futility, frustration, anger, and sadness as they faced the moral and ethical dilemma of deciding who could be saved and who was beyond saving. Often, both physical and emotional exhaustion ensued. Life was a continuous roller-coaster ride, and they were not able to get off.

Many nurses reflected on the nature of their relationships while deployed. Relationships with colleagues were often viewed as significant, intense, and long lasting. Nurses spoke of closeness, cohesion, oneness against all odds, professionalism, camaraderie, and togetherness. People depended on each other, and coworkers became one's military family. Relationships with patients varied with the nature and severity of injuries and the time spent in a hospital or clinic or on a medical evacuation flight. Therefore, some relationships were short lived, whereas others were meaningful, and a therapeutic alliance was forged. With serious life-threatening injuries, nurses often worked quickly to stabilize patients and ready them for a flight to Germany. However, when this was the case, there was often a void in the channels of communication, and the nurses did not always hear if the patient survived, made it to surgery, had a good outcome, and eventually made it to a rehabilitation unit or home. This lack of feedback proved to be incredibly frustrating for the nurses. They needed some type of closure or sustained hope or simply to put their concern to rest with a prayer for the loss of life.

Homecoming was fraught with a myriad of emotions according to most of the nurses. It was more difficult than most anticipated. Although the nurses embraced the safety and security of home, many had feelings of guilt about leaving colleagues behind and a sense of unfinished work. This was because as they returned to the United States, the fighting continued in Iraq and Afghanistan. Reintegration into their families and into society was stressful in many instances.

Lessons learned proved to be significant for the nursing profession. First of all, nurses involved in military or disaster nursing need to be clinically prepared with solid medical–surgical and trauma nursing skills prior to being deployed to a combat zone or disaster site. With the realization that it is impossible to predict the occurrence of a natural or man-made disaster, terrorist attack, or hostile action in our complex world of diverse national security interests, all military nurses and a large number of civilian nurses need to be ready to care for mass casualties. Additionally, all levels and types of nursing education programs need to emphasize that the emotional sequelae of catastrophic events and wartime deployment last a long time after the experience. Thus, memories may be extremely painful and disruptive for years to come. Fortunately, the military services and the Veteran's Administration have made significant strides in recent years to screen all returning service members for posttraumatic stress disorder. This screening is performed incrementally because the disorder frequently has a delayed manifestation of symptoms. The wars in Iraq and Afghanistan, as well as Vietnam, have made an incredibly strong case for the aforementioned initiative. In our opinion, this is long overdue. Yet, we are immensely grateful that mental health services for veterans have improved and will continue to do so.

Returning nurses need to be encouraged to share and talk freely about their wartime experiences within a supportive environment. Methods of caring for the emotional needs of health care providers after wartime deployment should be considered as important as taking care of the physical victims of war. Similarly, nurses who have deployed to these war theaters are in strategic positions to prepare future nurses for deployment. Anticipatory guidance from seasoned veteran nurses will offer a particularly valuable insight and credibility about what to expect on a wartime deployment.

The study of nurses' experiences in war and disaster needs to be a priority in future nursing research in a sustained effort to take care of the caregivers. This is of paramount importance with the reality of nurses returning to Iraq and Afghanistan for two, three, or four deployments.

Just as the nurses we interviewed for three research studies will never forget the memories of nursing in war, we will never forget these compassionate, patriotic, courageous, selfless, and dedicated nurses. Their voices were heard loud and clear. They touched our hearts with their words and their spirit. We savored the sharing that occurred as the nurses told their stories and greatly appreciated the opportunity to view wartime nursing through their lens.

After transcribing the tape-recorded interviews and listening to the nurses' voices over and over again, we believe we learned what it was like to be a nurse in Iraq or Afghanistan. We gained a valuable understanding of the totality of the experience as much as is possible without actually being there. The nurses we interviewed and their stories had a much more profound effect on our lives than we anticipated. We gained increased respect, appreciation, and admiration for our nursing profession.

Their voices are important for the United States and for the nursing profession. The purpose of this book was to document the experiences of U.S. military nurses who served in Iraq or Afghanistan during the war years 2003 through 2010 and life after returning from war. We sought to inform our readers of the unique contributions these brave nurses made as well as to tell of their challenges, hardships, stresses, and triumphs. Mission accomplished!

REFERENCES

Tilghman, A. (2011, September 12). Our decade at war. Air Force Times, p. 3.

Van Devanter, L., & Morgan, C. (1983). Home before morning. New York, NY: Warner Communications.

Afterword

I visited countless medical units over my tenure as the 14th chief nurse of the Air Force Nurse Corps. I was humbled by the perseverance, endurance, and total commitment of the nurses and medical technicians I had the privilege to meet all over the globe, especially in Iraq and Afghanistan.

I can resoundingly validate the accounts of the 37 nurses in this book as true, whether in the deployment setting or on aeromedical evacuation missions, having flown with aeromedical evacuation nurses and technicians between December 2007 and March 2008. What an experience to bring the wounded home. While in Afghanistan, I slept in a wooden hooch (a kind of thatched hut) on the troop compound and experienced the 3-minute shower rule, and I can confirm that the walk from the hooch to the bathrooms/shower trailer was lonesome and scary in the middle of the night. One morning, I walked into the women's trailer to brush my teeth, and everyone went to attention. One of the women finally had the courage to ask me why a two-star general was not given better living arrangements. I told her it was my choice.

In Iraq, I listened to the sounds of war all night while the trailer shook with the nonstop sounds of combat. The blowing up of assigned targets echoed through the trailer. Our medics worked through the noise during their shift while mortars fall around and above the medical tentage/hardened facility. Of course, it is the responsibility of all the medics working on the injured to shield the patient by protecting them from falling debris with the medics' own bodies. First, do no harm. After their shift was complete, medics attempted to find rest at night as the war waged onward very close to them. From observing Air Force medics save the life of an Iraqi child hit by a car off base to hearing our wounded crying out in pain, it was an honor to spend my tour of duty as nurse corps chief, seeing it with my own eyes, listening to their stories, and feeling it deeply in my soul.

Early in my time spent as the assistant surgeon general for nursing services and assistant surgeon general for medical force development, I opened my phone lines and email to those deployed and encouraged them to be in continuous contact with me. The real-time accounts of what they faced were heart wrenching, and thus, "telling your story" was born. A standing, open-door invitation was given to any deployers who wished to sit down and talk about their deployment. These stories are forever etched in my memory.

Moreover, it became clear that a new set of issues was emerging related to steady-state deployments. These emerging issues included maintaining a high level of personal readiness, finding inner resilience to sustain the mission despite its wartime tragedies, enduring prolonged exposure to secondary trauma, and most importantly, finding the ability to rejuvenate upon returning home from deployment and ultimately regain a sense of personal and professional balance.

Every member of the nursing force, officer and enlisted, active duty, Air National Guard, and Air Force Reserves told me that their deployment to take care of America's precious sons and daughters has been the most professionally rewarding experience of their lives. Those experiences, though, took a toll on them as a result of extended, repeated deployments with little time to revitalize upon return from caring for the casualties of war.

For a combat troop to lose his buddies in the midst of battle is truly a devastating moment, an unforgettable point in time for many of them for years to come—if they are ever able to recover from it. There is quite another kind of sustained, unrelenting devastation that nurses and medical technicians experience when they feel, hear, smell, and see the carnage of wounded warriors over and over again, day after day. I learned from many that the tours of duty in the deployed setting were an all-consuming, 24/7 experience. They explained to me that, despite their shift with the wounded having ended, when they heard choppers landing with the injured, they arose from their bunks regardless of the hour and returned to caring for the new casualties. I asked all of them why they felt compelled to report for work. To a person, each said it was their mission and duty and what they were sent to the war zone to fulfill.

I will never forget the nurse who came to my office in Washington, DC, after her deployment. She returned on a weekend and came to me first thing Monday morning wearing her formal dress blue uniform and ready to share the story of her time in Iraq with me. She recalled for me the night a trooper was brought to Balad Air Force Hospital so severely burned that his ethnic background could not be discerned, and death was approaching. All who cared for him then knew his life could not be saved. He was sent to a separate medical tent to await death with other medics and the chaplain alongside him. The nurses and technicians, who were on duty when he arrived, were heading home at the end of their shift and saw the lights still on in the tent where he was sent. They knew he had not yet passed away. These medics entered the tent and rotated turns touching a small patch of skin on his upper arm that was the only flesh not burned. They all continued to give consoling, soothing words to him. His heart remained strong. At one point in their solace to him, the chaplain said the only thing they could do was to sing to him. They sang "Just As I Am" until he died.

It is not my story, but I remember it every time I think something in my life is too big to handle or overcome. I stop and recall that nothing is as poignant as losing one of these warriors who willingly gave their lives for us. They are our nation's treasure, and so are those who willingly care for them.

Nursing services recognized and acknowledged early on that strong collegial bonds held us together no matter how dire the situation. A growing realization emerged that, as caregivers, we also needed to take care of ourselves and each other. Many voiced their concerns about feeling weak or causing additional burden to teammates if they allowed themselves to talk about the down side of their assignments in Iraq or Afghanistan. Nurses and medical technicians believed, then and now, that it is part of their job to be "strong." A common misperception persists that sharing thoughts and feelings signals that one cannot handle the stresses of war and thus is not strong enough to be in nursing.

The realization of having someone acknowledge that the raw emotions exposed were a normal human response to an abnormal situation can be deeply comforting. Even when the deployer was able to rationalize that a normal healing process was underway, it can often take much longer for the heart to catch up and fully appreciate the journey. It is important to feel validated and shored up by others who understand what deployed medics have encountered.

As a nursing team, we heard one another's stories of difficult and challenging patient care situations, quiet acts of heroism, and doing whatever is needed to comfort patients, even if there was nothing more that could be done for the wounded, other than "just being there." It became critical for all to share their ordeal and feelings about what they suffered, lived through, and endured. Nurses work hard to help their patients heal from their wounds and get on with their lives as best they can. But the caregiver cannot be forgotten either. Healing one's self is hard work. Listening to each other and taking a turn to tell your story begins the sojourn toward healing.

This book may have been a first step and pivotal part of the healing process for the 37 subjects of this nursing research. I applaud heartily the efforts of the researchers, Elizabeth "Beth" Scannell-Desch and Mary Ellen Scannell Doherty, for giving a voice to the tragedies these nurses faced daily during their deployments. The lived experience is exactly as the research subjects portrayed it. This book by these two nurse researchers, whom I call colleagues and friends, will sit in the most esteemed position of honor on my bookshelf and will be cherished in a special place in my heart. It has been through the myriad of speaking engagements since I retired in which I shared accounts of military nursing in Iraq and Afghanistan that I began taking the first steps toward telling my story. Thanks to Beth and Mary Ellen for sending me drafts of this book's chapters and conversing with me over email on the book's contents. Immersing myself in the accounts of the 37 nurses triggered more personal memories. The work requested of me by the researchers contributed immensely to my own continued healing.

Dear Reader, It is my hope you will always remember, as you absorb the riveting memoirs in this book, that more nurses and enlisted medics, at this very moment, are feeling, hearing, smelling, and seeing for the first time the images of war. Let us all trust they will eventually find the courage and stamina to step forward and tell us their story.

Melissa A. Rank, Major General (Retired), USAF, NC, NEA-BC

Glossary

AK47:	A Russian made machine gun
Battle Rattle:	Slang term for full body armor, Kevlar helmet, individual issued weapon
CCATT:	Critical Care Air Transport Team
CRNA:	Certified registered nurse anesthetist
EPW:	Enemy prisoner of war
FOB:	Forward Operating Base
FST:	Forward Surgical Team
ICU:	Intensive care unit
IED:	Improvised Explosive Device
MOPP Gear:	Mission oriented protective posture gear; protective clothing worn when under the threat of chemical weapon attack consisting of gas mask, gas mask filter, protective hood, battle dress over-garment, rubber over-boots, heavy butyl rubber gloves
Mortar:	An explosive projectile fired from a distant site
MRE:	Meal ready to eat
RPG:	Rocket Propelled Grenade
TRAC2ES:	An automated system that helps coordinate and monitor patient movement between medical treatment facilities during peacetime, contingencies and war including mass casualty situations. It is designed to support the patient movement process, combining both a manual/human component as well as an information technology component.

Index